Encyclopedia of Drug Discovery and Development: Cancer Treatment and Anti-Infectives

Volume III

Encyclopedia of Drug Discovery and Development: Cancer Treatment and Anti-Infectives
Volume III

Edited by **Ned Burnett**

FOSTER
A C A D E M I C S

New Jersey

Published by Foster Academics,
61 Van Reypen Street,
Jersey City, NJ 07306, USA
www.fosteracademics.com

Encyclopedia of Drug Discovery and Development:
Cancer Treatment and Anti-Infectives
Volume III
Edited by Ned Burnett

International Standard Book Number: 978-1-63242-138-8 (Hardback)

Contents

Preface

This book has been a concerted effort by a group of academicians, researchers and scientists, who have contributed their research works for the realization of the book. This book has materialized in the wake of emerging advancements and innovations in this field. Therefore, the need of the hour was to compile all the required researches and disseminate the knowledge to a broad spectrum of people comprising of students, researchers and specialists of the field.

Significant information regarding cancer treatment has been provided in this insightful book. It describes a case study based analysis of several distinct aspects of drug development, ranging from target recognition and characterization to chemical enhancement for efficiency and security, as well as bioproduction of natural products. Special aspects of the formal drug development process are also described. Since drug development is an extremely complicated integrative process, case studies are a distinguished device to acquire insight in this field. The whole book represents an uncommon compilation of distinct facets providing insight in the complexity of drug development covering two sections: 'Novel Approaches to Cancer Treatment' and 'Anti-Infectives'.

At the end of the preface, I would like to thank the authors for their brilliant chapters and the publisher for guiding us all-through the making of the book till its final stage. Also, I would like to thank my family for providing the support and encouragement throughout my academic career and research projects.

Editor

Part 1

Novel Approaches to Cancer Treatment

Discovery and Optimization of Inhibitors of DNA Methyltransferase as Novel Drugs for Cancer Therapy

Jakyung Yoo and José L. Medina-Franco
Torrey Pines Institute for Molecular Studies
USA

1. Introduction

The genome contains genetic and epigenetic information. While the genome provides the blueprint for the manufacture of all the proteins required to create a living thing, the epigenetic information provides instruction on how, where, and when the genetic information should be used (Robertson, 2001). The major form of epigenetic information in mammalian cells is DNA methylation that is the covalent addition of a methyl group to the 5-position of cytosine, mostly within the CpG dinucleotide (Robertson, 2001). DNA methylation is involved in the control of gene expression, regulation of parental imprinting and stabilization of X chromosome inactivation as well as maintenance of the genome integrity. It is also implicated in the development of the immune system, cellular reprogramming and brain function and behaviour (Jurkowska et al., 2011). DNA methylation is mediated by a family of DNA methyltransferase enzymes (DNMTs). In mammals, three DNMTs have been identified so far in the human genome, including the two *de novo* methyltransferases (DNMT3A and DNMT3B) and the maintenance methyltransferase (DNMT1), which is generally the most abundant and active of the three (Goll and Bestor, 2005; Robertson, 2001; Yokochi and Robertson, 2002). DNMT3L is a related protein that has high sequence similarity with DNMT3A, but it lacks any catalytic activity owing to the absence of conserved catalytic residues. However, DNMT3L is required for the catalytic activity of DNMT3A and 3B (Cheng and Blumenthal, 2008). The protein DNMT2 can also be found in mammalian cells. Despite the fact that the structure of DNMT2 is very similar to other DNMTs, its role is comparably less understood (Schaefer and Lyko, 2010). It has been reported that DNMT2 does not methylate DNA but instead methylates aspartic acid transfer RNA (tRNA[Asp]) (Goll et al., 2006). Recent evidence suggests that DNMT2 activity is not limited to tRNA[Asp] and that DNMT2 represents a noncanonical enzyme of the DNMT family (Schaefer and Lyko, 2010).

DNMT1 is responsible for duplicating patterns of DNA methylation during replication and is essential for mammalian development and cancer cell growth (Chen et al., 2007). These enzymes are key regulators of gene transcription, and their roles in carcinogenesis have been the subject of considerable interest over the last decade (Jones and Baylin, 2007; Robertson, 2001). Therefore, specific inhibition of DNA methylation is an attractive and novel approach for cancer therapy (Kelly et al., 2010; Lyko and Brown, 2005; Portela and

Esteller, 2010; Robertson, 2001). It is worth noting that DNA methylation inhibitors have also emerged as a promising strategy for the treatment of immunodeficiency and brain disorders (Miller et al., 2010; Zawia et al., 2009).

The structure of mammalian DNMTs can be divided into two major parts, a large N-terminal regulatory domain of variable size, which has regulatory functions, and a C-terminal catalytic domain which is conserved in eukaryotic and prokaryotic carbon-5 DNMTs. The N-terminal domain guides the nuclear localization of the enzymes and mediates their interactions with other proteins, DNA, and chromatine. The smaller C-terminal domain harbors the active center of the enzyme and contains ten amino acids motifs diagnostic for all carbon-5 DNMTs (Jurkowska et al., 2011). Motifs I-III form the cofactor binding pocket, motif IV has the catalytic cysteine, motifs VI, VIII, and X compose the substrate binding site, and motifs V and VII form the target recognition domain (Sippl and Jung, 2009). Human DNMT1 has 1616 amino acids for which limited three-dimensional structural information is available. For example, just recently a crystal structure of human DNMT1 bound to duplex DNA containing unmethylated cytosine-guanine (CG) sites was published (Song et al., 2011). Further details of the structure of DNMTs and other available crystal structures of DNMTs are extensively reviewed elsewhere (Cheng and Blumenthal, 2008; Lan et al., 2010; Sippl and Jung, 2009).

The proposed mechanism of DNA cytosine-C5 methylation is summarized in Fig. 1 (Schermelleh et al., 2005; Sippl and Jung, 2009; Vilkaitis et al., 2001). DNMT forms a complex with DNA, and the cytosine which will be methylated flips out from the DNA. The thiol of the catalytic cysteine from motif IV acts as a nucleophile that attacks the 6-position of the target cytosine to generate a covalent intermediate. The 5-position of the cytosine is activated and conducts a nucleophilic attack on the cofactor S-adenosyl-L-methionine (AdoMet) to form the 5-methyl covalent adduct and S-adenosyl-L-homocysteine (AdoHcy). The attack on the 6-position is assisted by a transient protonation of the cytosine ring at the endocyclic nitrogen atom N3, which is stabilized by a glutamate residue from motif VI. The same residue also contacts the exocyclic N4 amino group and stabilizes the flipped base. The carbanion may also be stabilized by resonance, where an arginine residue from motif VIII may participate in the stabilization of the cytosine base. The covalent complex between the methylated base and the DNA is resolved by deprotonation at the 5-position to generate the methylated cytosine and the free enzyme.

DNA methylation inhibitors have been well characterized and tested in clinical trials (Issa and Kantarjian, 2009). To date, only 5-azacytidine and 5-aza-2'-deoxycytidine (Fig. 2) have been developed clinically. These two drugs are nucleoside analogues, which, after incorporation into DNA, cause covalent trapping and subsequent depletion of DNA methyltransferases (Schermelleh et al., 2005; Stresemann and Lyko, 2008). Aza nucleosides are approved by the Food and Drug Administration of the United States for the treatment of myelodysplastic syndrome, where they demonstrate significant, although usually transient improvement in patient survival and are currently being tested in many solid cancers (Issa et al., 2005; Schrump et al., 2006). Despite the clinical successes achieved with DNA methylation inhibitors, there is still need for improvement since aza nucleosides have relatively low specificity and are characterized by substantial cellular and clinical toxicity (Stresemann and Lyko, 2008). Their exact mechanism of antitumor action – demethylation of aberrantly silenced growth regulatory genes, induction of DNA damage, or other mechanism also remains unclear (Fandy et al., 2009; Issa, 2005; Palii et al., 2008).

Consequently, there is clear need to identify novel and more specific DNMT inhibitors that do not function via incorporation into DNA.

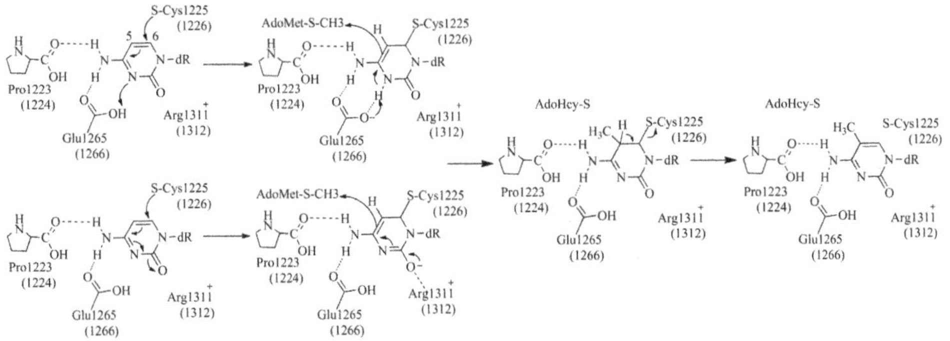

Fig. 1. Mechanism of DNA cytosine-C5 methylation. Amino acid residue numbers are based on the homology model. Equivalent residue numbers in parentheses correspond to the crystal structure.

There is now an increasing number of substances that are reported to inhibit DNMTs (Lyko and Brown, 2005). Selected DNMT inhibitors and other candidate demethylating agents are depicted in Fig. 2. Some of these compounds are approved drugs for other indications; i.e., the antihypertensive drug hydralazine (Segura-Pacheco et al., 2003), the local anaesthetic procaine (Villar-Garea et al., 2003), and the antiarrhythmic drug procainamide (Lee et al., 2005a). Others like the L-tryptophan derivative RG108, NSC 14778 (Fig. 2) have been identified by docking-based virtual screening (Kuck et al., 2010a; Siedlecki et al., 2006). Several natural products have been implicated in DNA methylation inhibition. Selected examples are the main polyphenol compound from green tea, (-)-epigallocathechin-3-gallate (EGCG) (Fang et al., 2003; Lee et al., 2005b), other tea polyphenols such as catechin and epicatechin, and the bioflavonoids quercetin, fisetin, and myricetin. Curcumin, the major component of the Indian curry spice turmeric, has been reported to inhibit the DNA cytosine C5 methyltransferase M.SssI, an analogue of DNMT1 (Liu et al., 2009). However, more recent studies showed that curcumin did not cause DNA demethylation in three arbitrarily chosen human cancer cell lines (Medina-Franco et al., 2011). Mahanine, a plant-derived carbazole alkaloid, and a fluorescent carbazole analogue, has been reported to induce the Ras-association domain family 1 (RASSF1) gene in human prostate cancer cells, presumably by inhibiting DNMT activity (Jagadeesh et al., 2007; Sheikh et al., 2010). Nanaomycin A, a quinone antibiotic isolated from a culture of *Streptomyces*, has been described as the first non S-adenosyl-L-homocysteine (AdoHcy/SAH) analogue acting as a DNMT3B-selective inhibitor that induces genomic demethylation. Nanaomycin A treatment reduced the global methylation levels in three cell lines and reactivated transcription of the RASSF1A tumor suppressor gene (Kuck et al., 2010b). These and several other natural products as putative demethylating agents are extensively reviewed elsewhere (Gilbert and Liu, 2010; Hauser and Jung, 2008; Li and Tollefsbol, 2010; Medina-Franco and Caulfield, 2011). While the substantial number of recent reports may suggest that many natural products inhibit DNA methylation, it should be noted that only a few reports provide compelling evidence for DNMT inhibition in biochemical and in cellular assays. As such, it remains possible that many of these compounds have an indirect and fortuitous effect on DNA methylation, but do not show a pharmacologically relevant activity that can be developed further for therapeutic purposes (Medina-Franco et al., 2011).

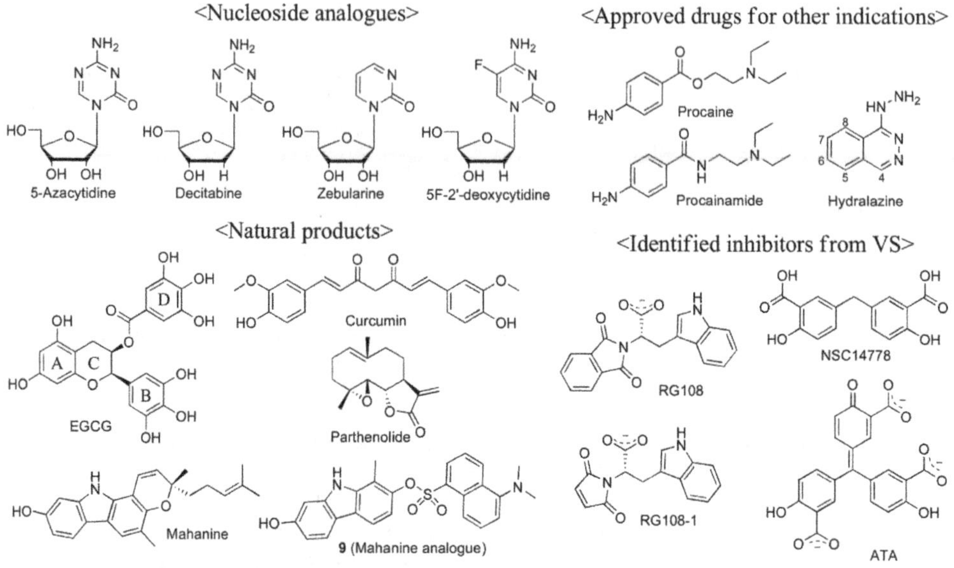

Fig. 2. Chemical structures of selected DNA methyltransferase inhibitors and other compounds with putative demethylating activity.

Until now most compounds associated with DNA methylation inhibition have been identified fortuitously. Remarkable exceptions are RG108 and 5,5′-methylenedisalicylic acid (NSC 14778) that were identified by computational screening followed by experimental evaluation (Kuck et al., 2010a; Siedlecki et al., 2006). In order to accelerate the discovery and optimization of new DNMT inhibitors, rational approaches are increasingly being used. To this end, *in silico* studies have significantly helped to understand the structure and function of DNMTs and the mechanism of DNMT inhibition (Medina-Franco and Caulfield, 2011). This chapter focuses on the different strategies ongoing in our and other research groups for the discovery and optimization of inhibitors of DNMTs with particular emphasis on *in silico* screening (section two) and *in silico* design (section three).

2. *In silico* screening of compound collections to identify novel inhibitors

In silico screening, also called in the literature, computational or virtual screening, consists of the computational evaluation of databases aiming to select a small number of reliable and experimentally testable candidate compounds that have a high probability of being active (Muegge, 2008; Shoichet, 2004). *In silico* screening is one of the most common rational approaches to guide the identification of new hits from large compound libraries. Hit identification using this approach requires several interactive steps that include (1) the compound collection, (2) the computational methods used for screening, and (3) the analysis of the output (López-Vallejo et al., 2011).

2.1 Screening databases

A number of compound databases from different sources can be used in *in silico* screening. These libraries may contain existing or hypothetical; i.e., virtual compounds. Libraries of existing compounds may be proprietary; e.g., in-house libraries, commercial, or public. The sources of screening libraries, with emphasis on libraries in the public domain, have been reviewed (Bender, 2010; Scior et al., 2007). Currently, the ZINC database is one of the most used libraries (Irwin and Shoichet, 2005). The type of screening library utilized should be closely associated with the objective of the particular screening campaign (Shelat and Guy, 2007). Chemically diverse libraries are particular attractive for identifying novel scaffolds for new or relatively unexplored targets such as DNMTs. If the goal is lead optimization, e.g., optimize the activity of known DNMT inhibitors (Fig. 2), focused libraries or collections with high inter-molecular similarity (highly dense libraries) are an attractive source.

2.1.1 Natural product databases

The presence of DNMT inhibitors in dietary products and commonly used herbal remedies (Gilbert and Liu, 2010; Hauser and Jung, 2008; Li and Tollefsbol, 2010) demonstrates the feasibility of identifying additional inhibitors of natural origin. Natural products have unique characteristics attractive for drug discovery. For example, the chemical structures of natural products are, in general, different from the chemical structures of synthetic compounds occupying different areas of chemical space (Ganesan, 2008; Medina-Franco et al., 2008; Singh et al., 2009b). In addition, natural products may be drug candidates themselves or may be the starting point for an optimization program (Ganesan, 2008; Hauser and Jung, 2008). Indeed several natural products are bioavailable, and the rationale of these observations has been recently provided (Ganesan, 2008). Fig. 3 shows a visual representation of the chemical space of natural products, drugs, and DNMT inhibitors. To compare the chemical space, a subset of 1,000 compounds was randomly selected from each database. The visual representation was obtained with principal component analysis (PCA) of the similarity matrix of the databases computed using Molecular ACCess System (MACCS) keys (166 bits) and the Tanimoto coefficient (Maggiora and Shanmugasundaram, 2011). The first three principal components are displayed in Fig. 3 and account for 79% of the variance. This figure clearly shows that most of the DNMT inhibitors, e.g., nucleoside analogues, RG108, RG108-1, procaine, procainamide, SG1027, and hydralazine, share the same chemical space of drugs. This observation is expected from inhibitors such as procaine, procainamide, and hydralazine. In contrast, NSC14778 and DNMT inhibitors from natural origin, EGCG and curcumin, are in a less-dense populated area of the chemical space of drugs. These compounds are characterized by containing one or more hydroxyl groups. Fig. 3b shows that most of the compounds in the natural product database also occupy this second region. Before conducting virtual and experimental screening, it is feasible to filter out natural products with potential toxicity issues using drug- or lead-like filters (Charifson and Walters, 2002).

2.1.2 Combinatorial libraries

Combinatorial libraries, either existing or virtual, are important sources of compound collections that can be used for *in silico* screening (López-Vallejo et al., 2011). Advances in synthetic approaches can generate *libraries from libraries, target-oriented* libraries, and *diversity-oriented* libraries which explore the chemical space in different ways (López-Vallejo et al., 2011) and can be used in lead optimization or hit-identification, depending on the goals of the screening campaign.

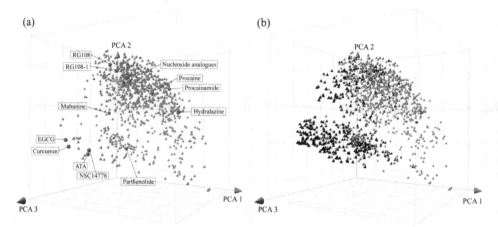

Fig. 3. Comparison of 486 natural products (black triangles), 1,000 drugs (red triangles), and 14 DNMT1 inhibitors (blue spheres). Depiction of a visual representation of the chemical space obtained by PCA of the similarity matrix computed using MACCS keys and Tanimoto similarity. The first three PCs account for 79% of the variance. (a) Comparison of drugs and DNMT1 inhibitors. (b) Comparison of drugs, natural products, and DNMT inhibitors.

2.2 Development and validation of computational approaches

In silico screening can be divided into two general strategies: ligand-based and structure-based (Medina-Franco et al., 2006; Ooms, 2000). Ligand-based approaches use the structural information and biological activity data from a set of known active compounds to select promising candidates for experimental screening. When the three-dimensional structure of the target is known, structure-based methods can be used. Three-dimensional structure information of the target is usually obtained from X-ray crystallography or nuclear magnetic resonance. In the absence of three-dimensional structural information of the receptor, homology models have been successfully used (Grant, 2009; Villoutreix et al., 2009). Perhaps the most common structure-based approach is molecular docking. Docking aims to find the best position and orientation of a molecule within a binding site and gives a score for each docked pose (Hernández-Campos et al., 2010; Kitchen et al., 2004; Villoutreix et al., 2009). Ligand- and structure-based methods can be combined if information for both the experimentally active compounds and the three-dimensional structure of the target are available (Sperandio et al., 2008). The selection of a particular method is generally based on the goal of the project, the information available for the system, and the computational resources available. For structure-based and ligand-based methods, it is highly advisable to validate the virtual screening protocol prior to the selection of compounds for experimental testing. However, the experimental results of the tested candidates will provide full validation of the virtual screening approach.

2.2.1 Structure-based screening

Structure-based screening for novel DNMT inhibitors performed so far has been conducted with homology models of the catalytic domain (Kuck et al., 2010a; Siedlecki et al., 2006). The construction of useful homology models has been facilitated by the extensive conservation of the catalytic domain of DNMTs (Kumar et al., 1994). Crystal structures of other methyltransferases such as bacterial DNA cytosine C5 methyltransferase from *Haemophilus hemolyticus* (M.HhaI), bacterial cytosine C5 methyltransferase M.HaeIII, and the human DNMT2 (Siedlecki et al., 2003; Yoo and Medina-Franco, 2011) have been used as templates (Medina-Franco and Caulfield, 2011).

We have recently developed two homology models of the catalytic domain of DNMT1. In one model (Yoo and Medina-Franco, 2011), the crystal structures of the DNMTs M.HhaI, M.HaeIII, and DNMT2 were used as templates. The first structure is a ternary complex of M.HhaI, *S*-adenosyl methionine (AdoMet), and DNA containing flipped 4'-thio-2'-deoxcytidine with partial methylation at C5. The crystal structure of M.HaeIII is bound covalently to DNA. In this complex, the substrate cytosine is extruded from the DNA and it is inserted into the active site. The structure of human DNMT2 complexed with *S*-adenosyl-L-homocysteine (AdoHcy/SAH) has high similarities to methyltransferases of both prokaryotes and eukaryotes. A second homology model was developed using only the structure of M.HhaI as template. Both models contain DNA and the conserved residues which are involved in the catalytic mechanism. The target cytosine which is flipped out of the embedded DNA is inserted into the active site. The catalytic loop containing the catalytic cysteine is located above the cytosine as an active site "lid". The target cytosine lies between the nucleophile cysteine residue (Cys1225) and the sulfur atom of AdoHcy. The distance of cytosine C6 to the sulfur atom of Cys1225 is 3.3 Å. The cytosine C5 atom is 3.0 Å away from the sulfur atom of AdoHcy. In the reactive state of Cys1225, the distance between $O^{\varepsilon 1}$ of Glu1265 and N3 of cytidine is 2.8 Å, where the N3 atom is proposed to be protonated making a hydrogen bond with the acidic side chain of Glu1265. In addition, the N3 protonated form of cytosine can make hydrogen bonds with Arg1311 and Pro1223. These key interactions in the catalytic site are commonly observed in both homology models. More specifically, in the first homology model, the α-phosphate backbone and 3'-OH of the sugar moiety of deoxycytidine make a hydrogen bond network with Arg1311, Arg1461, Ser1229, Gly1230, and Gln1396; in the second model, the interactions are observed with the following residues: Gln1226, Ser1229, Gly1230, Arg1268, and Arg1310.

Fig. 4 shows a superimposition of the first homology model of the catalytic site of hDNMT1 (Yoo and Medina-Franco, 2011) with the recently published crystal structure of unmethylated human DNMT1 (Song et al., 2011). The catalytic cores of their methyltransferase domains have similar features, but unmethylated DNA in the crystallographic structure is positioned further away from the active site. In the crystal structure of the human DNMT complex, the key amino acid residues Glu1265 and Arg1311 are positioned in very similar place. In contrast, the catalytic loop adopts a different conformation with respect to the homology model. The catalytic loop has an open conformation, and the catalytic cysteine is far from the binding site, e.g., the distance of superimposed cytosine C6 to the sulfur atom of Cys1225 is 9.5 Å. Taken together, the structural characterization of the catalytic site supports that our homology model is in full agreement with the proposed catalytic mechanism of DNA methylation.

In silico screening has been successfully used to identify novel small molecule inhibitors of DNMT1. In one study, 1990 compounds in the Diversity Set available from the National Cancer Institute were the starting point of a screening using docking with a validated homology model of human DNMT1. Compounds with undesirable size, hydrophobicity, and uncommon atom types were filtered out. Two of the top scoring compounds were tested experimentally showing activity both *in vitro* and *in vivo*, probably by binding into the DNMT1 catalytic pocket (Siedlecki et al., 2006). In that work, RG108 (Fig. 2) showed an IC_{50} = 0.60 μM with M.SssI (Siedlecki et al., 2006). Additional characterization showed that this L-tryptophan derivative did not cause covalent enzyme trapping and that the carboxylate group plays an essential role in the binding with the enzyme since the analogue without this moiety is inactive (Brueckner et al., 2005).

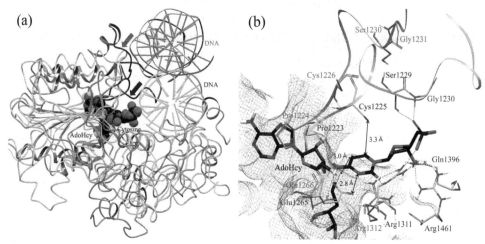

Fig. 4. (a) Superposition of the homology model (green) of the catalytic domain of human DNMT1 with the crystallographic structure (pink) of the unmethylated human DNMT1. The catalytic loops are marked with arrows. AdoHcy and the flipped cytosine in the homology model are shown in space-filling view. (b) Binding model of deoxycytidine (black) with key amino acid residues of homology model (carbon atoms in green) and crystal structure (carbon atoms in pink). Hydrogen bonding interactions are represented by dotted lines.

In a follow-up study, our group screened a larger set of the National Cancer Institute database containing more than 260,000 compounds (Kuck et al., 2010a). In order to focus the screening on compounds that could be promising for further development, we selected a subset of approximately 65,000 lead-like molecules (Charifson and Walters, 2002). The lead-like set was further filtered using a high-throughput *in silico* screening. As part of the screening, three docking programs were used. Favorable docking scores from all three docking approaches were combined to create a total of 24 consensus compounds. Of the 24 molecules that were identified, thirteen were obtained for experimental testing. Seven out of the thirteen consensus hits had detectable DNMT1 inhibitory activity in biochemical assays. Further experimental characterization of active compounds showed that six out of the seven inhibitors appeared selective for DNMT1. The methylenedisalicylic acid derivative, NSC 14778 (Fig. 2), showed an IC_{50} = 92 μM with DNMT1 and an IC_{50} = 17 μM with DNMT3B. The observed potency was comparably low for most test compounds, which was partially attributed to the high amount of protein used in the biochemical assay. In fact, it is well-known that DNMTs are weak catalysts and are difficult to assay (Hemeon et al., (2011 - ASAP)). Despite the low potency, the *in silico* screening was successful in that it identified diverse scaffolds that were not previously reported for DNMT inhibitors. The new scaffolds represent excellent candidates for optimizing their inhibitory activity and selectivity.

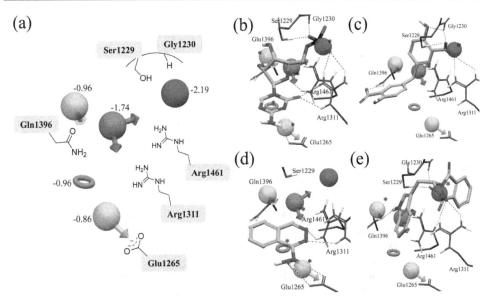

Fig. 5. (a) Structure-based pharmacophore model proposed for human DNMT1 inhibitors. *Red sphere*: negative ionizable, *pink sphere*: hydrogen bond acceptor, *blue sphere*: hydrogen bond donors, and *orange ring*: aromatic ring. Selected amino acid residues in the catalytic site of homology model are schematically depicted for reference. Comparison between the binding mode and pharmacophore hypothesis for representative DNMT inhibitors, (b) 5-azacytidine, (c) NSC14778, (d) hydralazine, and (e) RG108.

Recently, our group developed a structure-based pharmacophore hypothesis for inhibitors of DNMT1 (Yoo and Medina-Franco, 2011). Using the energy optimized hypothesis, 'e-pharmacophore' method (Salam et al., 2009) the pharmacophore model was developed based on the scores and predicted binding modes of 14 known DNMT1 inhibitors docked with a homology model of DNMT1. Fig. 5a shows the pharmacophore model for the 14 DNMT1 inhibitors. The model contains five features which represent the most important interactions of the inhibitors with the catalytic domain. The energetic value assigned to each pharmacophoric feature is displayed in the figure. Nearby amino acids are schematically depicted for reference. The best-scoring feature is a negative charge which is close to the side chains of Ser1229, Gly1230, and Arg1311. The second most favorable feature is an acceptor site that is in close proximity with the side chains of Arg1311 and Arg1461. The third ranked features are an aromatic ring that stabilizes the binding conformation of ligands between AdoHcy and Cys1225, and a donor site that is close to the side chain of Gln1396. The fifth-ranked feature is a donor site that is nearby the side chain of Glu1265 which is a residue implicated in the methylation mechanism. Fig. 5b shows the alignment of representative DNMT inhibitors to the pharmacophore hypothesis. It remains to evaluate the performance of the pharmacophore model in prospective *in silico* screening.

2.2.2 Ligand-based screening

Ligand-based screening can be performed as an alternative approach when the relevant crystal structures are not available on the molecular target. Ligand-based approaches include similarity searching, substructure, clustering, quantitative structure-activity relationships (QSAR), pharmacophore-, or three-dimensional shape matching techniques (Villoutreix et al., 2007). Several ligand-based methods, including similarity searching and QSAR, can roughly be divided into two- or three-dimensional approaches. Ligand-based virtual screening may be applied even if a single known-ligand has been identified through similarity-based screening. Interestingly, although many more successful structure-based than ligand-based virtual screening applications are reported to date, recent reviews indicate that the potency of hits identified by ligand-based approaches is on average considerably higher than for structure-based methods (Ripphausen et al., 2011; Ripphausen et al., 2010).

If multiple active compounds are known, it is possible to apply QSAR using two- or three-dimensional information of the ligands. One of the main goals of QSAR is to derive statistical models that can be used to predict the activity of molecules not previously tested in the biological assay. Despite the fact that QSAR is a valuable tool, there are potential pitfalls to develop predictive QSAR models (Scior et al., 2009). A major pitfall can occur when the compounds were assayed using different experimental conditions. Other major pitfall is due to the presence of "activity cliffs," i.e., compounds with very high structural similarity but very different biological activity (Maggiora, 2006). Activity cliffs give rise to QSAR with poor predictive ability (Guha and Van Drie, 2008).

3. *In silico* design and optimization of established inhibitors

Concerns about severe toxicity of nucleoside analogues have strongly encouraged not only identifying novel DNMT inhibitors but also developing further established non-nucleoside inhibitors. To this end, medicinal chemistry approaches, either alone or in combination with *in silico* strategies, are being pursued.

3.1 Optimization of RG108, procaine, and mahanine

As mentioned above, procaine, a local anesthetic drug, and procainamide, a drug for the treatment of cardiac arrhythmias, have been reported as inhibitors of DNA methylation (Fig. 2). In a recent report, constrained analogues of procaine were synthesized and tested for their inhibition against DNMT1 (Castellano et al., 2008). Procaine as a lead structure was modified to partially reduce the high flexibility which can have a detrimental effect for drug-likeness. The most potent inhibitor in an *in vitro* methylation assay also showed demethylation activity in HL60 human myeloid leukemia cells, and it was suggested as a lead compound for further studies (Castellano et al., 2008).

In a separate work, a series of maleimide derivatives of RG108 were reported (Suzuki et al., 2010). In that work, design, chemical synthesis, inhibitory activity assays, and automated docking methods were used. The most active compound of the series was RG108-1 (Fig. 2). A binding model of RG108-1 with the crystal structure of bacterial M.HhaI suggested that this compound could be a covalent blocker of the catalytic cysteine. A more recent molecular modelling study using a model of human DNMT1 (Yoo and Medina-Franco, 2011) supported this hypothesis. Interestingly, in the model obtained with human DNMT, the maleimide moiety of RG108-1 interacts with Arg1311, Arg1461, and lies next to Cys1225, where the conjugate addition of the thiol group of the catalytic cysteine to the maleimide can occur. In addition, the carboxylate anion of RG108-1 overlaps with that of RG108 and has the same interaction with Arg1311, Ser1229, and Gly1230 (Yoo and Medina-Franco, 2011).

The natural product mahanine (Fig. 2) has the ability to restore RASSF1A expression, and it is a potent inhibitor of androgen dependent (LNCaP) and androgen independent (PC-3) human prostate cancer cell proliferation (Jagadeesh et al., 2007). The antiproliferative activity of mahanine is associated with inhibition of the DNMT activity. Recently, fluorescent carbazole analogues of mahanine were designed and synthesized to find a novel and more potent small molecule with a mechanistic profile similar to that of the parent compound. Compound '9' in Fig. 2 inhibited human prostate cancer cell proliferation at 1.5 μM and also showed DNMT inhibition activity without the cytotoxic effects seen with mahanine treatment. Inhibition of DNMT was proposed as the event leading to the restoration of RASSF1A expression (Sheikh et al., 2010).

3.2 Structure-based optimization of hydralazine

Hydralazine, a potent arterial vasodilator, has been used for the management of hypertensive disorders and heart failure. Using a drug repurposing strategy (Duenas-Gonzalez et al., 2008), clinical trials have demonstrated the antitumor effect of the combination of hydralazine with valporic acid (a histone deacetylase inhibitor). Hydralazine and procainamide were first reported to have DNA methylation inhibition effect in 1988. Despite the fact that numerous studies were conducted with hydralazine, its molecular mechanism has remained unknown. In order to help understand the activity of hydralazine at the molecular level, we developed a binding mode of this compound with a validated homology model of the catalytic domain of DNMT1 using docking and molecular dynamics (Singh et al., 2009a; Yoo and Medina-Franco, 2011).

In molecular modeling studies, hydralazine showed similar interactions within the binding pocket as nucleoside analogues including a complex network of hydrogen bonds with arginine and glutamic acid residues that play a major role in the mechanism of DNA methylation (Yoo and Medina-Franco, 2011). Fig. 6 shows the comparison of the binding modes of hydralazine with 5-azacytidine. The amino group of hydralazine matched well with the amino group of 5-azacytidine, and it is capable of making hydrogen bonds with Glu1265 and Pro1223. The nitrogen of the phthalazine ring overlapped with the carbonyl oxygen of 5-azacytidine and formed hydrogen bonds with Arg1311 and Arg1461. We also identified that the small structure of hydralazine could not occupy the site of the sugar ring and phosphate backbone of nucleoside analogues. This result also suggests that hydralazine can be substituted at the C4 position to yield analogues with enhanced affinity with the enzyme. In contrast, there is a small empty pocket nearby the carbocyclic aromatic ring of hydralazine (C5-C8) that can be occupied by a substituent (Yoo and Medina-Franco, 2011). The molecule shown in Fig. 6 was designed based on the structure and binding mode of hydralazine. Molecular modeling indicates that the addition of a phenyl group in the C4 position of hydralazine improves the calculated binding affinity with DNMT1. Moreover, adding polar substituents at various positions of the phenyl group can provide additional favorable interactions with the catalytic site. Also based on our molecular modeling analysis, the binding affinity is expected to increase by the addition of polar groups to the carbocyclic aromatic ring of phthalazine. It is *expected* that new compounds with increased calculated affinity with the enzyme will show increased potency in the DNMT1 enzyme inhibition assays.

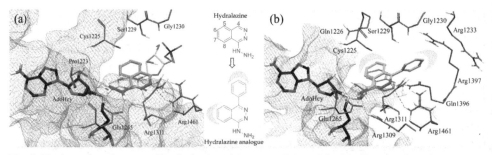

Fig. 6. Design of analogues of hydralazine. (a) comparison of the binding modes of hydralazine (carbon atoms in pink) with 5-azacytidine (carbon atoms in green) (b) structure-guided design of a representative hydralazine analogue (carbon atoms in green).

3.3 Design of focused combinatorial libraries

Computer-assisted combinatorial library design is a powerful tool frequently used in the discovery and optimization of new lead compounds. Molecular diversity has played a critical role in designing combinatorial libraries for screening (Tommasi and Cornella, 2006; Zheng and Johnson, 2008). However, the core chemical scaffolds of some currently used diverse libraries might be inadequate to provide drug-like compounds for new targets. Library design based on bioisosteric replacement or scaffold hopping methods can be used as an alternative to diversity oriented synthesis. Bioisostere searching involves swapping functional groups of a molecule with other functional groups that have similar biological properties. Scaffold hopping is an approach to discover structurally novel compounds starting from known active compounds by modifying the central core structure of the molecule (Brown and Jacoby, 2006). Scaffold hopping is an important drug design strategy to develop novel molecules with potent activity, altered physicochemical attributes, and Absorption, Distribution, Metabolism, Excretion and Toxicity –ADMET- properties. An example of application is phosphodiesterase 5 inhibitors for the treatment of erectile dysfunction. Sildenafil and vardenafil represent a case of heteroaromatic core scaffolds hopping with a small change in the scaffold (Jordan and Roughley, 2009). In contrast, tadalafil has a very different core scaffold, but it has the same biological activity. Computational design of focused libraries or compounds designed using any other strategy has to be in agreement with the experimental synthetic feasibility of the compounds proposed. Ideally, synthetic routes should follow short and easy steps.

Fig. 7 shows additional hydralazine analogues that have been proposed based on the knowledge gained in our previous molecular modeling studies of DNMT inhibitors. Starting from the 1-hydrazinyl-4-phenylphthalazine, polar groups are introduced into the carbocyclic aromatic ring of phthalazine. Based on molecular modeling analysis, substitution at ortho-, meta-, and para- position of the phenyl group with e.g., carboxyl, cyanide, and acetyl, showed a significant improvement in the calculated binding of the new compounds with DNMT1. A carboxyl group introduced into the ortho position plays a key role to make hydrogen bonds with Ser1229 or Gly1230. In contrast, substitution at C8 position of the phthalazine did not fit well into the catalytic site because of the narrow pocket size. Addition of polar groups to other positions slightly increases the predicted binding affinity with the enzyme. Further chemical modifications to the structures of the lead DNMT inhibitors will be suggested toward the improvement of the *in vitro* and *in vivo* demethylating activity.

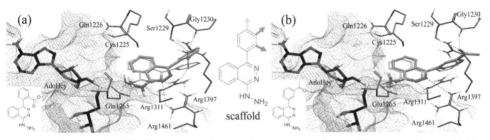

Fig. 7. Binding mode of hydralazine analogues (carbon atoms in pink) designed by scaffold hopping. The carbon atoms of new core scaffold are in green. Analogues with (a) ortho-carboxylate substitution and (b) meta-acetyl substitution on the phenyl moiety.

3.4 Characterization of structure-activity relationships

Currently, DNMT inhibitors have been screened in different assays using different conditions, and QSAR studies may not be reliable. However, once quality activity data has been gathered for several compounds assayed under comparable experimental conditions, it is feasible to conduct structure-activity relationships (SAR) of the compounds tested. When there is a significant amount of data, for example, activity data for more than 100 or 200 compounds, systematic analysis of the SAR can be performed via chemoinformatic approaches using the concept of "activity landscape modelling" (Wawer et al., 2010). The goal of activity landscape modeling of molecular data sets is to help rationalize the underlying SAR identifying key compounds and structural features for further exploration. The concept of activity landscape is strongly associated with the basic relationships between molecular structure and biological activity. While predictive SAR methods, such as pharmacophore modelling and traditional QSAR, focus on specific molecular descriptors or arrangements of substructures or functional groups associated with activity, descriptive activity landscape models rely on the "similarity property principle," i.e., similar structures should have similar biological properties (Bender and Glen, 2004; Maggiora and Shanmugasundaram, 2011) and employ whole-molecular similarity measures (Wawer et al., 2010). Systematic approaches to model activity landscapes and to detect "activity cliffs" using multiple representations are published elsewhere (Medina-Franco et al., 2009; Pérez-Villanueva et al., 2010; Pérez-Villanueva et al., 2011).

4. Conclusion

DNA methyltransferases are promising epigenetic targets for the treatment of cancer and other diseases. Clinical data demonstrates the potential of DNMT inhibitors for the therapeutic treatment of cancer. This is evidenced by the two DNMT inhibitors approved by the Food and Drug Administration of the United States for the treatment of patients with high-risk myelodysplastic syndrome. However, current approved drugs are nucleoside analogues that are not specific and still present issues such as cellular and clinical toxicity. A wide range of computational approaches are being used to assist in the discovery and development of novel DNMT inhibitors. Molecular docking, pharmacophore modelling and molecular dynamics have been used to better understand the mechanism of action of established DNMT inhibitors; *in silico* screening of large compound libraries followed by experimental testing has been successful in identifying non-nucleoside inhibitors with novel chemical scaffolds; structure-based design is being used to guide the optimization of inhibitors such as hydralazine. Homology models of the catalytic domain of DNMT1 has played an important role to conduct the computational approaches that rely on the three dimensional structure of the target. It is expected that the recently published crystal structure of human DNMT1 bound to duplex DNA containing unmethylated CG sites will be the starting point of future structure-based studies with inhibitors of DNA methylation. It is also anticipated that the synergistic combination of computational approaches with combinatorial chemistry, and the systematic *in silico* and experimental screening of natural products will boost the discovery and optimization of inhibitors of DNMT for cancer therapy.

5. Acknowledgment

Discussions with Dr. Fabian López-Vallejo and other members of the group are highly appreciated. Authors are also very grateful to Karen Gottwald for proofreading the chapter. This work was supported by the State of Florida, Executive Office of the Governor's Office of Tourism, Trade, and Economic Development. J.L.M-F. also thanks the Menopause & Women's Health Research Center for funding.

6. References

Bender, A., 2010. Databases compound bioactivities go public. *Nat. Chem. Biol.* 6, 309-309.

Bender, A., Glen, R.C., 2004. Molecular similarity: A key technique in molecular informatics. *Org. Biomol. Chem.* 2, 3204-3218.

Brown, N., Jacoby, E., 2006. On scaffolds and hopping in medicinal chemistry. *Mini-Rev. Med. Chem.* 6, 1217-1229.

Brueckner, B., Boy, R.G., Siedlecki, P., Musch, T., Kliem, H.C., Zielenkiewicz, P., Suhai, S., Wiessler, M., Lyko, F., 2005. Epigenetic reactivation of tumor suppressor genes by a novel small-molecule inhibitor of human DNA methyltransferases. *Cancer Res.* 65, 6305-6311.

Castellano, S., Kuck, D., Sala, M., Novellino, E., Lyko, F., Sbardella, G., 2008. Constrained analogues of procaine as novel small molecule inhibitors of DNA methyltransferase-1. *J. Med. Chem.* 51, 2321-2325.

Charifson, P.S., Walters, W.P., 2002. Filtering databases and chemical libraries. *J. Comput.-Aided Mol. Des.* 16, 311-323.

Chen, T.P., Hevi, S., Gay, F., Tsujimoto, N., He, T., Zhang, B.L., Ueda, Y., Li, E., 2007. Complete inactivation of DNMT1 leads to mitotic catastrophe in human cancer cells. *Nat. Genet.* 39, 391-396.

Cheng, X.D., Blumenthal, R.M., 2008. Mammalian DNA methyltransferases: A structural perspective. *Structure* 16, 341-350.

Dueñas-González, A., García-López, P., Herrera, L.A., Medina-Franco, J.L., González-Fierro, A., Candelaria, M., 2008. The prince and the pauper. A tale of anticancer targeted agents. *Mol. Cancer* 7, 33.

Fandy, T.E., Herman, J.G., Kerns, P., Jiemjit, A., Sugar, E.A., Choi, S.H., Yang, A.S., Aucott, T., Dauses, T., Odchimar-Reissig, R., Licht, J., Mcconnell, M.J., Nasrallah, C., Kim, M.K.H., Zhang, W.J., Sun, Y.Z., Murgo, A., Espinoza-Delgado, I., Oteiza, K., Owoeye, I., Silverman, L.R., Gore, S.D., Carraway, H.E., 2009. Early epigenetic changes and DNA damage do not predict clinical response in an overlapping schedule of 5-azacytidine and entinostat in patients with myeloid malignancies. *Blood* 114, 2764-2773.

Fang, M.Z., Wang, Y.M., Ai, N., Hou, Z., Sun, Y., Lu, H., Welsh, W., Yang, C.S., 2003. Tea polyphenol (-)-epigallocatechin-3-gallate inhibits DNA methyltransferase and reactivates methylation-silenced genes in cancer cell lines. *Cancer Res.* 63, 7563-7570.

Ganesan, A., 2008. The impact of natural products upon modern drug discovery. *Curr. Opin. Chem. Biol.* 12, 306-317.

Gilbert, E.R., Liu, D., 2010. Flavonoids influence epigenetic-modifying enzyme activity: Structure-function relationships and the therapeutic potential for cancer. *Curr. Med. Chem.* 17, 1756-1768.

Goll, M.G., Bestor, T.H., 2005. Eukaryotic cytosine methyltransferases. *Annu. Rev. Biochem.* 74, 481-514.

Goll, M.G., Kirpekar, F., Maggert, K.A., Yoder, J.A., Hsieh, C.-L., Zhang, X., Golic, K.G., Jacobsen, S.E., Bestor, T.H., 2006. Methylation of tRNAAsp by the DNA methyltransferase homolog Dnmt2. *Science* 311, 395-398.

Grant, M.A., 2009. Protein structure prediction in structure-based ligand design and virtual screening. *Comb. Chem. High Throughput Screening* 12, 940-960.

Guha, R., Van Drie, J.H., 2008. Assessing how well a modeling protocol captures a structure-activity landscape. *J. Chem. Inf. Model.* 48, 1716-1728.

Hauser, A.T., Jung, M., 2008. Targeting epigenetic mechanisms: Potential of natural products in cancer chemoprevention. *Planta Med.* 74, 1593-1601.

Hemeon, I., Gutierrez, J.A., Ho, M.-C., Schramm, V.L., (2011). Characterizing DNA methyltransferases with an ultrasensitive luciferase-linked continuous assay. *Anal. Chem.*, 83, 4996-5004.

Hernández-Campos, A., Velázquez-Martínez, I., Castillo, R., López-Vallejo, F., Jia, P., Yu, Y., Giulianotti, M.A., Medina-Franco, J.L., 2010. Docking of protein kinase B inhibitors: Implications in the structure-based optimization of a novel scaffold. *Chem. Biol. Drug Des.* 76, 269-276.

Irwin, J.J., Shoichet, B.K., 2005. ZINC - A free database of commercially available compounds for virtual screening. *J. Chem. Inf. Model.* 45, 177-182.

Issa, J.-P., 2005. Optimizing therapy with methylation inhibitors in myelodysplastic syndromes: Dose, duration, and patient selection. *Nat. Clin. Pract. Oncol.* 2 Suppl 1, S24-9.

Issa, J.-P.J., Kantarjian, H.M., 2009. Targeting DNA methylation. *Clin. Cancer Res.* 15, 3938-3946.

Issa, J.P.J., Kantarjian, H.M., Kirkpatrick, P., 2005. Azacitidine. *Nat. Rev. Drug Discovery* 4, 275-276.

Jagadeesh, S., Sinha, S., Pal, B.C., Bhattacharya, S., Banerjee, P.P., 2007. Mahanine reverses an epigenetically silenced tumor suppressor gene RASSF1A in human prostate cancer cells. *Biochem. Biophys. Res. Commun.* 362, 212-217.

Jones, P.A., Baylin, S.B., 2007. The epigenomics of cancer. *Cell* 128, 683-692.

Jordan, A.M., Roughley, S.D., 2009. Drug discovery chemistry: A primer for the non-specialist. *Drug Discovery Today* 14, 731-744.

Jurkowska, R.Z., Jurkowski, T.P., Jeltsch, A., 2011. Structure and function of mammalian DNA methyltransferases. *ChemBioChem* 12, 206-222.

Kelly, T.K., De Carvalho, D.D., Jones, P.A., 2010. Epigenetic modifications as therapeutic targets. *Nat. Biotechnol.* 28, 1069-1078.

Kitchen, D.B., Decornez, H., Furr, J.R., Bajorath, J., 2004. Docking and scoring in virtual screening for drug discovery: Methods and applications. *Nat. Rev. Drug Discov.* 3, 935-949.

Kuck, D., Singh, N., Lyko, F., Medina-Franco, J.L., 2010a. Novel and selective DNA methyltransferase inhibitors: Docking-based virtual screening and experimental evaluation. *Bioorg. Med. Chem.* 18, 822-829.

Kuck, D., Caulfield, T., Lyko, F., Medina-Franco, J.L., 2010b. Nanaomycin A selectively inhibits DNMT3B and reactivates silenced tumor suppressor genes in human cancer cells. *Mol. Cancer Ther.* 9, 3015-23.

Kumar, S., Cheng, X.D., Klimasauskas, S., Mi, S., Posfai, J., Roberts, R.J., Wilson, G.G., 1994. The DNA (cytosine-5) methyltransferases. *Nucleic Acids Res.* 22, 1-10.

Lan, J., Hua, S., He, X.N., Zhang, Y., 2010. DNA methyltransferases and methyl-binding proteins of mammals. *Acta Biochim. Biophys. Sin.* 42, 243-252.

Lee, B.H., Yegnasubramanian, S., Lin, X.H., Nelson, W.G., 2005a. Procainamide is a specific inhibitor of DNA methyltransferase 1. *J. Biol. Chem.* 280, 40749-40756.

Lee, W.J., Shim, J.Y., Zhu, B.T., 2005b. Mechanisms for the inhibition of DNA methyltransferases by tea catechins and bioflavonoids. *Mol. Pharmacol.* 68, 1018-1030.

Li, Y., Tollefsbol, T.O., 2010. Impact on DNA methylation in cancer prevention and therapy by bioactive dietary components. *Curr. Med. Chem.* 17, 2141-2151.

Liu, Z.F., Xie, Z.L., Jones, W., Pavlovicz, R.E., Liu, S.J., Yu, J.H., Li, P.K., Lin, J.Y., Fuchs, J.R., Marcucci, G., Li, C.L., Chan, K.K., 2009. Curcumin is a potent DNA hypomethylation agent. *Bioorg. Med. Chem. Lett.* 19, 706-709.

López-Vallejo, F., Caulfield, T., Martínez-Mayorga, K., Giulianotti, M.A., Nefzi, A., Houghten, R.A., Medina-Franco, J.L., 2011. Integrating virtual screening and combinatorial chemistry for accelerated drug discovery. *Comb. Chem. High Throughput Screening* 14, 475-487.

López-Vallejo, F., Nefzi, A., Bender, A., Owen, J.R., Nabney, I.T., Houghten, R.A., Medina-Franco, J.L., 2011. Increased diversity of libraries from libraries: Chemoinformatic analysis of bis-diazacyclic libraries. *Chem. Biol. Drug Des.* 77, 328-342.

Lyko, F., Brown, R., 2005. DNA methyltransferase inhibitors and the development of epigenetic cancer therapies. *J. Natl. Cancer Inst.* 97, 1498-1506.

Maggiora, G.M., 2006. On outliers and activity cliffs-why QSAR often disappoints. *J. Chem. Inf. Model.* 46, 1535-1535.

Maggiora, G.M., Shanmugasundaram, V., 2011. Molecular similarity measures, In: *Chemoinformatics and Computational Chemical Biology, Methods in Molecular Biology,* J. Bajorath, (Ed.), pp. 39-100, Springer, New York.

Medina-Franco, J., López-Vallejo, F., Kuck, D., Lyko, F., 2011. Natural products as DNA methyltransferase inhibitors: A computer-aided discovery approach. *Mol. Diversity* 15, 293-304.

Medina-Franco, J.L., Caulfield, T., 2011. Advances in the computational development of DNA methyltransferase inhibitors. *Drug Discovery Today* 16, 418-425.

Medina-Franco, J.L., López-Vallejo, F., Castillo, R., 2006. Diseño de fármacos asistido por computadora. *Educ. Quim.* 17, 452-457.

Medina-Franco, J.L., Martínez-Mayorga, K., Giulianotti, M.A., Houghten, R.A., Pinilla, C., 2008. Visualization of the chemical space in drug discovery. *Curr. Comput.-Aided Drug Des.* 4, 322-333.

Medina-Franco, J.L., Martínez-Mayorga, K., Bender, A., Marín, R.M., Giulianotti, M.A., Pinilla, C., Houghten, R.A., 2009. Characterization of activity landscapes using 2D and 3D similarity methods: Consensus activity cliffs. *J. Chem. Inf. Model.* 49, 477-491.

Miller, C.A., Gavin, C.F., White, J.A., Parrish, R.R., Honasoge, A., Yancey, C.R., Rivera, I.M., Rubio, M.D., Rumbaugh, G., Sweatt, J.D., 2010. Cortical DNA methylation maintains remote memory. *Nat. Neurosci.* 13, 664-666.

Muegge, I., 2008. Synergies of virtual screening approaches. *Mini-Rev. Med. Chem.* 8, 927-933.

Ooms, F., 2000. Molecular modeling and computer aided drug design. Examples of their applications in medicinal chemistry. *Curr. Med. Chem.* 7, 141-158.

Palii, S.S., Van Emburgh, B.O., Sankpal, U.T., Brown, K.D., Robertson, K.D., 2008. DNA methylation inhibitor 5-aza-2'-deoxycytidine induces reversible genome-wide DNA damage that is distinctly influenced by DNA methyltransferases 1 and 3B. *Mol. Cell. Biol.* 28, 752-771.

Pérez-Villanueva, J., Santos, R., Hernández-Campos, A., Giulianotti, M.A., Castillo, R., Medina-Franco, J.L., 2010. Towards a systematic characterization of the antiprotozoal activity landscape of benzimidazole derivatives. *Bioorg. Med. Chem.* 18, 7380-7391.

Pérez-Villanueva, J., Santos, R., Hernandez-Campos, A., Giulianotti, M.A., Castillo, R., Medina-Franco, J.L., 2011. Structure-activity relationships of benzimidazole derivatives as antiparasitic agents: Dual activity-difference (DAD) maps. *Med. Chem. Comm.* 2, 44-49.

Portela, A., Esteller, M., 2010. Epigenetic modifications and human disease. *Nat. Biotechnol.* 28, 1057-1068.

Ripphausen, P., Nisius, B., Bajorath, J., 2011. State-of-the-art in ligand-based virtual screening. *Drug Discovery Today* 16, 372-376.

Ripphausen, P., Nisius, B., Peltason, L., Bajorath, J.R., 2010. *Quo vadis*, virtual screening? A comprehensive survey of prospective applications. *J. Med. Chem.* 53, 8461-8467.

Robertson, K.D., 2001. DNA methylation, methyltransferases, and cancer. *Oncogene* 20, 3139-3155.

Salam, N.K., Nuti, R., Sherman, W., 2009. Novel method for generating structure-based pharmacophores using energetic analysis. *J. Chem. Inf. Model.* 49, 2356-2368.

Schaefer, M., Lyko, F., 2010. Solving the dnmt2 enigma. *Chromosoma* 119, 35-40.

Schermelleh, L., Spada, F., Easwaran, H.P., Zolghadr, K., Margot, J.B., Cardoso, M.C., Leonhardt, H., 2005. Trapped in action: Direct visualization of DNA methyltransferase activity in living cells. *Nat. Methods* 2, 751-756.

Schrump, D.S., Fischette, M.R., Nguyen, D.M., Zhao, M., Li, X.M., Kunst, T.F., Hancox, A., Hong, J.A., Chen, G.A., Pishchik, V., Figg, W.D., Murgo, A.J., Steinberg, S.M., 2006. Phase I study of decitabine-mediated gene expression in patients with cancers involving the lungs, esophagus, or pleura. *Clin. Cancer Res.* 12, 5777-5785.

Scior, T., Bernard, P., Medina-Franco, J.L., Maggiora, G.M., 2007. Large compound databases for structure-activity relationships studies in drug discovery. *Mini-Rev. Med. Chem.* 7, 851-860.

Scior, T., Medina-Franco, J.L., Do, Q.T., Martinez-Mayorga, K., Yunes Rojas, J.A., Bernard, P., 2009. How to recognize and workaround pitfalls in QSAR studies: A critical review. *Curr. Med. Chem.* 16, 4297-4313.

Segura-Pacheco, B., Trejo-Becerril, C., Perez-Cardenas, E., Taja-Chayeb, L., Mariscal, I., Chavez, A., Acuña, C., Salazar, A.M., Lizano, M., Dueñas-Gonzalez, A., 2003. Reactivation of tumor suppressor genes by the cardiovascular drugs hydralazine and procainamide and their potential use in cancer therapy. *Clin. Cancer Res.* 9, 1596-1603.

Sheikh, K.D., Banerjee, P.P., Jagadeesh, S., Grindrod, S.C., Zhang, L., Paige, M., Brown, M.L., 2010. Fluorescent epigenetic small molecule induces expression of the tumor suppressor Ras-association domain family 1a and inhibits human prostate xenograft. *J. Med. Chem.* 53, 2376-2382.

Shelat, A.A., Guy, R.K., 2007. The interdependence between screening methods and screening libraries. *Curr. Opin. Chem. Biol.* 11, 244-251.

Shoichet, B.K., 2004. Virtual screening of chemical libraries. *Nature* 432, 862-865.

Siedlecki, P., Boy, R.G., Musch, T., Brueckner, B., Suhai, S., Lyko, F., Zielenkiewicz, P., 2006. Discovery of two novel, small-molecule inhibitors of DNA methylation. *J. Med. Chem.* 49, 678-683.

Siedlecki, P., Boy, R.G., Comagic, S., Schirrmacher, R., Wiessler, M., Zielenkiewicz, P., Suhai, S., Lyko, F., 2003. Establishment and functional validation of a structural homology model for human DNA methyltransferase 1. *Biochem. Biophys. Res. Commun.* 306, 558-563.

Singh, N., Dueñas-González, A., Lyko, F., Medina-Franco, J.L., 2009a. Molecular modeling and dynamics studies of hydralazine with human DNA methyltransferase 1. *ChemMedChem* 4, 792-799.

Singh, N., Guha, R., Giulianotti, M.A., Pinilla, C., Houghten, R.A., Medina-Franco, J.L., 2009b. Chemoinformatic analysis of combinatorial libraries, drugs, natural products, and molecular libraries small molecule repository. *J. Chem. Inf. Model.* 49, 1010-1024.

Sippl, W., Jung, M., 2009. DNA methyltransferase inhibitors, In: *Epigenetic Targets in DrugDiscovery*, W. Sippl, and M. Jung (Eds.), pp. 163-183, Wiley-VCH, Weinheim.

Song, J., Rechkoblit, O., Bestor, T.H., Patel, D.J., 2011. Structure of DNMT1-DNA complex reveals a role for autoinhibition in maintenance DNA methylation. *Science* 331, 1036-1040.

Sperandio, O., Miteva, M.A., Villoutreix, B.O., 2008. Combining ligand- and structure-based methods in drug design projects. *Curr. Comput.-Aided Drug Des.* 4, 250-258.

Stresemann, C., Lyko, F., 2008. Modes of action of the DNA methyltransferase inhibitors azacytidine and decitabine. *Int. J. Cancer* 123, 8-13.

Suzuki, T., Tanaka, R., Hamada, S., Nakagawa, H., Miyata, N., 2010. Design, synthesis, inhibitory activity, and binding mode study of novel DNA methyltransferase 1 inhibitors. *Bioorg. Med. Chem. Lett.* 20, 1124-1127.

Tommasi, R., Cornella, I., 2006. Focused libraries: The evolution in strategy from large-diversity libraries to the focused library approach, In: *Exploiting Chemical Diversity for Drug Discovery*, A. Bartlett and M. Entzeroth, (Eds.), pp. 163-183, The Royal Society of Chemistry, Cambridge.

Vilkaitis, G., Merkiene, E., Serva, S., Weinhold, E., Klimasauskas, S., 2001. The mechanism of DNA cytosine-5 methylation. Kinetic and mutational dissection of HhaI methyltransferase. *J. Biol. Chem.* 276, 20924-20934.

Villar-Garea, A., Fraga, M.F., Espada, J., Esteller, M., 2003. Procaine is a DNA-demethylating agent with growth-inhibitory effects in human cancer cells. *Cancer Res.* 63, 4984-4989.

Villoutreix, B.O., Eudes, R., Miteva, M.A., 2009. Structure-based virtual ligand screening: Recent success stories. *Comb. Chem. & High Throughput Screening* 12, 1000-1016.

Villoutreix, B.O., Renault, N., Lagorce, D., Sperandio, O., Montes, M., Miteva, M.A., 2007. Free resources to assist structure-based virtual ligand screening experiments. *Curr. Protein Pept. Sci.* 8, 381-411.

Wawer, M., Lounkine, E., Wassermann, A.M., Bajorath, J., 2010. Data structures and computational tools for the extraction of SAR information from large compound sets. *Drug Discovery Today* 15, 630-639.

Yokochi, T., Robertson, K.D., 2002. Preferential methylation of unmethylated DNA by mammalian de novo DNA methyltransferase dnmt3a. *J. Biol. Chem.* 277, 11735-11745.

Yoo, J., Medina-Franco, J.L., 2011. Homology modeling, docking, and structure-based pharmacophore of inhibitors of DNA methyltransferase. *J. Comp.-Aided Mol. Des.* 25, 555-567.

Zawia, N.H., Lahiri, D.K., Cardozo-Pelaez, F., 2009. Epigenetics, oxidative stress, and Alzheimer disease. *Free Radical Biol. Med.* 46, 1241-1249.

Zheng, W., Johnson, S.R., 2008. Compound library design - principles and applications, In: *Chemoinformatics Approaches to Virtual Screening*, A. Varnek and A. Tropsha, (Eds.), pp. 268-294, Royal Society of Chemistry, Cambridge.

2

Development of Novel Secondary Hormonal Therapies for Castrate-Resistant Prostate Cancer

Rahul Aggarwal and Charles J. Ryan
University of California San Francisco
United States of America

1. Introduction

Androgen deprivation therapy (ADT), initially via surgical orchiectomy and more contemporarily with medical castration through the use of luteinizing hormone-releasing hormone (LHRH) agonists, has been the mainstay of treatment for advanced prostate cancer for more than 60 years (Huggins and Hodges, 1941). Though initially effective in decreasing serum PSA, lessening pain from bone metastases, and delaying clinical progression, almost all men develop disease progression despite ADT within 2-3 years. Initially, this disease state was considered hormone-refractory and androgen-independent. However, more recent research has led to the understanding that many prostate cancers continue to depend on androgen receptor (AR) signalling in this state of low but still detectable circulating androgens. Thus, a more appropriate term for this disease state is castrate resistant prostate cancer (CRPC). In this chapter we will discuss the biology behind continued AR signalling in CRPC, traditional non-selective secondary hormonal therapies, and the development of novel secondary hormonal agents which selectively and potently target the AR axis in CRPC.

2. Androgen Receptor signalling in Castrate Resistant Prostate Cancer

In many cases, CRPC retains the ability to activate the AR to stimulate prostate cancer growth and progression, despite low circulating levels of testosterone induced by medical or surgical castration (i.e. less than 50 ng/dL). Various research efforts have sought to understand the mechanism through which this occurs, both as a means of understanding tumor biology and as a means of developing new targeted therapies exploiting the AR axis in CRPC. Signalling can be conceptually divided into efforts to understand ligand production and AR modification.

2.1 Ligand production in Castrate Resistant Prostate Cancer
2.1.1 Endocrine ligands
Current ADT strategies using LHRH agonists suppress gonadal androgen production, resulting in a decrease in circulating serum testosterone to castrate levels (less than 50 ng/dL). Despite gonadal androgen suppression, low levels of circulating androgens persist

in CRPC, often via production of adrenal androgens, such as dihydroepiandrostenedione (DHEA), DHEA-sulfate (DHEA-S), and androstenedione, which are then converted to testosterone in peripheral tissues. Figure 1 below displays the steroid biosynthetic pathway and several secondary hormonal agents which block various steps of steroidogenesis, to be discussed in the following sections.

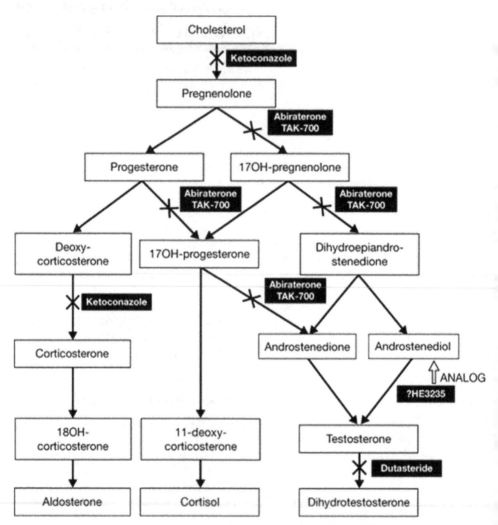

Fig. 1. Steroid Biosynthetic Pathway. Adapted from Aggarwal R and Ryan C, 2011.

Due to the peripheral conversion of adrenal steroids, low levels of circulating testosterone persists, and may account for levels up to 10% of that of pre-castrate levels (Puche, C et al. 2002). Low levels of circulating testosterone, along with circulating adrenal androgens, are hypothesized to subsequently stimulate CRPC progression through activation of the AR.

2.1.2 Intracrine ligands

More recently, research has shown that CRPC tissue has the ability to convert adrenal steroids to androgens, thereby creating an intracrine signalling system capable of converting steroid precursors to testosterone and dihydrotestosterone (DHT) which leads to continued stimulation of the AR and prostate cancer progression. The evidence for this comes from various lines of research. Direct measurements of intra-prostatic androgens including DHT demonstrates that levels of androgens in CRPC tissue is not significantly different compared with normal prostate tissue, despite significantly lower levels of circulating testosterone in the castrate men (Nishiyama T, et al. 2004). This finding implies that CRPC tissue acquires the ability to produce testosterone and DHT in an intracrine fashion, a finding which has been supported by further studies showing up-regulation of many of the steroid enzymes involved in androgen synthesis (see figure 1).

For example, Stanbrough et al. analysed oligonucleotide microarrays from 33 CRPC bone metastasis samples and compared their gene expression with samples from 22 hormone-sensitive primary cancers. The CRPC bone metastases demonstrated up-regulated expression of several enzymes involved in the steroid synthetic pathway: 17-beta hydroxysteroid dehydrogenase which converts androstenedione to testosterone; 3-beta hydroxysteroid dehydrogenase, which converts DHEA to androstenedione, and increased ratio of 5-alpha reductase isoform 1 to 2, which converts testosterone to DHT (Stanbrough M, et al 2006).

In a follow up study, Montgomery et al. evaluated androgen levels and transcripts encoding steroidogenic enzymes in benign prostate tissue, untreated primary prostate cancer, metastases from patients with castration-resistant prostate cancer, and xenografts derived from castration-resistant metastases. In this study, castrate-resistant tissues displayed increased expression of several key enzymes involved in androgen synthesis, including: CYP17A1 (C17,20 lyase), a key enzyme which converts progesterone and pregnenolone to 17-hydroxyprogesterone and 17-OH pregnenolone, as well as subsequent conversion of these steroids to androstenedione and DHEA respectively; 3-beta hydroxysteroid dehydrogenase as in the prior study. Furthermore, metastatic prostate cancers from CRPC patient samples express transcripts encoding androgen-synthesizing enzymes and maintain intratumoral androgens at concentrations capable of activating AR target genes and maintaining tumor cell survival in a xenograft model (Montgomery R et al, 2008). Finally, in an innovative study by Locke et al., it was demonstrated that tumor explants isolated from CRPC progression are capable of de novo conversion of [14C] acetic acid to dihydrotestosterone and that uptake of [3H] progesterone allows detection of the production of six other steroids upstream of dihydrotestosterone.

This cumulative body of evidence suggests that CRPCs are capable of adapting to lower circulating levels of androgens induced by castration, in which steroid enzymes involved in the synthetic pathway are upregulated, and thereby maintain high levels of intra-tumor androgens capable of stimulating the AR and driving prostate cancer progression. Understanding this mechanism of castration resistance has led to the development of targeted secondary hormonal therapies which specifically inhibit key enzymes of the androgen synthetic pathway, as will be discussed in the later section.

2.2 Androgen Receptor modification in Castrate Resistant Prostate Cancer

In addition to modification in the enzymes involved in steroid hormone production, the AR itself undergoes adaptation in the castrate state, and is implicated in disease progression to

CRPC. Mechanisms by which the AR adapts to the castrate state have been extensively studied in the past several decades, and include: (1) AR amplification and overexpression (2) heightened AR sensitivity to ligand activation through increased AR stabilization, enhanced nuclear localization, and overexpression of nuclear co-activators (3) increased AR promiscuity through various point mutations (4) ligand-independent activation of the AR through various signal transduction pathways, (5) AR splice variants with constitutive activity. In the following sections we will examine some of the evidence behind these modifications to the AR.

2.2.1 Androgen Receptor gene amplification and overexpression

In the late 1990s, research was starting to show that AR activation continued to play an important role in prostate cancer progression despite low circulating testosterone levels, and a potential mechanism through which this might occur was AR gene amplification and overexpression. In a study by Koivisto, et al, AR gene amplification was analyzed in 54 patient tumor samples at the time of recurrence after prior therapy, as well as in 26 cases, paired primary tumor samples prior to any therapy. In this study, 28% of the recurrent therapy-resistant tumors, versus none of the primary tumor samples, displayed AR gene amplification. Furthermore, through genomic analysis, the AR gene was wild type in all but one of the 15 AR gene amplified tumor samples. Interestingly, this study went on to show a clinicopathologic correlation between AR gene amplification and prior responsiveness to ADT, as well as improved subsequent prognosis (Koivisto P et al. 1997). In a follow up study by Linja et al., in which real-time quantitative reverse transcriptase polymerase chain reaction (RT-PCR) was used to analyze AR expression levels in eight benign prostate hyperplasias, 33 untreated and 13 castrate-resistant locally recurrent carcinomas, as well as 10 prostate cancer xenografts. All castrate-resistant tumors showed on average, 6-fold higher expression than androgen-dependent tumors or benign prostate hyperplasias (P < 0.001). Four of 13 (31%) castrate-resistant tumors contained AR gene amplification detected by fluorescence in situ hybridization. Finally, and equally as important, two of the ten prostate cancer xenograft models displayed AR overexpression, thus providing a key model for testing future drugs targeting the AR in the AR-amplified disease state (Linja MJ, et al. 2001).

Early studies such as these provided compelling evidence that AR gene amplification and thus overexpression may represent an important mechanism by which prostate cancers overcome low circulating androgen levels. Given this, a logical therapeutic strategy is the development of potent AR antagonists which would have activity in this AR-amplified disease state, and indeed, there are several novel potent, AR antagonists which are in clinical phase of drug development (see section below).

2.2.2 Androgen Receptor stabilization and heightened activity

In addition to numerical increase in the number of ARs per cancer cell, increased stabilization and nuclear localization of the AR may also factor into the mechanism of prostate cancer progression in the castrate resistant disease state. In a prior study by Gregory et al, recurrent prostate cancer cell lines had an AR degradation half-life that was 2-4 times longer than that of androgen-sensitive cancer cell lines. Furthermore, IHC staining showing that AR localization was entirely nuclear in the recurrent cancer cell lines; while localizing to both the cytoplasm and nucleus in the androgen sensitive cell lines (Gregory

CW, et al. 2001). This data suggests that AR activation and subsequent AR-mediated gene expression may in part be stimulated in CRPCs by mechanisms to prevent AR degradation and enhance localization to the nucleus. The mechanism of AR stabilization in CRPCs may in part related to increased cyclin-dependent kinase 1, which has been shown to phosphorylate and stabilize the AR and is also upregulated in castrate-resistant cell lines in prior pre-clinical study (Chen S, et al. 2006).

2.2.3 Androgen Receptor point mutations

Estimating the true frequency of acquired point mutations with functional significance in advanced prostate cancer has been difficult, due to various factors including patient selection, tumor heterogeneity, tissue source (prostate gland v metastases), method of tissue preservation, and molecular methods. They appear to be fairly uncommon in early prostate cancer and more prevalent in advanced prostate cancer. In a correlative analysis of bone marrow samples from patients with CRPC being treated with first generation anti-androgen withdrawal (CALGB study 9663), 10% of the patient samples had an AR point mutation, which was found within the hormone binding domain involved with transcription factor binding (Taplin M, et al. 2003). From a functional standpoint, it appears that certain AR point mutations lead to a more promiscuous AR, capable of being activated by a wider range of ligands. In a prior study of a mutant AR transfected into various cell lines, the adrenal androgen DHEA was capable of inducing greater AR-mediated transcriptional activity in the mutant AR cell line compared with wild type AR (Tan J, et al. 1997).

In this way, the increase in AR promiscuity may complement the changes in ligand production as outlined in the previous section, in which point mutations in the AR confer a greater ability for the AR to be activated by alternative ligands in the presence of low circulating testosterone levels, including the adrenal androgens such as DHEA. Mutations in the AR may also lead to partial agonistic activity of the first generation anti-androgens, such as flutamide, nilutamide, and bicalutamide, as will be discussed in the following section.

2.2.4 Ligand-independent activation of the Androgen Receptor

There is a wide-ranging body of evidence which suggests that for a subset of prostate cancers, ligand-independent activation of the AR, via activation from other signal transduction pathways, can independently activate the AR and lead to disease progression in the absence of hormone binding to the AR. Though not the focus of the current book chapter, the various signaling pathways that have been implicated in such a manner include the insulin-like growth factor pathway, epidermal growth factor receptor, and keratinocyte growth factor pathways, among others (Feldman B & Feldman D, 2001).

2.2.5 Androgen Receptor splice variants

Over the past several years a growing body of research implicates the generation of AR splice variants as a potential mechanism of driving disease progression to CRPC. Such AR splice variants have "hidden exons" within introns that are not normally transcribed in the wild type AR. The alternate splicing that incorporates such hidden exons into the variant mRNA transcripts creates pre-mature stop codons prior to the translation of the C-terminal ligand binding domain. Thus, variant AR proteins are created which lack the traditional ligand binding domain (see figure 2 below). In a seminal paper by Hu et al. prostate cancer tissue from primary hormone-sensitive and metastatic CRPC cancer tissue was analyzed by *in silico* DNA sequencing for the presence of AR splice variants. In total, 7 variant AR transcripts were discovered, AR-V1 through AR-V7. The two most abundantly expressed were AR-V1 and AR-V7. On average, there was 20-fold higher expression of these two variant transcripts in CRPC as opposed to hormone-sensitive prostate cancer. Functionally, AR-V7 was found to localize to the nucleus of prostate cancer cell line under androgen depleted conditions, and most importantly, was constitutively active in driving the expression of androgen-responsive genes (Hu, R, et al. 2009).

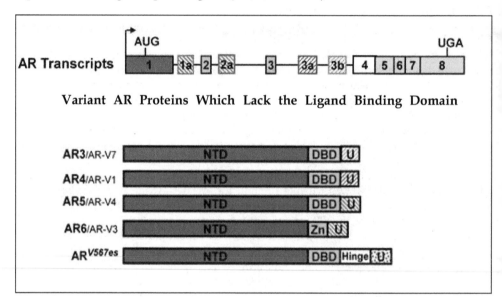

Fig. 2. Androgen Receptor Transcript and Splice Variants. NTD = N terminal domain. DBD = DNA binding domain. The hatched areas represent "hidden" exons spliced into the DNA biding domain exons (2 and 3), thus creating variant AR transcripts. The hidden exons of the variant AR transcripts encode stop codons, leading to premature termination and exclusion of the C-terminal ligand binding domain (exons 5-8 in green). Figure adapted from Guo, Z & Qiu, Y, 2011.

The exciting discovery of AR splice variants represents another potential mechanism by which cancer cells modify AR processing to adapt to a low circulating testosterone environment, creating AR splice variants which are not dependent on hormone binding to drive gene expression and cancer cell division and metastasis. Targeting the variant AR proteins, perhaps at the more ubiquitous N-terminal domain, represents a potential therapeutic approach to overcome this mechanism of resistance.

3. Traditional secondary hormonal therapies for Castrate Resistant Prostate Cancer

Traditional hormonal manipulations can be of some benefit to patients with CRPC; however significant responses are not seen in the majority of patients, and responses tend to be short-lived. Furthermore, the response duration and magnitude of benefit tend to diminish with each successive hormonal manipulation. Chemotherapy has traditionally been the mainstay of treatment for CRPC patients who have failed secondary hormonal therapy; however the median increase in overall survival with first line docetaxel chemotherapy is a modest 3 months, and fewer than 20% of patients with CRPC live beyond 3 years (Tannock, et al. 2004; Petyrlak DP, et al. 2004). Clearly, novel therapies are needed which applied together or in succession can lead to meaningful improvement in the quality and quantity of time for patients with CRPC. In the following sections we will first discuss the traditional secondary hormonal agents which have been used to treat CRPC. We will then continue onwards with a discussion of the novel secondary hormonal therapies currently in clinical development, which more selectively and potently inhibit either steroid ligand production or AR activation.

3.1 First generation antiandrogens

First generation antiandrogens, which competitively inhibit the binding of androgens to the ligand binding doman of the AR, remain in widespread use in the treatment of prostate cancer of various disease stages. The addition of a first generation antiandrogen (i.e. flutamide, nilutamide, or bicalutamide) to medical castration (combined androgen blockade) demonstrates only modest benefits in the hormone-sensitive disease population, with a small absolute survival benefit of less than 5% in most studies and meta-analyses. Similarly, the addition of an anti-androgen after ADT fails has demonstrated only modest benefit in prior clinical studies. In a prior clinical trial of flutamide 250 mg orally three times daily versus prednisone 5 mg orally four times per day, the median time to symptomatic progression on flutamide was only 2.3 months (as compared to 3.4 months with prednisone), and the proportion of patients with a greater than 50% decline in PSA or greater was 23% in the flutamide group vs. 21% in the prednisone group (Fossa SD, et al. 2001).

Similar rates of biochemical response were noted in a trial of 232 men who received either flutamide 375 mg/day or bicalutamide 80 mg/day after disease progression on combined androgen blockade. The percentage of men with a greater than 50% decline in PSA was 35.8%; the response duration was a little over 6 months (Suzuki H, et al. 2008). In another small trial of 31 men with CRPC treated with high dose bicalutamide 150 mg/day, only 22.5% of men had a PSA decline of > 50% for more than 2 months, almost all in men without prior treatment with flutamide (Joyce R, et al. 1998).

The modest efficacy and limited duration of response of first generation anti-androgens may in part be due to the fact that these molecules can act as partial agonists of the AR, especially AR which develop point mutations as a mechanism of resistance to these anti-androgens. Clinically, this partial agonist effect is observed with the phenomenon of anti-androgen withdrawal, a therapeutic maneuver in which the anti-androgen is discontinued in a patient who is progressing despite combined androgen blockade. In a prior study of anti-androgen withdrawal, 11% of patients demonstrated a decline of 50% or more in serum PSA after anti-androgen withdrawal (Small E, et al. 2004). Presumably, in these small subsets of patients who respond to antiandrogen withdrawal, the AR may have developed mutations which confer the ability to be activated by the antiandrogen.

Novel second generation antiandrogens which lack any agonist activity against the AR and demonstrate markedly more potent AR inhibition, including MDV-3100, will be discussed in the upcoming section.

3.2 Estrogens

Estrogens have long known to have been active in the treatment of prostate cancer; however the exact mechanism of actions remains uncertain. Putative mechanisms include inhibition of LH hormone release from the pituitary gland, inhibition of adrenal androgen production, and a direct cytotoxic effect on prostate cancer cells (Robertson CN, et al. 1996). In a prior phase randomized phase II trial comparing the estrogenic herbal compound PC-SPES with diethylstilbestrol, a greater than 50% decline in baseline PSA was noted in 40% and 24% of patients respectively; median time to progression was 5.5 vs. 2.9 months respectively (Oh W, et al. 2004).

There is clearly a modest degree of activity of estrogenic compounds in the treatment of CRPC; however current use of these agents (i.e. diethylstilbestrol, Premarin, etc.) is limited by the small but not insignificant risk of venous thromboembolic events and possibly increased risk of myocardial infarction and stroke; these particular co-morbidities are especially concerning in a disease population of elderly men. Concomitant prophylactic anticoagulation is recommended when using these agents.

3.3 Ketoconazole

Ketoconazole is a broad, non-specific inhibitor of multiple cytochrome p450 enzymes involved in androgen biosynthesis, including the conversion of cholesterol to pregnenolone, 11-beta hydroxylation, and 17-alpha hydroxylase/C17, 20 lyase (CYP17) activity. In a previously referred to randomized phase II study of 260 men with CRPC, with progressive disease despite combined androgen blockade, randomized to treatment with antiandrogen withdrawal alone or in combination with ketoconazole, 27% of patients assigned to the ketoconazole arm had a 50% or greater decline in serum PSA level, and 20% of patients had an objective response (Small EJ, et al. 2004). Interestingly, at the time of disease progression on ketoconazole, levels of adrenal androgens including DHEA, DHEA-S, and androstenedione had all increased compared to month 1 levels, which suggest that ketoconazole resistance may in part reflect inadequate androgen production suppression. This mechanism of resistance has implications for the development of novel androgen synthetic enzyme inhibitors such as abiraterone acetate. In an intriguing analysis of adrenal androgen hormone levels from the study by Small et al., patients who had higher baseline levels of androstenedione had a higher likelihood of response to treatment with ketoconazole (Ryan CJ, et al. 2007). This suggests that baseline adrenal androgen levels may be used as predictive biomarker for the use of adrenal androgen blockade as a therapeutic maneuver for CRPC; however this hypothesis requires prospective validation in larger studies.

Ketoconazole is a relatively non-specific inhibitor of multiple enzymes involved in the steroid synthetic pathway, and as such, as blocks normal corticosteroid production and causes iatrogenic adrenal insufficiency. Accordingly, side effects of this medication include lethargy, rash, nausea, and liver toxicity. Supplementation with physiologic replacement doses of hydrocortisone (i.e. 20 mg in the morning, 10 mg in the evening) is required while patients are taking ketoconazole. Furthermore, given the relatively non-specific CYPP450 inhibition, ketoconazole interacts with a wide number of other medications. Its oral absorption and bioavailability can be variable, depending on the acidity of the stomach and fed/fasting state and use of acid suppressing medications.

Despite these potential side effects and drug interactions, ketoconazole represents a viable and widely used secondary hormonal agent for CRPC, especially in the patient population with asymptomatic or minimally symptomatic bone-only metastatic or rising PSA-only disease.

4. Novel secondary hormonal therapies for Castrate Resistant Prostate Cancer

Insights into the mechanisms of continued AR signaling in CRPC, as discussed above, including (1) adrenal and intra-tumoral androgen ligand production, and (2) modifications of the AR, including gene amplification, over-expression, point mutations, ligand-independent activation, and splice variants, have led to the development of novel secondary hormonal therapies for CRPC. These new therapies are more selective and potent than their traditional counterparts. In the following subsections we will discuss the clinical development of several of the new hormonal therapies for CRPC.

4.1 Selective inhibition of CYP17

As displayed in figure 1, CYP17 (17-alpha hydroxylase/C17, 20 lyase) catalyzes two key steps of androgen synthesis within the steroid biosynthetic pathway: the 17-hydroxylation of progesterone and pregnenolone and subsequent conversion to DHEA and androstenedione respectively. Inhibition of this enzyme would divert cholesterol derivatives away from androgen production, and towards mineralocorticoid production (corticosterone and aldosterone). As outlined above, intra-tumoral upregulation of CYP17 has been previously implicated in the progression to CRPC. Logically then, selective inhibition of CYP17 represents an attractive strategy for inhibiting adrenal and intra-tumor androgen production in CRPCs and thereby slowing disease progression.

4.1.1 Abiraterone acetate

Abiraterone acetate is the prodrug of abiraterone, a potent, highly selective, irreversible inhibitor of CYP17. In pre-clinical in vivo study using WHT mice, this compound was able to markedly decrease the level of serum testosterone to less than 0.1 nanomolar concentration, despite 3-4 fold increase in serum LH concentration (Barrie SE, et al. 1994). In the first phase 1 study of abiraterone, O'Donnell et al. studied various dosing schedules ranging from 10 to 500 mg x 1 dose in castrate resistant men. At a dose level of 500 mg, there was suppression of serum testosterone to less than lower limit of detection (< 0.14 nmol/L) with parallel reduction androstenedione levels, supporting its mechanism of action of CYP17 inhibition. The duration of testosterone suppression after a single dose was variable, but generally ranged from days 2-5 post-dose (O'Donnell A, et al. 2004). In a follow up phase I trial by Attard and colleagues, 21 patients with CRPC and progression through multiple prior traditional secondary hormonal therapies were treated with abiraterone with doses ranging from 250 mg to 2000 mg/day. Pharmacodynamic effects on serum hormone levels showed a plateau at a dose of 1000 mg/day, which was the dose level of an expanded cohort of 9 patients and the subsequent recommended phase II/III dose. There were no treatment-related grade 3 or 4 adverse events from this trial. As expected, increases in levels of ACTH, corticosterone, and 11-deoxycorticosterone were observed, and there were adverse events related to subsequent mineralocorticoid excess, namely hypokalemia and hypertension. This was effectively managed with the use of eplerenone, a mineralocorticoid antagonist. The median baseline serum testosterone level was 7 ng/mL in this study; at all dose levels serum testosterone was decreased to < 1 ng/mL within 8 days of treatment initiation.

In a separate phase I dose escalation study of abiraterone acetate in 33 men, including 19 with prior ketoconazole treatment, daily dosing from 250 mg to 1000 mg was well tolerated with no dose-limiting toxicities (DLTs) (Ryan CJ, et al. 2010). Hypertension and hyperkalemia, signs of mineralocorticoid excess, as might be expected by the mechanism of action, were the most common serious toxicities (grade 3 or higher 12% and 9% respectively), which responded to medical management including low dose corticosteroids or mineralocorticoid receptor antagonists such as eplerenone. Spironolactone was avoided given its potential androgenic properties. Overall, 55% of patients in this study had a confirmed 50% or greater decline in serum PSA level at 12 weeks. In the subset of 19 patients with prior ketoconazole exposure, 46% had a greater than or equal to 50% decline in serum PSA at 12 weeks. Importantly, this data suggests that CRPCs which are resistant to ketoconazole may still be sensitive to the effects of abiraterone, which is a more potent and selective inhibitor of androgen synthesis compared to ketoconazole. In contrast to prior studies of ketoconazole in CRPC, in which adrenal androgens levels rose at the time of disease progression, serum hormone levels including testosterone and DHEA-S did not rise at the time of disease progression on abiraterone. This data suggests the mechanism of resistance to abiraterone may be unrelated to a rise in androgen levels. The phase II portion of this study included added prednisone 5 mg orally twice daily, and excluded patients with prior chemotherapy or ketoconazole (Ryan CJ, et al. 2009). Preliminary results indicated a 50% or greater decrease in PSA in 88% of patients; median time to PSA progression was 337 days.

Subsequent various phase II studies have evaluated abiraterone as monotherapy and combined with low dose prednisone in men with CRPC and prior docetaxel chemotherapy. In a two stage phase II trial by Reid and colleagues of 47 men with CRPC and previous treatment with docetaxel, treated with abiraterone 1000 mg/day monotherapy, 51% of patients demonstrated a 50% or greater decline in serum PSA level. Furthermore, the median time to PSA progression was 169 days; the objective response rate was 28% among men with measurable disease at baseline. 8 patients had prior ketoconazole treatment; all but one had prior treatment with a first generation antiandrogen. Adverse events were as expected due to secondary mineralocorticoid excess, including 55% with hypokalemia, 17% with hypertension, and 15% with fluid retention. In a phase II trial of abiraterone 1000 mg/day + prednisone 5 mg twice daily in 58 men with CRPC and prior docetaxel treatment, a confirmed ≥ 50% decline in PSA was observed in 36% of patients, including 27% of patients with prior ketoconazole treatment (Danila DC, et al. 2010). The median time to PSA progression was 169 days. The addition of prednisone decrease the incidence of clinical mineralocorticoid excess, and no patients required treatment with eplerenone while on study.

Results of the follow up confirmatory randomized phase III trial of abiraterone in the post-docetaxel CRPC population were recently reported (de Bono JS, et al. 2011). In this trial, 1195 patients with CRPC and prior docetaxel were randomized in a 2:1 fashion to receive either the combination of abiraterone 1000 mg/day + prednisone 5 mg twice daily versus placebo + prednisone 5 mg twice daily. After a median follow up of 12.8 months, overall survival was longer in the abiraterone group vs. the placebo group (median overall survival of 14.8 vs. 10.9 months; HR = 0.65, p < 0.0001). The data was unblinded at the time of interim analysis, as the results exceeded the pre-planned stopping rule for efficacy. All secondary endpoints, including progression-free survival, objective response rate, and PSA response rate favored the abiraterone treatment arm. Hypokalemia was noted in 17% of abiraterone group patients, and 10% of patients experienced hypertension of any grade severity. As a result of the overall survival benefit demonstrated in this phase III trial, abiraterone acetate was granted FDA approval on April 28th, 2011 for use in men with metastatic CRPC who had received prior chemotherapy containing docetaxel. An ongoing phase III trial of prednisone with or without abiraterone in men with metastatic CRPC without prior chemotherapy has finished accrual; study results are expected within the next year (NCT00887198).

The drug development of abiraterone acetate has unfolded rapidly over the past decade, based on a strong scientific rationale, pre-clinical and early clinical phase data indicating potent blockade of CYP17, a rational phase II/III dose selection, and the selection of clinically relevant endpoints for confirmatory phase III trials. Development of this drug remains ongoing, and many questions remain to be answered, including: (1) mechanisms of abiraterone resistance (2) optimal sequencing in the therapy of men with CRPC (e.g. before or after docetaxel?) (3) potential combination with other secondary hormonal agents (4) activity in patients with prior ketoconazole (patients treated with ketoconazole were excluded from the above mentioned phase III trials) (5) population pharmacokinetic analysis, and (6) development of predictive biomarkers that might allow for individualized patient selection for those most likely to benefit from abiraterone. This last issue is likely to become increasingly more relevant in an era of rising medical costs and the choice of multiple new agents for the treatment of CRPC. Preliminary data suggests that patients with higher levels of baseline adrenal androgen levels are more likely to respond to abiraterone, similar to the results obtained with prior studies of ketoconazole (Logothetis CJ, et al. 2008).

4.1.2 TAK-700 and TOK-001

Orteronel (TAK-700) is a selective CYP17 inhibitor which has reached clinical development in CRPC. Preliminary phase 1 data of 26 men with CRPC treated with dose levels ranging from 100 through 600 mg twice daily as well as 400 mg twice daily + low dose prednisone were recently presented (Dreicer R, et al. 2010). No dose limiting toxicities were seen. Fatigue was the most common adverse event, seen in 62% of patients, including 3 patients with grade 3 fatigue at the 600 mg twice daily dose. Other common adverse events included nausea, vomiting, anorexia, and constipation. Doses at or above 300 mg twice daily produced a 50% or greater decline in PSA in 70% of patients, of whom 29% had an impressive > 90% decline in serum PSA. Phase 3 trials of orteronel in men with metastatic CRPC pre and post docetaxel are ongoing (NCT01193244 and NCT01193257 respectively).

TOK-100, in a pre-clinical model, selectively inhibits CYP17 enzymatic activity and down regulates AR expression. In the LAPC4 xenograft model, TOK-100 combined with castration inhibited tumor growth and down-regulated AR expression, in contrast to treatment with castration or bicalutamide alone, in which AR expression was up-regulated (Vasaitis T, et al. 2008). Phase I/II trials of TOK-001 are underway in CRPC. The potential for down regulation of AR expression in addition to CYP17 inhibition may lead to more potent suppression of AR-mediated disease progression in CRPC, a hypothesis that warrants testing in current and future clinical trials of this compound.

4.2 Selective and potent inhibition of the Androgen Receptor

AR gene amplification and over-expression appears to be a relatively common phenomenon as tumors adapt to a low circulating testosterone environment, and may lead to progression to CRPC. First generation AR antagonists such as flutamide or bicalutamide inhibit ligand binding to the AR and thereby decrease nuclear localization and activation of AR-mediated gene expression. However, in the AR-amplified state, the first generation antiandrogens may not block the AR in a potent enough manner to block ligand-mediated AR activation. Furthermore, acquired point mutations in the AR may cause first generation antiandrogens to exhibit partial agonistic activity towards the AR, as supported by the clinical phenomenon of response to antiandrogen withdrawal. Pre-clinically, first generation antiandrogens exhibit partial agonist activity towards the AR in prostate cancer cell lines engineered to expression higher amounts of AR. More potent AR antagonists, which are capable of inhibiting the AR even in cells with AR overexpression, and do not possess any agonistic activity towards the AR, would be highly desirable as a hormonal therapy in CRPC, a potentially AR-amplified disease state.

4.2.1 MDV3100

MDV3100 was developed pre-clinically in an iterative screening process of various compounds that retain AR antagonistic activity in an AR-overexpressed cell line. MDV3100 binds to AR with 5-8 fold greater affinity compared to the first generation antiandrogen bicalutamide (Tran C, et al. 2009), impairs AR nuclear translocation, and inhibits AR binding to DNA, and blocks binding of AR to co-activators to a greater degree than bicalutamide. In tumor xenograft models known to overexpress AR, treatment with MDV3100 led to substantial tumor shrinkage.

MDV3100 was studied in a phase I/II clinical trial of 140 men with CRPC, including 45% of patients with prior ketoconazole and 54% with prior chemotherapy, in doses ranging from 30 mg to 600 mg/day. The maximum tolerated dose for ≥ 28 days was 240 mg/day. At doses of 360 mg/day and higher, 13% of patients discontinued treatment due to an adverse event, including three patients with seizures and one patient with a myocardial infarction. In contrast, at doses of 240 mg/day or lower, 1% of patients (1 out of 87 patients) discontinued treatment due to an adverse event. The most common grade 3 or higher dose-limiting toxicity was fatigue, which generally resolved with dose reduction. Anti-tumor activity was noted at all dose levels. In total, 56% of patients showed a 50% or greater reduction in serum PSA level; 22% of patients had an objective radiographic response among those with measurable disease at baseline, and conversion from unfavorable to favorable circulating tumor cell (CTC) count in 49% of patients. Similar PSA response rates were seen in patients with and without prior chemotherapy, though among patients with prior ketoconazole exposure, there was a lower percentage of patients with a 50% or greater decline in serum PSA (37% vs. 71% for those with and without prior ketoconazole respectively). The median time to radiographic progression was 47 weeks. Based on the encouraging results of this phase I/II clinical trial, ongoing phase III trials of MDV3100 vs. placebo, at a dose of 160 mg/day, are ongoing in patients with metastatic CRPC with and without prior docetaxel treatment (NCT00974311 and NCT01212991 respectively).

4.2.2 Other Androgen Receptor antagonists

Several other second generation, highly potent, pure AR antagonists have reached clinical development in CRPC. BMS-641988 is a highly potent AR inhibitor was designed based on

AR crystal structure. In pre-clinical study, this AR antagonist showed a > 1 log increase in potency of AR inhibition compared with bicalutamide, both in regards to AR binding and inhibition of AR-mediated gene expression (Attar RM, et al. 2009). Furthermore, in a human xenograft model, BMS-6419888 displayed greater growth inhibition compared with bicalutamide. Based on the encouraging pre-clinical data, this compound was subsequently tested in a phase I dose escalation study (Rathkopf D, et al. 2010). In this trial, doses of BMS-6419888 were escalated from 5 mg to 150 mg. In total, 61 men were treated. One patient experienced an epileptic seizure at a dose of 60 mg twice daily. Antitumor activity was limited to one partial response, and partial agonism was seen as evidenced by a decrease in serum PSA upon drug withdrawal. Based the limited anti-tumor activity despite achieving target therapeutic levels, as well as the epileptic seizure, the study was closed prematurely and further clinical development of this compound discontinued.

ARN-509 is a potent AR antagonist in the early phases of clinical development. It inhibits AR nuclear translocation and DNA binding, thereby modulating expression of genes which drive prostate cancer growth. It is currently being tested in a phase I/II clinical trial of men with metastatic CRPC with up to two prior chemotherapy regimens (NCT01171898). The primary endpoint is maximum tolerated dose; secondary endpoints include change in PSA, number of new bone lesions, and objective response by RECIST criteria. Enrollment began in July of 2010 and results are expected in 2012. Likely due to the several seizure events during prior clinical trials of MDV3100 and BMS-6419888, patients with a history of seizures or potentially lower seizure threshold are excluded from this phase I/II trial of ARN-509.

5. Future directions

The clinical activity of the novel secondary hormonal therapies which attack the AR axis continues to lend credence to the now widely held hypothesis that continued activation of the AR plays an important role in the progression of disease to CRPC and ultimately to prostate cancer death. Much progress has been made over the past several decades in the drug development of secondary hormonal therapies for CRPC. However, there are many questions that remain yet to be answered, including: (1) optimal timing and sequence of hormonal therapies in relation to chemotherapy and each other (2) relative risks and benefits of combination versus sequential hormonal monotherapy (3) mechanisms of resistance (4) patterns of disease progression on these novel therapies (5) potential predictive biomarkers to help individualize patient therapy, including the molecular characterization of circulating tumor cells (6) pharmacokinetic studies across various study populations and ethnicities (7) pharmacogenomics analysis of potential associations between germ line mutations and response (8) long term safety data, and (9) optimal phase II/III clinical trial endpoints to assess efficacy of these agents, including the potential use of surrogate markers such as change in number of circulating tumor cells.

Furthermore, there are new treatment strategies which target the AR axis that are in the infancy of drug discovery and development. Among them is EPI-001, a compound which inhibits transactivation of the N-terminal domain of the AR, without interacting with the AR ligand-binding doman, and thus may serve as a potential inhibitor of the AR splice variants that are hypothesized to play a role in the resistance to androgen ablation therapy (Andersen et al, 2010). Additionally, inhibitors of heat shock proteins, which act to stabilize the AR among other proteins, are also in clinical development.

6. Conclusions

AR activation continues to play a role in the progression of CRPC, despite low circulating serum testosterone levels in this disease state. This is accomplished through endocrine ligand production via adrenal androgen synthesis, intracrine ligand formation via up-regulation of the enzymes involved in androgen synthesis, including CYP17, AR overexpression and point mutations which confer receptor promiscuity and promote agonistic activity of traditional antiandrogen therapy, ligand-independent AR activation, and generation of constitutively active AR splice variants, among others. Pre-clinical drug discovery and development targeting specific steps in these mechanisms has led to the clinical development of numerous secondary hormonal agents which specifically and potently target the AR axis. Ongoing research is directed at optimizing and personalizing the use of the current novel secondary hormonal therapies as well as developing new therapeutic strategies to overcome treatment resistance in CRPC.

7. References

Aggarwal, R & Ryan, CJ. (2011). Castration-resistant prostate cancer: targeted therapies and individualized treatment. *The Oncologist*, Vol. 16, No. 3 (March 2011), pp. 264-275.

Andersen, RJ; Mawji, NR; Wang, J; et al. Regression of castrate-recurrent prostate cancer by a small-molecule inhibitor of the amino-terminus domain of the androgen receptor. *Cancer Cell*, Vol. 17 (June 2010), pp. 535-546.

Attar, RM; Jure-Kunkel, M; Balog, A; et al. Discovery of BMS-641988: a novel and potent inhibitor of androgen receptor signaling for the treatment of prostate cancer. *Cancer Research*, Vol. 69, No. 16 (August 2009), pp. 6522-6530.

Attard, G; Reid, AHM; Yap, TA; et al. Phase I clinical trial of a selective inhibitor of CYP17, abiraterone acetate, confirms that castration-resistant prostate cancer commonly remains hormone driven. *Journal of Clinical Oncology*, Vol. 28, No. 28 (October 2008), pp. 4563-4571.

Barrie, SE; Potter, GA; Goddard, PM; et al. (1994). Pharmacology of novel steroidal inhibitors of cytochrome P450 (17) alpha (17 alpha-hydroxylase/C17-20 lyase). *Journal of Steroid Biochemical Molecular Biology*, Vol. 50, No. 5/6 (2004), pp. 267-273.

Chen, S; Xu, Y; Yuan, X; et al. Androgen receptor phosphorylation and stabilization in prostate cancer by cyclin-dependent kinase 1. *Proceedings of the National Academy of Sciences*, Vol. 103, No. 43 (October 2006), pp. 15969-15974.

Danila, DC; Morris, MJ; de Bono, J; et al. Phase II multicenter study of abiraterone acetate plus prednisone in patients with docetaxel-treated castration-resistant prostate cancer. *Journal of Clinical Oncology*, Vol. 28, No. 9 (March 2010), pp. 1496-1501.

de Bono, JS; Logothetis, CJ; Molina, A; et al. Abiraterone and increased survival in metastatic prostate cancer. *New England Journal of Medicine*, Vol. 364, No. 21 (May 2011), pp. 1995-2005.

Dreicer, R; Agus, DB; MacVicar, GR; et al. Safety, pharmacokinetics, and efficacy of TAK-700 in castration-resistant metastatic prostate cancer: a phase I/II open label study. ASCO Genitourinary Cancer Symposium 2010, abstract 103.

Feldman, BJ & Feldman D. (2001). The development of androgen independent prostate cancer. *Nature Reviews: Cancer*, Vol. 1 (October 2001), pp. 34-45.

Fossa, SD; Slee, PH; Brausi, M; et al. (2001). Flutamide versus prednisone in patients with prostate cancer symptomatically progressing after androgen-ablative therapy: a phase III study of the European Organization for Research and Treatment of Cancer Genitourinary Group. *Journal of Clinical Oncology*, Vol. 19, No. 1 (January 2001), pp. 62-71.

Gregory, CW; Johnson, RT; Mohler, JL; et al. (2006). Androgen receptor stabilization in recurrent prostate cancer is associated with hypersensitivity to low androgen. *Cancer Research*, Vol. 61 (April 2001), pp. 2892-2898.

Guo, Z & Qiu, Y. A New Trick of an Old Molecule: Androgen Receptor Splice Variants Taking the Stage?!. *International Journal of Biological Sciences*, Vol. 7, No. 6 (July 2011), pp. 815-822.

Hu, R; Dunn, TA; Wei, S; et al. (2009). Ligand-independent androgen receptor variants derived from splicing of cryptic exons signify hormone-refractory prostate cancer. *Cancer Research*, Vol. 69, No. 1 (January 2009), pp. 16-22.

Huggins, C; Stevens Jr, RE; & Hodges, CV. (1941). Studies on prostatic cancer: The effect of castration on advanced carcinoma of the prostate gland. *Archives of Surgery,*Vol. 43 (1941), pp. 209-223.

Joyce, R; Fenton, MA; Rode, P; et al. High dose bicalutamide for androgen independent prostate cancer: effect of prior hormonal therapy. *Journal of Urology*, Vol. 159, No. 1 (January 1998), pp. 149-153

Koivisto, P; Kononen, J; Palmberg, C; et al. (1997). Androgen receptor gene amplification: a possible molecular mechanism for androgen deprivation therapy failure in prostate cancer. *Cancer Research*, Vol. 57 (January 1997), pp. 314-319.

Linja, MJ; Savinainen, KJ; Saramaki, OR; et al. (2001). Amplification and overexpression of androgen receptor gene in hormone-refractory prostate cancer. *Cancer Research*, Vol. 61 (May 2001), pp. 3550-3555.

Logothetis, CJ; Wen, S; Molina, A; et al. Identification of an androgen withdrawal responsive phenotype in castrate resistant prostate cancer patients treated with abiraterone acetate. *Journal of Clinical Oncology*, Vol. 26, supplement, abstract 5017.

Montgomery, RB; Mostaghel, EA; Vessella R, et al. (2008). Maintenance of intratumoral androgens in metastatic prostate cancer: a mechanism for castration-resistant tumor growth. *Cancer Research*, Vol. 68, No. 11 (June 2008), pp. 4447-4454.

Nishiyama, T; Hashimoto, Y & Takahashi, K. (2004). The influence of androgen deprivation therapy in dihydrotestosterone levels in the prostate tissue of patients with prostate cancer. *Clinical Cancer Research*, Vol. 10 (2004), pp. 7121-7126.

O'Donnell, A; Judson, I; Dowsett, M; et al. (2004). Hormonal impact of the 17 alpha-hydroxylase/C(17,20) lyase inhibitor abiraterone acetate (CB7630) in patients with prostate cancer. *British Journal of Cancer*, No. 90 (May 2004), pp. 2317-2325.

Oh, WK; Kantoff, PW; Weinberg, V; et al. (2004). Prospective, multicenter, randomized phase II trial of the herbal supplement, PC-SPES, and diethylstilbestrol in patients with androgen-independent prostate cancer. *Journal of Clinical Oncology*, Vol. 22, No. 18 (September 2004), pp. 3705-3712.

Petyrlak, DP; Tangen, CM; Hussain, MH; et al. (2004). Docetaxel and estramustine compared with mitoxantrone and prednisone for advanced refractory prostate cancer. *New England Journal of Medicine*, Vol. 351 (October 2004), pp. 1513-1520.

Puche, C; Jose, M; Cabero, A; et al. (2002). Expression and enzymatic activity of the P450c17 gene in human adipose tissue. *European Journal of Endocrinology*, Vol. 146 (February 2002), pp. 223-229.

Reid, AH; Attard, D; Danila, D; et al. Significant and sustained antitumor activity in post-docetaxel, castration-resistant prostate cancer with the CYP17 inhibitor abiraterone acetate. *Journal of Clinical Oncology*, Vol. 28, No. 9 (March 2010), pp. 1489-1495.

Robertson, CN; Roberson, KM; Padilla, GM; et al. (1996). Induction of apoptosis by diethylstilbestrol in hormone-insensitive prostate cancer cells. *Journal of the National Cancer Institute*, Vol. 88, No. 13 (April 1996), pp. 908-917.

Ryan, CJ; Halabi, S; Ou, S; et al. (2007). Adrenal androgen levels as predictors of outcome in prostate cancer patients treated with ketoconazole plus antiandrogen withdrawal: results from a Cancer and Leukemia Group B Study. *Clinical Cancer Research*, Vol. 13, No. 7 (April 2007), pp. 2030-2037.

Ryan, CJ; Smith, MR; Fong, L; et al. Phase I clinical trial of the CYP17 inhibitor abiraterone acetate demonstrating clinical activity in patients with castration-resistant prostate cancer who received prior ketoconazole. *Journal of Clinical Oncology*, Vol. 28, No. 9 (March 2010), pp. 1481-1488.

Ryan, CJ; Efstathiou, E; Smith, M; et al. Phase II multicenter study of chemotherapy (chemo)-naïve castration resistant prostate cancer (CRPC) not exposed to ketoconazole, treated with abiraterone acetate plus prednisone. *Journal of Clinical Oncology*, Vol. 27, No. 15s (June 2009), abstract 5046.

Small, EJ; Halabi, S; Dawson, NA; et al. (2004). Antiandrogen withdrawal alone or in combination with ketoconazole in androgen-independent prostate cancer patients. *Journal of Clinical Oncology*, Vol. 22, No. 6 (March 2004), pp. 1025-1033.

Stanbrough, M; Bubley, GJ; Ross K, et al. (2006). Increased expression of genes converting adrenal androgens to testosterone in androgen-independent prostate cancer. *Cancer Research*, Vol. 66, No. 5 (March 2006), pp. 2815-2825.

Suzuki, H; Okihara, K; Miyake, H; et al. (2008). Alternative nonsteroidal antiandrogen therapy for advanced prostate cancer that relapsed after initial maximum androgen blockade. *Journal of Urology*, Vol. 180, No. 3 (September 2008), pp. 921-927.

Tan, J; Sharief, Y; Hamil, KG; et al. (1997) Dehydroepiandrosterone activates mutant androgen receptors expressed in the androgen- dependent human prostate cancer xenograft CWR22 and LNCaP cells. *Molecular Endocrinology*, Vol. 11, No. 4 (April 1997), pp. 450-459.

Tannock, IF; de Wit, R; Berry, WR; et al. (2004) Docetaxel plus prednisone or mitoxantrone plus prednisone for advanced prostate cancer. *New England Journal of Medicine*, Vol. 351 (October 2004), pp. 1502-1512.

Taplin, M; Rajeshkumar, B; Halabi, S; et al. Androgen receptor mutations in androgen-independent prostate cancer: Cancer and Leukemia Group B Study 9663. *Journal of Clinical Oncology*, Vol. 21 (July 2003), pp. 2673-2678.

Tran, C; Ouk, S; Clegg, NJ; et al. Development of a second-generation antiandrogen for treatment of advanced prostate cancer. *Science*, Vol. 324 (May 2009), pp. 787-790.

Vasaitis, T; Belosay, A; Schayowitz, A; et al. Androgen receptor inactivation contributes to antitumor efficacy of 17-alpha hydroxylase/17,20-lyase inhibitor 3beta-hydroxy-17-(1H-benzimidazole-1-yl)androsta-5,16-diene in prostate cancer. *Molecular Cancer Therapeutics*, Vol. 7, No. 8 (August 2008), pp. 2348-2357.

3

Histamine Receptors as Potential Therapeutic Targets for Cancer Drug Development

Vanina A. Medina[1,2], Diego J. Martinel Lamas[1], Pablo G. Brenzoni[1],
Noelia Massari[1], Eliana Carabajal[1] and Elena S. Rivera[1]
*[1]Laboratory of Radioisotopes, School of Pharmacy and Biochemistry,
University of Buenos Aires*
*[2]National Scientific and Technical Research Council (CONICET)
Argentina*

1. Introduction

Although research over the last decade has led to new and improved therapies for a variety of different diseases, anticancer drug therapy continues to have undesirable outcomes, including both poor response and severe toxicity. In addition to the critical need to discover new drugs, it is important to optimize existing therapies in order to minimize adverse reactions and maximize efficacy.

In the context of the complexity of cancer disease processes, future anticancer treatments will have to take into account the tumour microenvironment and aim to target the different cellular and molecular participants encompassed in a tumour, as well as their specific interactions.

In the present chapter we aimed to briefly summarize current knowledge on histamine and histamine receptors involvement in cancer, focusing on some recent evidence that points them out as a promising molecular targets and avenue for cancer drug development. On the basis of the role on immune system, it has been reported the efficiency of histamine as an adjuvant to tumour immunotherapy. In addition, we present here novel findings, suggesting the potential application of histamine and its ligands as adjuvants to tumour radiotherapy.

2. Histamine receptors

It is generally acknowledged that histamine is an important regulator of a plethora of (patho) physiological conditions and exerts its actions through the interaction with four histamine receptor subtypes. All these receptors belong to the family of heptahelical G-protein coupled receptors (GPCR) and they are the H_1, H_2, H_3 and H_4 histamine receptors (H_1R, H_2R, H_3R, H_4R). Based on the classical pharmacological analysis H_1R was proposed in 1966 by Ash and Schild (Ash & Schild, 1966) and H_2R was described in 1972 by Black et al. (Black et al., 1972). The third histamine receptor was discovered in 1983 by a traditional pharmacological approach, consisting of assessing the inhibitory effect of histamine on its own release from depolarized rat brain slices (Arrang et al., 1983). It was not until 2000-2001 that by using the H_3R DNA sequence, several independent research groups identified the novel H_4R highly expressed in immune cells (Coge et al. 2001b; Lui et al., 2001; Morse et al. 2001; Nakamura et al., 2000; Nguyen et al. 2001; Oda et al., 2000).

Recent studies employing human genetic variance and mice lacking specific receptors or the ability to generate histamine, have shown functions for the histamine pathway that extend well beyond the established roles. As a result, antihistamines may have wider applications in the future than previously predicted (Smuda & Bryce, 2011).

	Agonists	Antagonists/ Inverse agonists
H_1R	Histaprodifens, 2-(3-trifluoromethylphenyl) histamine	Mepyramine, cetirizine, terfenadine diphenhydramine, loratadine
H_2R	Amthamine, impromidine, arpromidine	Famotidine, ranitidine, cimetidine, roxatidine, zolantidine
H_3R	R-(α)-methylhistamine, imetit, immepip	Clobenpropit, thioperamide, iodoproxyfan
H_4R	Clobenpropit, VUF 8430, imetit, 4-methylhistamine, R-(α)-methylhistamine, OUP-16, clozapine	Thioperamide, JNJ7777120, VUF 6002, A-987306, A-940894

Table 1. Compounds most widely used in histamine receptor investigation

Like most other GPCR, histamine receptors exist as equilibrium between their inactive and active conformations. Constitutive activity has now been shown for all four types of histamine receptors, leading to the reclassification of some antagonists as inverse agonists. These members of the GPCR family may exist as homo- and hetero-oligomers at the cell surface, which could have different pharmacological and physiological effects (Bongers et al., 2007; Fukushima et al., 1997; Hancock et al., 2003; Leurs et al., 2002, 2009). Moreover, the affinity of histamine binding to different histamine receptors varies significantly. Thus, the effects of histamine and receptor ligands upon receptor stimulation are rather complex. Pharmacologic agents are summarized in table 1.

2.1 Histamine H_1R

Since histamine is considered to be the most important mediator in allergies such as allergic rhinitis, conjunctivitis, atopic dermatitis, urticaria, asthma and anaphylaxis, the most commonly used drugs to treat these pathological disorders are antihistamines acting on the H_1R. In the lung, it mediates bronchoconstriction and increased vascular permeability. The H_1R is expressed in a wide variety of tissues, including airway and vascular smooth muscle, endothelia, gastrointestinal tract, liver, genitourinary and cardiovascular systems, central nervous system (CNS), adrenal medulla, chondrocytes and in various immune cells including neutrophils, monocytes, eosinophils, dendritic cells (DC), as well as T and B lymphocytes, in which it mediates the various biological manifestations of allergic responses. The coding sequence of the human H_1R is intronless and is located in the chromosome 3 (Bakker et al., 2001; Dy & Schneider, 2004; Leurs et al., 1995). The human H_1R

contains 487 amino acids and is a Gαq/11-coupled protein with a very large third intracellular loop and a relatively short C-terminal tail. The most important signal induced by ligand binding is the activation of phospholipase C (PLC)-generating inositol 1,4,5-triphosphate (Ins (1,4,5) P3) and 1,2-diacylglycerol leading to increased cytosolic calcium. In addition to the inositol signalling system, H_1R activation could lead to additional secondary signalling pathways. This rise in intracellular calcium levels seems to account for the various pharmacological activities promoted by the receptor, such as nitric oxide production, vasodilatation, liberation of arachidonic acid from phospholipids and increased cyclic guanosine-3',5'-monophosphate (cGMP). Additionally, it was reported that H_1R can directly increase the cyclic adenosine-3',5'-monophosphate (cAMP) levels (Davio et al., 1995). H_1R also activates NF-kB through Gαq11 and Gβγ upon agonist binding, while constitutive activation of NF-kB occurs only through the Gβγ (Bakker et al., 2001; Leurs et al., 1995; Smit et al., 1999). Recently, it was reported that the stimulation of H_1R induced H_1R gene expression through protein kinase C δ (PKCδ) activation, resulting in receptor upregulation (Mizuguchi et al., 2011).

2.2 Histamine H₂R

The H_2R principal action from a clinical point of view is its role in stimulating gastric acid secretion, thus H_2R antagonists are used in the relief of symptoms of gastro-oesophageal reflux disease treatment. The human H_2R intronless gene, encodes a protein of 359 amino acids and is located on chromosome 5. The H_2R has a ubiquitous expression as the H_1R. It is expressed in gastric parietal cells, heart, endothelial cells, nerve cells, airway and vascular smooth muscle, hepatocytes, chondrocytes and immune cells, such as neutrophils, monocytes, eosinophils, DC, and T and B lymphocytes (Black et al., 1972; Dy & Schneider, 2004; Leurs et al., 1995). The H_2R is coupled both to adenylate cyclase via a GTP-binding protein G_s, and phosphoinositide second messenger systems by separate GTP-dependent mechanisms. However, H_2R-dependent effects of histamine are predominantly mediated by cAMP that activates protein kinase A (PKA) enzymes phosphorylating a wide variety of proteins involved in regulatory processes. Activation of H_2R is also associated with other additional signal transduction pathways including activation of c-Fos, c-Jun, PKC and p70S6kinase (Davio et al., 1995; Fitzsimons et al., 2002; Fukushima et al., 1997).

2.3 Histamine H₃R

The H_3R has initially been identified in both central and peripheral nervous system as a presynaptic receptor controlling the release of histamine and other neurotransmitters (dopamine, serotonine, noradrenalin, γ-aminobutyric acid and acetylcholine) (Arrang et al., 1983; Bongers et al., 2007; Leurs et al., 2005; Lovenberg et al., 1999). The H_3R has gained pharmaceutical interest as a potential drug target for the treatment of various important disorders like obesity, myocardial ischemia, migraine, inflammatory diseases and several CNS disorders like Alzheimer's disease, attention-deficit hyperactivity disorder and schizophrenia. Pitolisant (BF2.649, 1-{3-[3-(4-chlorophenyl)propoxy]propyl} piperidine, hydrochloride) is the first H_3R inverse agonist to be introduced in the clinics. Its wake-promotion activity was evidenced in excessive diurnal sleepiness of patients with narcolepsy, Parkinson's disease or obstructive sleep apnea/hypopnea (Bongers et al., 2007; Lebois et al., 2011; Leurs et al., 2005; Schwartz, 2011). The human H_3R gene consists of either three exons and two introns, or four exons and three introns spanning 5.5 kb on chromosome 20. Alternatively, the most 3' intron has been proposed to be a pseudo-intron as it is retained in the $hH_3R(445)$ isoform, but deleted in the $hH_3R(413)$ isoform. Overall similarity between the H_3R and the H_1R and H_2R amounts to only 22% and 20%, respectively (Bongers et al., 2007; Coge et al., 2001a; Dy & Schneider, 2004; Leurs et al., 2005; Tardivel-Lacombe et al., 2001; Wellendorph et al., 2002).

The cloning of the human H_3R has led to the discovery of many H_3R isoforms generated through alternative splicing of the H_3R mRNA. H_3R can activate several signal transduction pathways, including Gi/o-dependent inhibition of adenylate cyclase that leads to inhibition of cAMP formation, activation of mitogen activated protein kinase pathway (MAPK), phospholipase A2, and Akt/protein kinase B, as well as the inhibition of the Na+/H+ exchanger and inhibition of K+-induced Ca2+ mobilization (Bongers et al., 2007; Coge et al., 2001a; Leurs et al., 2005; Wellendorph et al., 2002). A negative coupling to phosphoinositide turnover in the human gastric cell line HGT has also been described (Cherifi et al., 1992). Moreover, at least 20 isoforms of the human H_3R have been described and they vary in the length of the third intracellular loop, their distinct CNS localization, differential signalling pathways and ligand binding affinity, which contribute to the heterogeneity of H_3R pharmacology (Bongers et al., 2007; Coge et al., 2001a; Hancock et al., 2003; Leurs et al., 2005).

2.4 Histamine H_4R

The identification by genomics-based approach of the human H_4R by several groups has helped refine our understanding of histamine roles. It appeared to have a selective expression pattern restricted to medullary and peripheral hematopoietic cells including eosinophils, mast cells, DC, T cells and monocytes. Therefore, growing attention is directed towards the therapeutic development of H_4R ligands for inflammation and immune disorders. Several lines of evidence suggest a role of the H_4R in chronic inflammatory skin disease and the H_4R might be a therapeutic target for diseases such as atopic dermatitis (Gutzmer et al., 2011). In addition, H_4R was reported to be present on other cell types including intestinal epithelium, spleen, lung, stomach, CNS, nerves of nasal mucosa, enteric neurons and interestingly in cancer cells (Cianchi et al., 2005; Coge et al. 2001b; Connelly et al., 2009; Leurs et al. 2009; Lui et al., 2001; Medina et al., 2006; Morse et al. 2001; Nakamura et al., 2000; Nguyen et al. 2001; Oda et al., 2000). The significance of the H_4R presence in various human tissues remains to be elucidated and therefore, new roles of H_4R are still unrevealed (Leurs et al., 2009; Zampeli & Tiligada, 2009). The H_4R cDNA was finally identified in the human genome database on the basis of its overall homology (37%, 58% in transmembrane regions) to the H_3R sequence and it has a similar genomic structure. On the other hand, the homology with H_1R and H_2R is of approximately 19%. The human H_4R gene that mapped to chromosome 18 is interrupted by two large introns and encodes a protein of 390 amino acids (Coge et al., 2001b; Leurs et al., 2009). H_4R is coupled to Gαi/o proteins, inhibiting forskolin-induced cAMP formation (Nakamura et al., 2000; Oda et al., 2000). Additionally, stimulation of H_4R leads to activation of MAPK and also increased calcium mobilization via pertussis toxin-sensitive pathway (Leurs et al., 2009; Morse et al., 2001).

Isoforms have been described for the H_4R which have different ligand binding and signalling characteristics. H_4R splice variants [H_4R (67) and H_4R (302)] have a dominant negative effect on H_4R (390) functionality, being able to retain it intracellularly and to inactivate a population of H_4R (390) presumably via hetero-oligomerization (Leurs et al.,

2009; van Rijn et al., 2008). In addition, H_4R dimeric structures that include homo- and hetero-oligomer formation and post-translational changes of the receptor might contribute to added pharmacological complexity for H_4R ligands (Leurs et al., 2009; van Rijn et al., 2006, 2008).

3. Histamine receptors in breast cancer

An estimated 1 million cases of breast cancer are diagnosed annually worldwide. Breast cancer is the most common neoplastic disease in women, and despite advances in early detection, about 30% of patients with early-stage breast cancer have recurrent disease, which is metastatic in most cases and whose cure is very limited showing a 5-year survival rate of 20% (Ferlay et al., 2010; Gonzalez-Angulo et al., 2007).

Histamine plays a critical role in the pathologic and physiologic aspects of the mammary gland, regulating cell growth, differentiation and functioning during development, pregnancy and lactation. Among monoamines, histamine demonstrates the greatest proliferative activity in breast cancer (Davio et al., 1994; Malinski et al., 1993; Wagner et al., 2003). Furthermore, histamine is increased in plasma and cancerous tissue derived from breast cancer patients compared to healthy group which is associated to an enhanced histidine decarboxylase (HDC) activity and a reduced diaminooxydase (DAO) activity that determine an imbalance between the synthesis and degradation of this monoamine. Histamine plasma level is dependent on the concentration of histamine in the tissues of ductal breast cancers, suggesting the participation of this monoamine in the development of this neoplasia (Reynolds et al., 1998; Sieja et al., 2005; von Mach-Szczypiński et al., 2009). A pilot study revealed that in samples of the same invasive ductal carcinoma patient, histamine peripheral blood levels tended to be reduced post-operatively (Kyriakidis et al., 2009). It was reported that in experimental mammary carcinomas, histamine becomes an autocrine growth factor capable of regulating cell proliferation via H_1R and H_2R, as one of the first steps responsible for the onset of malignant transformation. In this light, the *in vivo* treatment with H_2R antagonists produced the complete remission of 70% of experimental tumours (Cricco et al., 1994; Davio et al., 1995; Rivera et al., 2000). Many reports indicate the presence of H_1R and H_2R in normal and malignant tissues as well as in different cell lines derived from human mammary gland. H_2R produced an increase in cAMP levels while H_1R was coupled to PLC activation in benign lesions. On the other hand, H_1R was invariably linked to PLC pathway but H_2R stimulated both transductional pathways in carcinomas (Davio et al., 1993, 1996). However, the clinical trials with H_2R antagonists demonstrated controversial results for breast cancer (Bolton et al., 2000; Parshad et al., 2005).

Recently, it was demonstrated that H_3R and H_4R are expressed in cell lines derived from human mammary gland (Medina et al., 2006). Histamine is capable of modulating cell proliferation exclusively in malignant cells while no effect on proliferation or expression of oncogenes related to cell growth is observed in non-tumorigenic HBL-100 cells (Davio et al., 2002; Medina et al., 2006). Furthermore, histamine modulated the proliferation of MDA-MB-231 breast cancer cells in a dose-dependent manner producing a significant decrease at 10 $\mu mol.L^{-1}$ concentration whereas at lower concentrations increased proliferation moderately. The negative effect on proliferation was associated to the induction of cell cycle arrest in G2/M phase, differentiation and a significant increase in the number of apoptotic cells (Medina et al., 2006; Medina & Rivera, 2010b). Accordingly, by using pharmacological tools, results demonstrated that histamine increased MDA-MB-231 cell proliferation and also migration via H_3R. In contrast, clobenpropit and VUF8430 treatments significantly decreased proliferation. This outcome was associated to an induction of apoptosis determined by Annexin-V staining and TdT-mediated UTP-biotin Nick End labelling (TUNEL) assay, which was blocked by the specific H_4R antagonist JNJ7777120. Also H_4R agonists exerted a 2.5-fold increase in the cell senescence while reduced migration (Medina et al., 2008, 2010c, 2011b). Furthermore, histamine differentially regulates expression and activity of matrix metalloproteinases, cell migration and invasiveness through H_2R and H_4R in MDA-MB-231 cells modulating H_2O_2 intracellular levels (Cricco et al., 2011).

In addition, histamine at all doses tested, decreased the proliferation of a more differentiated breast cancer cell line, MCF-7, through the stimulation of the four histamine receptor subtypes exhibiting a higher effect through the H_4R. Treatment of MCF-7 cells with the H_4R agonists, inhibited cell proliferation and increased apoptosis and senescence (Medina et al., 2011b). These results represent the first report about the expression of H_3R and H_4R in human breast cells and interestingly show that the H_4R is involved in the regulation of breast cancer cell proliferation, apoptosis, senescence, migration and invasion.

Recent results obtained with the orthotopic xenograft tumours of the highly invasive human breast cancer line MDA-MB-231 in immune deficient nude mice indicate that the H_4R was the major histamine receptor expressed in the tumour. Remarkably, *in vivo* JNJ7777120 treatment (10 mg.kg^{-1}, *p.o.*, daily administration) significantly decreased lung metastases, indicating that H_4R may be involved in the metastatic process (Medina & Rivera, 2010b). In addition, *in vivo* clozapine treatment (1 mg.kg^{-1}, *s.c.*, daily administration) significantly decreased tumour growth while enhanced survival of bearing tumour mice (Martinel Lamas et al., unpublished data).

Recent data indicate that H_3R and H_4R are expressed in human biopsies of benign lesions and breast carcinomas being the level of their expression significantly higher in carcinomas, confirming that H_3R and H_4R are present not only in cell lines but also in the human breast tissue. Furthermore, the expression of H_3R is highly correlated with proliferation and histamine production in malignant lesions while the 50% of malignant lesions expressed H_4R, all of them corresponding to metastases or high invasive tumours (Medina et al., 2008). The identification of histamine receptor subtypes and the elucidation of their role in the development and growth of human mammary carcinomas may represent an essential clue for advances in breast cancer treatment. The presented evidences contribute to the identification of molecules involved in breast carcinogenesis and confirm the role of H_4R in the regulation of breast cancer growth and progression representing a novel molecular target for new therapeutic approach.

4. Histamine receptors in lymphomas and leukaemia

There is increasing evidence that histamine plays a role in cell differentiation and proliferation in several of normal tissues and in a wide range of tumours, including haematological neoplasias.

After an initial work in the late 1970s showing that histamine is able to induce haematopoietic stem cell proliferation via H_2R (Byron, 1977), a real rush broke out in searching for further effects of histamine in haematopoiesis and haematological neoplasias. The histamine levels were determined in lymph nodes of patients with malignant lymphomas, Hodking's disease (HD) or non-Hodking lymphomas (NHL), and in all cases the values were higher than in controls. In patients with NHL, these levels showed dependence on the grade of malignancy as they found to be significantly higher in those classified as high-grade malignant (Belcheva & Mishkova, 1995). Immunostaining and ELISA method also confirmed the presence of histamine in the cytoplasm of acute lymphocytic leukaemia (ALL) cells, and H_1R antihistamines inhibited their clonogenic growth. There was no correlation between the clonogenic growth of ALL cells and their histamine content, suggesting that while histamine may be important for the clonogenic growth of ALL cells; other factors also affect their clonogenity (Malaviya et al., 1996). Furthermore, leukaemia cell lines such as U937, expressed histamine receptors and a switch of histamine receptor expression from H_2R to H_1R during differentiation of monocytes into macrophages is observed (Wang et al., 2000).

Most patients with acute myeloid leukaemia (AML) achieve complete remission after induction chemotherapy. Despite ensuing courses of consolidation chemotherapy, a large fraction of patients will experience relapses with poor prospects of long-term survival. Interleukin-2 (IL-2) and interferon-alpha (IFN-alpha) are effective activators of lymphocytes with anti-neoplastic properties, such as T-cells or natural killer (NK) cells, constituting the basis for their widespread used as immunotherapeutic agents in human neoplastic disease. The functions of intratumoural lymphocytes in many human malignant tumours are inhibited by reactive oxygen species (ROS), generated by adjacent monocytes/macrophages. *In vitro* data suggest that those immunotherapeutic cytokines only weakly activate T cells or NK cells in a reconstituted environment of oxidative stress and inhibitors of ROS formation or ROS scavengers synergize with IL-2 and IFN-alpha to activate T cells and NK cells. Recently, IL-2 therapy for solid neoplastic diseases and haematopoietic cancers has been supplemented with histamine dihydrochloride (Ceplene), a synthetic derivative of histamine, with the aim of counteracting immunosuppressive signals from monocytes/macrophages. Histamine dihydrochloride inhibits the formation of ROS that suppress the activation of T cells and NK cells by suppressing the activity of NADPH oxidase via H_2R. When administered in addition to IL-2, histamine dihydrochloride enables the activation of these lymphocytes by the cytokine, resulting in tumour cell killing. This combination was recently approved within the EU as a remission maintenance immunotherapy in AML, as histamine dihydrochloride reduces myeloid cell-derived suppression of anti-leukemic lymphocytes, improving NK and T-cell activation. Further research in this area will shed light on the role of histamine with the aim to improve cancer immunotherapy efficacy (Hellstrand et al., 2000; Martner et al., 2010; Yang & Perry, 2011).

5. Histamine receptors in gynaecologic cancers

Gynaecologic cancers encompass a remarkably heterogeneous group of tumours: cervical, ovarian, uterine, vaginal, and vulvar cancer. It has been postulated that histamine plays a critical role in proliferation of normal and cancer tissues, including the mammary gland, ovarian and endometrium.

In the murine uterus, the rapidly dividing epithelial cells of the endometrium can be defined as the major sources of histamine. In these cells the level of HDC expression is controlled mainly by progesterone-mediated signals which, interestingly, induce maximal level of HDC expression on the day of implantation (Pós et al., 2004).

In vitro studies showed that histamine may play an important role in follicular development and ovulation via H_1R and H_2R in women, acting as apoptosis inducer, taking part in the selection process of the dominant follicle and stimulating ovulation (Szukiewicz et al., 2007).

Interestingly, histamine content increased unequivocally in ovarian, cervical and endometrial carcinoma in comparison with their adjoining normal tissues, suggesting the participation of histamine in carcinogenesis. Besides, exogenous histamine, at micromolar concentration, stimulated proliferation of human ovarian cancer cell line SKOV-3 (Batra & Fadeel, 1994; Chanda & Ganguly, 1995). Preliminary results show that H_4R is expressed in primary and metastatic ovarian carcinoma and also in gallbladder cancer (Medina & Rivera, 2010b).

Histamine levels within ovarian tissue during the oestrus may correspond to cyclic changes of mast cells content and distribution in the ovary, suggesting an involvement of these cells in local regulation of ovarian function (Adyin et al., 1998; Nakamura et al., 1987). Interestingly, mast cells can typically be found in the peritumoural stroma of cervix carcinomas, as well as in many other cancers. Furthermore, high numbers of active, degranulated mast cells have been described in HPV infections and cervical intraepithelial neoplasias (Cabanillas-Saez et al., 2002; Demitsu et al., 2002). Hence, a functional relationship between mast cells and tumour cells has been proposed, where mast cells are involved in stimulating tumour growth and progression by enhancing angiogenesis, immunosuppression, mitogenesis, and metastasis (Chang et al., 2006). Mast cell activation leads to the release of inflammatory mediators, including histamine. Increased histamine levels have been described in the cervix lesions, where they have been associated with tumour growth and progression. Moreover, histamine receptors have been reported in different cell lines and tissues derived from experimental and human cervical neoplasias. The functional significance of immune cell infiltration of a tumour, specifically of mast cells located at the periphery of several neoplasias, is still a matter of controversy. Histamine acting via H_1R in cervical cancer cells could be pro-migratory, but when acting via H_4R could inhibit migration. On the other hand, other results also showed that cervical carcinoma cell mediators can activate mast cells to degranulate, demonstrating an active and dynamic cross-talk between tumour cells and infiltrating mast cells as shown in morphologic studies of neoplastic tissues (Rudolph et al., 2008).

In the light of these results, further investigations have to be done in order to elucidate the physiological role of histamine receptors on cell proliferation, as well as its implication in gynaecologic cancer progression with a potential interest for cancer treatment.

6. Histamine receptors in colorectal cancer

Colorectal cancer is one of the leading causes of cancer death among both men and women worldwide (Ferlay et al., 2010). It has been previously described that the histamine catabolising enzymes, DAO or histamine N-methyltransferase (HNMT), activities were significantly lower in adenoma tissue than in healthy mucosa in the same patients (Kuefner et al., 2008). Furthermore, HDC expression and its activity are increased in many human tumours including colorectal cancer (Cianchi et al., 2005; Masini et al., 2005; Reynolds et al., 1997). The levels of histamine were elevated in colon carcinoma and this is directly related to an increase in HDC expression and a decrease in DAO activity (Chanda & Ganguly, 1987). Also, the distribution of histamine receptors in the normal intestinal tract was reported (Sander et al., 2006). It was showed the expression pattern of H_1R, H_2R and H_4R in intestinal tract, receptors that were over expressed in the colon of patients with irritable bowel syndrome and food allergies. Furthermore, the H_3R was not detected in intestinal tissue (Sander et al., 2006). This data was further confirmed by Boer K et al, that also demonstrated

a decreased of H_1R and H_4R protein levels in colorectal cancer while the levels of the H_2R were not modified compared to normal colon mucosa (Boer et al., 2008).
It was described that the H_1R antagonist, loratadine, inhibited proliferation and enhanced radiosensitivity in human colon cancer cells (Soule et al., 2010). Also the H_2R seems to be implicated in the proliferation of colon cancer. In 1994 Adams, showed that *in vivo* and in two human colonic adenocarcinoma cell lines, C170 and LIM2412, cell proliferation induced by histamine in a dose dependent manner was blocked by H_2R antagonist, cimetidine (Adams et al., 1994). Ranitidine, another H_2R antagonist, also showed to extend the survival of patients who were under surgery of colorectal cancer (Nielsen et al., 2002). It is well known the effects of histamine in the immune system, according to this it was demonstrated that patients receiving cimetidine or famotidine before curative resection augmented the probabilities of having tumour infiltrating lymphocytes in their tumours than control patients (Adams & Morris, 1996; Kapoor et al., 2005). Furthermore, earlier studies demonstrated that histamine induced *in vitro* and *in vivo* cell proliferation and this outcome was blocked by H_2R antagonists (Adams et al., 1994; Cianchi et al., 2005). This effect was associated with the attenuation of anti-tumour cytokine expression in the tumour microenvironment exerted by histamine, thus resulting in stimulated colorectal cancer growth (Takahashi et al., 2001; Tomita & Okabe, 2005). In addition, H_2R antagonist significantly suppressed the growth of tumour implants in mice by inhibiting angiogenesis via reducing VEGF expression (Tomita et al., 2003).
As it was described above, the expression of the H_4R seems to be suppressed in human colorectal cancer. It was also demonstrated that the levels of the H_4R are reduced in advanced colorectal cancer compared with those in an initiating state, which suggest that the H_4R expression is regulated during the progression of the disease (Fang et al., 2011). The stimulation *in vitro* of the H_4R by a specific agonist induced an augmented expression of the p21[Cip1] and p27 [Kip1] proteins, producing an increase of arrested cells in the G1 phase. It has been proposed that prostaglandin E2 (PGE-2), the main product of the cyclooxygenase-2 activity, is implicated in colorectal cancer development. In this line, it has been demonstrated that histamine is fully implicated in the production of PGE-2 by its two receptors H_2R and H_4R in two human colon carcinoma cell lines (Cianchi et al., 2005). Histamine effect can be blocked by zolantidine, an H_2R antagonist, and also by JNJ7777120, an H_4R antagonist, whereas mepyramine, an H_1R antagonist, has no effect on the production of PGE-2. Furthermore, JNJ7777120 inhibited the cell growth induced by histamine in three different human colon cancer cell lines and also inhibited the histamine-mediated increase in VEGF in two cell lines. Combined treatment with zolantidine (an H_2R antagonist) and JNJ7777120 determined an additive effect on reducing the histamine-induced VEGF production and histamine-stimulated proliferation (Cianchi et al., 2005), suggesting the involvement of H_4R in colon carcinogenesis (Boer et al., 2008).

7. Histamine receptors in melanoma

Malignant melanoma arises from epidermal melanocytes and despite being the cause of less than 5% of skin cancers, it is responsible for the large majority of skin cancer deaths (Ferlay et al., 2010). Early detection is vital for long-term survival, given that there is a direct correlation between tumour thickness and mortality (Cummins et al., 2006).
Melanoma cells but not normal melanocytes contain large amounts of histamine that has been found to accelerate malignant growth (Pós et al., 2004). The absence of expression of

HDC in Mel-5 positive melanocytes isolated from skin samples of healthy persons, suggest that the level of HDC is strongly associated with malignancy in the skin (Haak-Frendscho et al., 2000). As a functional consequence of the inhibition of HDC protein synthesis, specific antisense oligonucleotide strongly (> 50%) decreased the proliferation rate of both WM938/B and HT168/91 human melanoma cells. Similar effects were found with other two melanoma cell lines WM35 and M1/15, suggesting that endogenous histamine may act as an autocrine growth factor (Hegyesi et al., 2000). On the other hand, overexpression of HDC markedly accelerated tumour growth and increased metastatic colony-forming potential along with rising levels of local histamine production that was correlated with tumour H_2R and rho-C expression in mouse melanoma (Pós Z et al., 2005).

It has been previously reported the expression of H_1R, H_2R and H_3R in melanoma cell lines (Hegyesi et al., 2005). In addition, it was described that in human melanoma cells, histamine acting through the H_1R decreases cell proliferation, whereas it enhances growth when acting through the H_2R (Lázar-Molnar et al., 2002). Furthermore, there is no evidence of mitogenic signalling through the H_3R in human melanoma (Hegyesi et al., 2005).

H_1R function is involved in chemotaxis via PLC activation, and its subsequent intracellular calcium mobilization. Proliferation assays showed that histamine exerted a concentration dependent dual effect on proliferation of the WM35 primary melanoma cell line. High concentrations of histamine (10^{-5} M) had an inhibitory effect while lower concentrations (10^{-7} M) increased colony formation. Similar results were achieved when using H_1R agonist 2-(3-fluoromethylphenyl)histamine and H_2R agonist arpromidine, respectively. The use of ranitidine, famotidine and cimetidine, all H_2R specific antagonists, abolished the stimulatory effect of histamine on cell proliferation, indicating the participation of H2R in this mitogenic role of histamine. Second messenger measurement indicated that H_2R are linked to cAMP production, thus suggesting an involvement of PKA in the mitogenic pathway triggered in this system, which is corroborated by the fact that forskolin and permeable cAMP analogues also produce a dose-dependent increase on cell proliferation (Lázar-Molnar et al., 2002).

Numerous *in vivo* studies employing animal models bearing syngenic or xenogenic melanoma grafts demonstrated that both endogenous and exogenous histamine have the ability to stimulate tumour growth while H_2R antagonists (e.g. cimetidine, famotidine, roxatidine) inhibited this effect (Pós et al., 2005; Szincsák et al., 2002; Tomita et al., 2005; Uçar, 1991). Additionally, H_2R antagonists stimulated melanogenesis and inhibited proliferation in B16-C3 mouse melanoma cells (Uçar, 1991). It was also found that melanoma tumour growth was not modulated by *in vivo* histamine treatment while treatment with terfenadine, an H_1R antagonist, *in vitro* induced melanoma cell death by apoptosis and *in vivo* significantly inhibited tumour growth in murine models (Blaya et al., 2010).

Differences between melanoma cells in their capacity to produce and degrade histamine could explain the different sensitivities of melanoma cell types to exogenous histamine treatment. Moreover, there is evidence that cytokines can influence HDC expression and activity. It has been shown that there is a regulation loop between interleukin 6 (IL-6) and histamine: histamine increased IL-6 expression and secretion in metastatic lines via the H_1R, and IL-6 treatment increased the HDC and histamine content in primary melanoma lines (Lázar-Molnar et al., 2002). Interferon-gamma (IFN-gamma) produced by surrounding immune cells decreases HDC expression, affecting melanoma growth and also impairs antitumour activity of the immune system, then contributing to the escape of melanoma cells from immunosurveillance (Horváth et al., 1999; Heninger et al., 2000). Furthermore, mast cell activation initiates upon ultraviolet-B irradiation, which triggers histamine secretion acts as a cellular immunity suppressor (Chang et al., 2006).

Moreover, the role of histamine in local immune reactions was further supported by the results of Hellstrand et al., who found that histamine can inhibit the ROS formation of monocytes/macrophages in the tumour (Hellstrand et al., 2000). This may explain the clinical benefit demonstrated by histamine (Ceplene) as an adjuvant to immunotherapy with IL-2 in several phase II and III clinical trials in metastatic melanoma (Agarwala, 2002). The addition of histamine dihydrochloride to an outpatient regimen of IL-2 is safe and well tolerated and demonstrates a survival advantage over IL-2 alone (9.4 vs. 5.1 months) in melanoma patients with liver metastases (Agarwala, 2002). However, a second confirmatory phase III study failed to show any survival benefit for those patients (Naredi, 2002).

Besides, Medina et al. showed that exogenous histamine modulated the activity of the antioxidant enzymes, increasing superoxide dismutase while decreasing catalase activity in WM35 melanoma cells. Accordingly, histamine treatment markedly augmented the levels of hydrogen peroxide and diminished those of superoxide anion, indicating that the imbalance of antioxidant enzymes leads to the cell proliferation inhibition (Medina et al., 2009).

Furthermore, it was demonstrated that WM35 and M1/15 melanoma cells express H_4R at the mRNA and protein level. By using histamine agonists and antagonists it was shown that the inhibitory effect of histamine on proliferation was in part mediated through the stimulation of the H_4R. Treatment with a specific H_4R antagonist, JNJ7777120 and the use of siRNA specific for H_4R mRNA blocked the decrease in proliferation triggered by the H_4R agonists. Furthermore, the decrease in proliferation exerted by H_4R agonists was associated with a 2-fold induction of cell senescence and an increase in melanogenesis that is a differentiation marker on these cells (Massari et al., 2011). Current studies indicate that the H_4R is expressed in the 42% of human melanoma biopsies of different histopathological types, showing cytoplasmic localization and confirming that the H_4R is present not only in these cell lines but also in human melanoma tissue (Massari et al., 2011).

The in vivo subcutaneous daily 1 $mg.kg^{-1}$ histamine or 1 $mg.kg^{-1}$ clozapine (H_4R agonist) injections of M1/15 melanoma cell tumour bearing nude mice showed a survival increase vs. control group (treated with saline solution). Besides, results showed an antitumour effect of histamine and clozapine, including suppression of tumour growth (Massari et al., unpublished data). Further studies are needed to corroborate the H_4R importance as potential target for new drug development for the treatment of this disease.

8. Histamine as a potential adjuvant to radiotherapy

8.1 Radioprotectors

Radiotherapy is the most common modality for treating human cancers and relies on ionising radiation induced DNA damage to kill malignant cells. Eighty percent of cancer patients need radiotherapy at some time or other, either for curative or palliative purpose. To optimise results, a cautious balance between the total dose of radiotherapy delivered and the threshold limit of the surrounding normal critical tissues is required. In order to obtain better tumour control with a higher dose, the normal tissues should be protected against radiation damage. Therefore, the role of radioprotective compounds is of utmost importance in clinical radiotherapy (Hall & Giaccia, 2006; Mah et at., 2011). Ionising radiation causes damage to living tissues through a series of molecular events. DNA double-strand breaks (DSBs), which are exceptionally lethal lesions, can be formed either by direct energy deposition or indirectly through the radiolysis of water molecules, which generate clusters of ROS that react with DNA molecules. Because human tissues contain 80% water, the major radiation damage produced by low linear transfer energy (LET) radiation is due to the aqueous free radicals. DSBs are essentially two single stranded nicks in opposing DNA strands that occur in close proximity, severely compromising genomic stability (Grdina, 2002; Hall & Giaccia, 2006; Mah et at., 2011). A series of complex pathways collectively known as the DNA damage response (DDR) is responsible for the recognition, signalling and repair of DSBs in cells, ultimately resulting in either cell survival or cell death (Mah et at., 2011). These free radicals react not only with DNA but also with other cellular macromolecules, such as RNA, proteins, membrane, *etc*, and cause cell dysfunction and mortality. Unfortunately, these reactions take place in tumour as well as normal cells when exposed to radiation. Therefore, to improve the efficacy of radiotherapy there is an intense interest in combining this modality with ionising radiation modifiers, such as radioprotectors. These compounds mitigate damage to surrounding non-malignant tissue (Brizel, 2007; Grdina, 2002; Hall & Giaccia, 2006; Hosseinimehr, 2007).

The most remarkable group of true radioprotectors is the sulfhydryl compounds. The simplest is cysteine, a sulfhydryl compound containing a natural amino acid (Table 2). In 1948, Patt discovered that cysteine could protect mice from the effects of total-body exposure to X-rays if the drug was injected or ingested in large amounts before the radiation exposure. At about the same time, in Europe independently discovered that cysteamine could also protect animals from total-body irradiation (Table 2). However, cysteine is toxic and induces nausea and vomiting at the dose levels required for radioprotection. A developmental program was initiated in 1959 and conducted at the Walter Reed Institute of Research to identify and synthesize drugs capable of conferring protection to individuals in a radiation environment by the U.S. Army. Over 4.000 compounds were synthesized and tested and it was discovered that the covering of the sulfhydryl group by a phosphate group reduced toxicity (Grdina, 2002; Hall & Giaccia, 2006; Nucifora et al., 1972).

The concept of the therapeutic ratio is central to understanding the rationale for using radioprotectors. It relates tumour control probabilities and normal tissue complication probabilities to one another. An ideal radioprotector will reduce the latter without compromising the former and should also be minimally toxic itself. Radioprotective strategies can be classified under the categories of protection, mitigation, and treatment. Protectors are administered before radiotherapy and are designed to prevent radiation-induced injury. Amifostine is the prototype drug (Table 2). Amifostine is the only radioprotective agent that is approved by FDA for preventing of xerostomia induced by gamma irradiation in patients under radiotherapy (Grdina et al., 2009; Hall & Giaccia, 2006; Hosseinimehr, 2007; Kouvaris et al., 2007, Wasserman & Brizel, 2001). Its selectivity for normal tissue is due to its preferential accumulation in normal tissue compared to the hypoxic environment of tumour tissues with low pH and low alkaline phosphatase, which is required to dephosphorylate and activate amifostine (Calabro-Jones et al., 1985; Grdina, 2002; Mah et at., 2011). The active metabolite, WR-1065 scavenges free radicals and is oxidised, causing anoxia or the rapid consumption of oxygen in tissues. This sulfhydryl compound is one of the most effective radioprotectors known nowadays, but there are two main problems of its using. The first one is their toxicity and the second is the short-ranged activity. Amifostine is also the unique radioprotector widely used in clinic on chemotherapy applications (Grdina et al., 2009; Hall & Giaccia, 2006; Hosseinimehr, 2007).

COMPOUND	SIDE EFFECTS	CHEMICAL STRUCTURE
Amifostine (WR-2721)	Drowsiness, feeling of coldness, flushing/feeling of warmth; hiccups, nausea, sneezing, vomiting	
Cysteamine	Depression, stomach or intestinal ulcer and bleeding, liver problems, skin condition, decreased calcification of bone, seizures, broken bone, decreased white blood cells	
Palifermin	Skin rash, flushing, unusual sensations in the mouth (tingling, tongue thickness)	C_{721}-H_{1142}-N_{202}-O_{204}-S_9
Cysteine	Toxic, nausea, vomiting	
Tempol	Constipation; diarrhoea, severe allergic reactions (rash; hives; itching; difficulty breathing; tightness in the chest; swelling of the mouth, face, lips, or tongue), loss of appetite, muscle weakness, nausea, slow reflexes, vomiting	

Table 2. Radioprotectors. Extracted and modified from http://www.wolframalpha.com/ entities/chemicals/palifermin/hs/j8/6k/; http://www.drugs.com

Mitigants are administered after radiotherapy but before the phenotypic expression of injury and are intended to ameliorate injury. The keratinocyte growth factor (KGF), palifermin, has been approved as a new, targeted therapy for the prevention of severe oral mucositis in patients with head and neck cancer undergoing post-operative radiochemotherapy and can be considered as the prototype mitigant (Weigelt et at., 2011) (Table 2). Palifermin, like the natural KGF, helps maintain the normal structure of the skin and gastrointestinal surface (lining) by stimulating cells to divide, grow and develop (Le et at., 2011; Weigelt et at., 2011).

Treatment is a strategy that is predominantly palliative and supportive in nature. Pharmacologic radioprotective strategies should be integrated with physical strategies such as intensity-modulated radiotherapy to realize their maximum clinical potential (Hall & Giaccia, 2006; Le et al., 2011).

In addition, low-to-moderate doses of some agents such as nitroxides, adrenoceptor agonist, were found to have radioprotective activity in experiments but their application in clinic remains doubtful. Tempol (4-hydroxy-2,2,6,6-tetramethyl-piperidinyloxy) belongs to a class of water-soluble nitroxides which are membrane-permeable stable free radical compounds that confer protection against radiation-induced damage (Bennett et at., 1987; Mah et at., 2011; Muscoli et at., 2003) (Table 2). It is thought to elicit its effects through the oxidation of reduced transition metals, scavenging free radicals and mimicking superoxide dismutase activity (Jiang et al., 2007).

8.2 Histamine as a radioprotector

Despite many years of research there are surprisingly few radiation protectors in use today, whose clinical value is limited due to their toxicity; thus, the development of effective and nontoxic agents is yet a challenge for oncologists and radiobiologists (Hall & Giaccia, 2006).

The acute effects of irradiation result from the death of a large number of cells in tissues with a rapid rate of turnover. These include effects in the epidermal layer or skin, gastrointestinal epithelium, and haematopoietic system, in which the response is determined by a hierarchical cell lineage, composed of stem cells and their differentiating offspring. In clinical radiotherapy, the tolerance of normal tissues for radiation depends on the ability of clonogenic cells to maintain a sufficient number of mature cells suitably structured to preserve organ function (Hall & Giaccia, 2006). During radiotherapy for intra-abdominal and pelvic cancers, radiation seriously affects radiosensitive tissues such as small intestine and bone marrow (Erbyl et al., 2005; Hall & Giaccia, 2006). It was previously demonstrated that histamine treatment (daily subcutaneous injection, 0.1 mg.kg[-1]) significantly protects mouse small intestine against radiation-induced toxicity ameliorating histological injury and improving trophism of enterocytes (Medina et al., 2007). Histamine completely prevented the decrease in the number of crypts evoked by whole body irradiation, which is vital for small intestine restoration since the intestinal crypt contains a hierarchy of stem cells that preserve the potential to regenerate the stem cell population and the tissue after cytotoxic exposure (Potten et al., 2002). Histamine radioprotective effect on small intestine was related to an increased rate of proliferation as evidenced by the enhanced proliferation markers immunoreactivity [5-bromo-2'-deoxyuridine (BrdU), and proliferating cell nuclear antigen (PCNA)]. Additionally, this outcome was accompanied by a reduction in the number of apoptotic cells per crypt and a modification of antioxidant enzyme levels that could lead to enhance the antioxidant capacity of intestinal cells (Medina et al., 2007). Histamine also protects rat small intestine against ionising radiation damage and this effect was principally associated to a decrease in intestinal cell crypt apoptosis (Medina & Rivera, 2010a).

The bone marrow pluripotent stem cells, such as erythroblast, are particularly radiosensitive and, after whole body irradiation, an important grade of aplasia is observed increasing the possibility of haemorrhage and/or infection occurrence that could be lethal. The survival of stem cells determines the subsequent repopulation of bone marrow after irradiation (Hall & Giaccia, 2006). Results demonstrated that histamine (0.1 mg.kg[-1]) significantly reduced the grade of aplasia, ameliorating the oedema and vascular damage produced by ionising radiation while eliciting a significant conservation of the medullar progenies on bone marrow in mouse and rat species, increasing the number of megakaryocytes, myeloid, lymphoid and erythroid cells per mm^2. The histamine effect is mediated at least in part by an increase in the rate of proliferation, as evidenced by the enhanced PCNA protein expression and BrdU incorporation, and is associated with an enhanced HDC expression in irradiated bone marrow cells (Medina et al., 2010; Medina & Rivera, 2010a). In this line, it was reported that a faster bone marrow repopulation was observed in wild type in comparison with HDC-deficient mice and that intracellular HDC and histamine content in regenerating bone marrow populations is increased after total-body irradiation (Horvath et al., 2006).

Despite improvements in the technology for delivering therapeutic radiation, salivary glands are inevitably injured during head and neck cancer radiotherapy, causing devastating side-effects which results in salivary hypofunction and consequent xerostomia (Burlage et al., 2008; Hall & Giaccia, 2006; Nagler, 2002). Salivary glands of rat are quite similar to human salivary glands in which salivary flow is rapidly reduced after radiation exposure (Nagler, 2002). Recent results demonstrated that histamine markedly prevented radiation injury on submandibular gland, ameliorating the histological and morphological alterations. Radiation significantly decreased salivation by approximately 35-40%, which was associated with a reduction of submandibular gland wet weight and an alteration of epithelial architecture, vacuolization of acinar cells and partial loss of eosinophilic secretor granular material. It is worth noting that histamine treatment (0.1 mg.kg^{-1}) completely reversed the reduced salivation induced by radiation, preserving glandular function and mass with normal structure organization of acini and ducts. Histamine prevented radiation-induced toxicity in submandibular gland essentially by suppressing apoptosis of ductal and acinar cells, reducing the number of apoptotic cells per field (Medina et al., 2011a).

To summarize, histamine treatment can selectively modulate cellular damage produced by ionising radiation, thus preventing radiation induced damage on small intestine, bone marrow and salivary glands. Furthermore, histamine *in vitro* enhances the radiosensitivity of breast cancer cells (Medina et al., 2006) while does not modify that of melanoma (Medina et al., 2007). Despite histamine may be proliferative in some cancer cell types, it may still be beneficial as radioprotector in view of the fact that it is only administered for a short period of time to reduce the radiation induced damage. It is important to highlight that histamine radioprotective effect was demonstrated in two different rodent species, which suggests that histamine could exert a radioprotective action in other mammals. Also, no local or systemic side effects were observed upon histamine administration in both species.

The presented evidences indicate that histamine is a potential candidate as a safe radioprotective agent that might increase the therapeutic index of radiotherapy for intra-abdominal, pelvic, and head and neck cancers, and enhance patient quality of life by protecting normal tissue from radiation injury. However, the efficacy of histamine needs to be carefully investigated in prospective clinical trials.

9. Conclusions

In this chapter, we have presented major findings of the most recent research in histamine cancer pharmacology. These data clearly indicate that histamine plays a key role as a mediator in most human tumours. Interestingly, histamine is not only involved in cancer cell proliferation, migration and invasion, but also the tumour microenvironment and immune system responses are tightly affected. In human neoplasias H$_3$R and H$_4$R seemed to be the main receptors involved in the control of the metabolic pathways responsible for tumour growth and progression, suggesting that H$_3$R and H$_4$R represent potential molecular targets for cancer drug development. Finally, a novel role for histamine as a selective radioprotector is highlighted, indicative of the potential application of histamine and its ligands as adjuvants to radiotherapy.

10. Acknowledgment

This work has been supported by grants from the University of Buenos Aires 20020090300039 and 20020100100270, from the National Agency of Scientific and Technological Promotion PICT-2007-01022, and from the EU-FP7 COST Action BM0806.

11. References

Adams, W.J., Lawson, J.A., Morris, D.L. (1994). Cimetidine inhibits in vivo growth of human colon cancer and reverses histamine stimulated in vitro and in vivo growth. *British Medical Association,* Vol. 35, (11/94), pp. (1632-1636), ISSN 0017-5749

Adams, W., Morris, D. (1996). Cimetidine and colorectal cancer. *Diseases of the colon and rectum,* Vol. 39, No. 1, (01/96), pp. (111-2), ISSN 0012-3706

Agarwala, S.S., Glaspy, J., O'Day, S.J., Mitchell, M., Gutheil, J., Whitman, E., Gonzalez, R., Hersh, E., Feun, L., Belt, R., Meyskens, F., Hellstrand, K., Wood, D., Kirkwood, J.M., Gehlsen, K.R., & Naredi, P. (2002). Results from a randomized phase III study comparing combined treatment with histamine dihydrochloride plus interleukin-2 versus interleukin-2 alone in patients with metastatic melanoma. *Journal of clinical oncology* Vol. 20, No 1, (06/02), pp. (125–33), ISSN 0732-183X

Arrang, J.M., Garbarg, M., & Schwartz, J.C. (1983). Auto-inhibition of brain histamine release mediated by a novel class (H3) of histamine receptor. *Nature,* Vol. 302, No. 5911, (04/83), pp. (832-7), ISSN 0028-0836

Ash, A.S., & Schild, H.O. (1966). Receptors mediating some actions of histamine. *British journal of pharmacology and chemotherapy,* Vol. 27, No. 2, (08/96), pp. (427-39), ISSN 0366-0826

Aydin, Y., Tunçel, N., Gürer, F., Tuncel, M., Koşar, M. & Oflaz, G. (1998). Ovarian, uterine and brain mast cells in female rats: cyclic changes and contribution to tissue histamine. *Comparative biochemistry and physiology. Part A, Molecular & integrative physiology,* Vol. 120, No. 2, (06/98), pp. 255-62, ISSN 1095-6433

Bakker, R.A., Schoonus, S.B.J., Smit, M.J., Timmerman, H., & Leurs, R. (2001). Histamine H1-receptor activation of nuclear factor-KB; roles for G gamma- and G alpha/11 subunits in constitutive and agonist-mediated signaling. *Molecular pharmacology,* Vol. 60, No. 5, (11/01), pp. (1133-42), ISSN 0026-895X

Batra, S. & Fadeel, I. (1994). Release of intracellular calcium and stimulation of cell growth by ATP and histamine in human ovarian cancer cells (SKOV-3). *Cancer letters,* Vol. 77, No. 1, (02/94), pp. 57-63, ISSN 0304-3835

Belcheva, A. & Mishkova, R. (1995). Histamine content in lymph nodes from patients with malignant lymphomas. *Inflammation Research,* Vol. 44 Suppl 1, (04/95), pp. S86-7, ISSN 1023-3830

Bennett, H., Swartz, H., Brown, Rr., & Koenig, S. (1987). Modification of relaxation of lipid protons by molecular oxygen and nitroxides. *Investigative radiology,* No. 6, (06/87), pp. (502-507), ISSN 0020-9996

Black, J.W., Duncan, W.A., Durant, C.J., Ganellin, C.R., & Parsons, E.M. (1972).Definition and antagonism of histamine H2-receptors. *Nature,* Vol. 236, No. 5347, (04/72), pp. (385-90), ISSN 0028-0836

Blaya, B., Nicolau, G.F., Jangi, S.M., Ortega, M.I., Alonso, T.E., Burgos-Bretones, J, Pérez, Y.G., Asumendi, A., & Boyano, M.D. (2010). Histamine and histamine receptor antagonists in cancer biology. *Inflammation & allergy drug targets,* Vol. 9, No. 3 ,(07/10), pp. (146-57) ISNN 1871-5281

Boer, K., Helinger, E., Helinger, A., Pocza, P., Pos, Z., Demeter, P., Baranyai, Z., Dede, K., Darvas, Z., Falus, A. (2008). Decreased expression of histamine H1 and H4 receptors suggests disturbance of local regulation in human colorectal tumours by histamine. *European journal of cell biology,* Vol. 87, (04/08), pp. (227–236), ISSN 0171-9335

Bolton, E., King, J., & Morris, D.L. (2000). H2-antagonists in the treatment of colon and breast cancer. *Seminars in cancer biology*, Vol. 10, No. 1, (02/00), pp. (3-10), ISSN 1044-579X

Bongers, G., Bakker, R.A., & Leurs, R. (2007). Molecular aspects of histamine H3 receptor. *Biochemical pharmacology*, Vol. 73, No. 8, (04/07), pp. (1195-204), ISSN 0006-2952

Brizel, DM. (2007). Pharmacologic approaches to radiation protection. *World journal of clinical oncology*, Vol., 25, No. 26, (09/07), pp. (4084-9), ISSN 2218-4333

Burlage, F.R., Roesink, J.M., Kampinga, H.H., Coppes, R.P., Terhaard, C., Langendijk, J.A., van Luijk, P., Stokman, M.A., & Vissink, A. (2008). Protection of salivary function by concomitant pilocarpine during radiotherapy: a double-blind, randomized, placebo-controlled study. *International journal of radiation oncology, biology, physics*, Vol. 70, No. 1, (01/08), pp. (14-22), ISSN 0360-3016

Byron, J.W. (1977). Mechanism for histamine H2-receptor induced cell-cycle changes in the bone marrow stem cell. *Agents and actions*, Vol. 7, No. 2, (07/77), pp. 209-13, ISSN 0065-4299

Cabanillas-Saez, A., Schalper, J.A., Nicovani, S.M. & Rudolph, M.I. (2002). Characterization of mast cells according to their content of tryptase and chymase in normal and neoplastic human uterine cervix. *International journal of gynecological cancer*, Vol. 12, (01/02), pp. 92–98, ISSN 1048-891X

Calabro-Jones, P., Fahey, R., Smoluk, G., & Ward, J. (1985). Alkaline phosphatase promotes radioprotection and accumulation of WR-1065 in V79-171 cells incubated in medium containing WR-2721. *International journal of radiation biology*, Vol., 47, No. 1, (06/85), pp. (23-7), ISSN 0020-7616

Chanda, R., Ganguly, A.K. (1987). Diamineoxidase activity and tissue histamine content of human skin, breast and rectal carcinoma. *Cancer letters*, Vol. 34, No. 2, (02/87), pp. (207-12), ISSN 0304-3835

Chanda, R. & Ganguly, A.K. (1995). Diamine-oxidase activity and tissue di- and poly-amine contents of human ovarian, cervical and endometrial carcinoma. *Cancer letters, Vol.* 89, No. 1, (02/95), pp. 23-8, ISSN 0304-3835

Chang, S., Wallis, R.A., Yuan, L., Davis, P.F. & Tan, S.T. (2006). Mast cells and cutaneous malignancies. *Modern pathology*, Vol. 19, (01/06), pp. 149–159, ISSN 0893-3952

Cherifi, I., Pigeon, C., Le romancer, M., Bado, A., Reyl-Desmars, F., & Lewin, M.J.M. (1992). Purification of a histamine H3 receptor negatively coupled to phosphoinositide turnover in the human gastric cell line HGT1. *The Journal of biological chemistry*, Vol. 267, No. 35, (12/92), pp. (25315-20), ISSN 0021-9258

Cianchi, F., Cortesini, C., Schiavone, N., Perna, F., Magnelli, L., Fanti, E., Bani, D., Messerini, L., Fabbroni, V., Perigli, G., Capaccioli, S., & Masini, E. (2005). The role of cyclooxygenase-2 in mediating the effects of histamine on cell proliferation and vascular endothelial growth factor production in colorectal cancer. *Clinical cancer research*, Vol. 11, No. 19 Pt 1, (10/05), pp. (6807-15), ISSN 1078-0432

Coge, F., Guenin, S.P., Audinot, V., Renouard-Try, A., Beauverger, P., Macia, C., Ouvry, C., Nagel, N., Rique, H., Boutin, J.A., & Galizzi, J.P. (2001a). Genomic organization and characterization of splice variants of the human histamine H3 receptor. *The Biochemical journal*, Vol. 355, No. Pt 2, (04/01), pp. (279-88), ISSN 0264-6021.

Coge, F., Guenin, S.P., Rique, H., Boutin, J.A., & Galizzi, J.P. (2001b). Structure and expression of the human histamine H4-receptor gene. *Biochemical and biophysical research communications*, Vol. 284, No. 2, (06/01), pp. (301-9), ISSN 0006-291X

Cricco, G.P., Davio, C.A., Fitzsimons, C.P., Engel, N., Bergoc, R.M., & Rivera, E.S. (1994). Histamine as an autocrine growth factor in experimental carcinomas. *Agents and actions*, Vol. 43, No. 1-2, (11/94), pp. (17-20), ISSN 0065-4299

Cricco, G., Mohamad, N., Sáez, M.S., Valli, E., Rivera, E.S., & Martín, G. Histamine and Breast Cancer: a New Role for a Well Known Amine, In: *Breast Cancer Cells / Book 1*, Mehmet Gunduz, pp. in press, Okayama University, ISBN 979-953-307-137-3, Japan

Connelly, W.M., Shenton, F.C., Lethbridge, N., Leurs, R., Waldvogel, H.J., Faull, R.L., Lees, G., & Chazot, P.L. (2009). The histamine H4 receptor is functionally expressed on neurons in the mammalian CNS. *British journal of pharmacology*, Vol. 157, No. 1, (05/09), pp. (55-63), ISSN 0007-1188

Cummins, D.L., Cummins, J.M., Pantle, H., Silverman, M.A., Leonard, A.L., & Chanmugam, A. (2006). Cutaneous malignant melanoma. *Mayo Clinic proceedings*, Vol 81, No 4, (04/06), pp. (500-7), ISSN:0025-6196

Davio, C.A., Cricco, G.P., Andrade, N., Bergoc, R.M., & Rivera, E.S. (1993). H1 and H2 histamine receptors in human mammary carcinomas. *Agents and actions*, Vol. 38, (06/93), pp. (C172-C174), ISSN 0065-4299

Davio, C.A., Cricco, G.P., Martin, G., Fitzsimons, C.P., Bergoc, R.M., & Rivera, E.S. (1994). Effect of histamine on growth and differentiation of the rat mammary gland. *Agents and actions*, Vol. 41, (06/94), pp. (C115-C117), ISSN 0065-4299

Davio, C.A., Cricco, G.P., Bergoc, R.M., & Rivera, E.S. (1995). H1 and H2 histamine receptors in experimental carcinomas with an atypical coupling to signal transducers. *Biochemical pharmacology*, Vol. 50, No. 1, (06/95), pp. (91-6), ISSN 0006-2952

Davio, C., Madlovan, A., Shayo, C., Lemos, B., Baldi, A., & Rivera, E. (1996). Histamine receptors in neoplastic transformation. Studies in human cell lines. *Inflammation research*, Vol. 45, No. Suppl. 1, (03/96), pp. (S62-S63), ISSN 1023-3830

Davio, C., Mladovan, A., Lemos, B., Monczor, F., Shayo, C., Rivera, E., & Baldi, A. (2002). H1 and H2 histamine receptors mediate the production of inositol phosphates but not cAMP in human breast epithelial cells. *Inflammation research*, Vol. 51, No. 1, (01/02), pp. (1-7), ISSN 1023-3830

Demitsu, T., Inoue, T., Kakurai, M., Kiyosawa, T., Yoneda, K. & Manabe, M. (2002). Activation of mast cells within a tumor of angiosarcoma: ultrastructural study of five cases. *The Journal of dermatology*, Vol. 29, (05/02), pp. 280–289, ISSN 0385-2407

Dy, M., & Schneider, E. (2004). Histamine-cytokine connection in immunity and hematopoiesis. *Cytokine and growth factor reviews*, Vol. 15, No. 5, (10/04), pp. (393-410), ISSN 1359-6101

Erbil, Y., Oztezcan, S., Giris, M., Barbaros, U., Olgac, V., Bilge, H., Kücücük, H., & Toker, G. (2005). The effect of glutamine on radiation-induced organ damage. *Life sciences*, Vol. 78, No. 4, (12/05), pp. (376-820), ISSN 0024-3205

Fang, Z., Yao, W., Xiong, Y., Li, J., Liu, L., Shi, L., Zhang, W., Zhang, C., Nie, L., Wan, J. (2011). Attenuated expression of HRH4 in colorectal carcinomas: a potential influence on tumor growth and progression. *BMC Cancer*, Vol. 11, No. 1, (05/11), pp. (195), ISSN 1471-2407

Ferlay, J., Shin, H.R., Bray, F., Forman, D., Mathers, C., & Parkin, D.M. (2010). Estimates of worldwide burden of cancer in 2008: GLOBOCAN 2008. *International journal of cancer*, Vol. 127, No. 12, (12/10), pp. (2893-917), ISSN 0020-7136

Fukushima, Y., Asano, T., Saitoh, T., Anai, M., Funaki, M., Ogihara, T., Katagiri, H., Matsuhashi, N., Yazaki, Y., Sugano, K. (1997). Oligomer formation of histamine H2 receptors expressed in Sf9 and COS7 cells. *FEBS letters*, Vol. 409, No. 2, (06/97), pp. (283-6), ISSN 0014-5793

Fitzsimons, C., Engel, N., Policastro, L., Durán, H., Molinari, B., & Rivera, E. (2002). Regulation of phospholipase C activation by the number of H(2) receptors during Ca(2+)-induced differentiation of mouse keratinocytes. *Biochemical pharmacology* 2002; Vol. 63, No. 10, (05/02), pp. (1785-96), ISSN 0006-2952

Gonzalez-Angulo, A.M., Morales-Vasquez, F., & Hortobagyi, G.N. (2007). Overview of resistance to systemic therapy in patients with breast cancer. *Advances in experimental medicine and biology*, Vol. 608, pp. (1-22), ISSN 0065-2598

Grdina, D.J., Murley, J.S., & Kataoka, Y. (2002). Radioprotectans: current status and new directions. *Oncology*, Vol., 63, No. Suppl. 2-2 10, ISSN 0030-2414

Grdina, D.J., Murley, J.S., Kataoka, Y., Baker, K.L., Kunnavakkam, R., Coleman, M.C., & Spitz, D.R. (2009). Amifostine induces antioxidant enzymatic activities in normal tissues and a transplantable tumor that can affect radiation response. *International journal of radiation oncology, biology, physics*, Vol., 1-73, No. 3 (03/09), pp. (886-96), ISSN 0360-3016

Gutzmer, R., Gschwandtner, M., Rossbach, K., Mommert, S., Werfel, T., Kietzmann, M., & Baeumer, W. (2011). Pathogenetic and therapeutic implications of the histamine H4 receptor in inflammatory skin diseases and pruritus. *Frontiers in bioscience (Scholar edition)*, Vol. 3, (06/11), pp. (985-94), ISSN 1945-0516

Haak-Frendscho, M., Darvas, Z., Hegyesi, H., Kárpáti, S., Hoffman, R.L., László, V., Bencsáth, M., Szalai, C., Fürész, J., Timár, J., Bata-Csörgō, Z., Szabad, G., Pivarcsi, A., Pállinger, E., Kemény, L., Horváth, A., Dobozy, A., & Falus, A. (2000). Histidine decarboxylase expression in human melanoma. *The Journal of investigative dermatology*, Vol 115, No 3, (09/00), pp. (345-52), ISSN:0022-202X

Hall E.J., & Giaccia, A.J. (Eds.). (2006). *Radiobiology for the radiologist*, Lippincott Williams & Wilkins, ISBN 978-0-7817-4151-4, Philadelphia

Hancock, A.A., Esbenshade, T.A., Krueger. K,M., & Yao, B.B. (2003). Genetic and pharmacological aspects of histamine H3 receptor heterogeneity. *Life sciences*, Vol. 73, No. 24, (10/03), pp. (3043-72), ISSN 0024-3205

Hegyesi, H., Somlai, B., Varga, V.L., Toth, G., Kovacs, P., Molnar, E.L., Laszlo, V., Karpati, S., Rivera, E., Falus, A., & Darvas, Z. (2000). Suppression of melanoma cell proliferation by histidine decarboxylase specific antisense oligonucleotides. *The Journal of investigative dermatology*, Vol 117, No 1, (07/00), pp. (151-3), ISSN:0022-202X

Hegyesi, H., Horváth, B., Pállinger, E., Pós, Z., Molnár, V., & Falus, A. (2005). Histamine elevates the expression of Ets-1, a protooncogen in human melanoma cell lines through H2 receptor. *FEBS letters*, Vol 579, No 11, (04/05), pp. (2475-9), ISSN:0014-5793

Hellstrand, K., Brune, M., Naredi, P., Mellqvist, U.H., Hansson, M., Gehlsen, K.R. & Hermodsson, S. (2000). Histamine: a novel approach to cancer immunotherapy. *Cancer investigation*, Vol. 18, No. 4, pp. 347-55, ISSN 0735-7907

Heninger, E., Falus, A., Darvas, Z., Szalai, C., Zsinko, M., Pos, Z., & Hegyesi, H. (2000). Both interferon (IFN) alpha and IFN gamma inhibit histidine decarboxylase expression in the HT168 human melanoma cell line. *Inflammation research*, Vol. 49, No. 8, (08/00), pp. (393- 7), ISSN 1023-3830

Horváth, B.V., Szalai, C., Mándi, Y., László, V., Radvány, Z., Darvas, Z., & Falus, A. (1999). Histamine and histamine-receptor antagonists modify gene expression and biosynthesis of interferon gamma in peripheral human blood mononuclear cells and in CD19-depleted cell subsets. *Immunology letters*, Vol 70, No 2, (11/99), pp. (95-9), ISSN:0165-2478

Horvath, Z., Pallinger, E., Horvath, G., Jelinek, I., Falus, A., & Buzas, E.I. (2006). Histamine H1 and H2 receptors but not H4 receptors are upregulated during bone marrow regeneration. *Cellular immunology*, Vol. 244, No. 2, (12/06), pp. (110-5), ISSN 0008-8749

Hosseinimehr, S.J. (2007). Trends in the development of radioprotective agents. *Drug discovery today*, Vol., 12, No.19-20, (10/07), pp. (794-805), ISSN 1741-8364

Jiang, J., Kurnikov, I., Belikova, N.A., Xiao, J., Zhao, Q., Amoscato, A.A., Braslau, R., Studer, A., Fink, M.P., Greenberger, J.S., Wipf, P., & Kagan, V.E. (2007). Structural requirements for optimized delivery, inhibition of oxidative stress, and antiapoptotic activity of targeted nitroxides. *The Journal of pharmacology and experimental therapeutics*, Vol., 320, No. 3, (03/07), pp. (1050-60), ISSN 0022-3565

Kapoor, S., Pal, S., Sahni, P., Dattagupta, S., Kanti Chattopadhyay, T. (2005). Effect of pre-operative short course famotidine on tumor infiltrating lymphocytes in colorectal cancer: a double blind, placebo controlled, prospective randomized study. *The Journal of surgical research*, Vol. 129, No. 2, (12/05), pp. (172-5), ISSN 0022-4804

Kouvaris, J.R., Kouloulias, V.E., & Vlahos, L.J. (2007). Amifostine: the first selective-target and broad-spectrum radioprotector. *The oncologist*, Vol., 12, No. 6, (06/07), pp. (738-47), ISSN 1083-7159

Kuefner, M.A., Schwelberger, H.G., Hahn, E.G., Raithel, M. (2008). Decreased histamine catabolism in the colonic mucosa of patients with colonic adenoma. *Digestive diseases and sciences*, Vol. 53, No. 2, (02/08), pp. (436-42), ISSN 0163-2116

Kyriakidis, K., Zampeli, E., & Tiligada, E. (2009). Histamine levels in whole peripheral blood from women with ductal breast cancer: a pilot study *Inflammation research*, Vol. 58, No. Suppl. 1, (04/09), pp. (S73-4), ISSN 1023-3830

Lázár-Molnár, E., Hegyesi, H., Pállinger, E., Kovács, P., Tóth, S., Fitzsimons, C., Cricco, G., Martin, G., Bergoc, R., Darvas, Z., Rivera, E.S., & Falus, A. (2002). Inhibition of human primary melanoma cell proliferation by histamine is enhanced by interleukin-6. *European journal of clinical investigation*, Vol 32, No 10, (10/02), pp. (743-9), ISSN:0014-2972

Le, Q.T., Kim, H.E., Schneider, C.J., Muraközy, G., Skladowski, K., Reinisch, S., Chen, Y., Hickey, M., Mo, M., Chen, M.G., Berger, D., Lizambri, R., & Henke, M. (2011). Palifermin Reduces Severe Mucositis in Definitive Chemoradiotherapy of Locally

Advanced Head and Neck Cancer: A Randomized, Placebo-Controlled Study. *World journal of clinical oncology*, (06/11), ISSN 2218-4333

Lebois, E.P., Jones, C.K., & Lindsley, C.W. (2011). The evolution of histamine H3 antagonists/inverse agonists. *Current topics in medicinal chemistry*, Vol. 11, No. 6, pp. (648-60), ISSN 1568-0266

Leurs, R., Smits, M.J., & Timmerman, H. (1995). Molecular pharmacological aspects of histamine receptors. *Pharmacology & therapeutics*, Vol. 66, No. 3, (06/95), pp. (413-63), ISSN 0163-7258

Leurs, R., Church, M.K., & Taglialatela, M. (2002). H1-antihistamines: inverse agonism, anti-inflammatory actions and cardiac effects. *Clinical and experimental allergy*, Vol. 32, No. 4, (04/02), pp. (489-98), ISSN 0954-7894

Leurs, R., Bakker, R.A., Timmerman, H., & de Esch, I.J.P. (2005). The histamine H3 receptor: from gene cloning to H3 receptor drugs. *Nature reviews. Drug discovery*, Vol. 4, No. 2, (02/05), pp (107-22), ISSN 1474-1776

Leurs, R., Chazot, P.L., Shenton, F.C., Lim, H.D., & de Esch, I.J. (2009). Molecular and biochemical pharmacology of the histamine H4 receptor. *British journal of pharmacology*, Vol. 157, No. 1, (05/09), pp. (14-23), ISSN 0007-1188

Liu, C., Ma, X.J., Jiang, X., Wilson, S.J., Hofstra, C.L., Blevitt, J., Pyati, J., Li, X., Chai, W., Carruthers, N., & Lovenberg, T.W. (2001). Cloning and pharmacological characterization of a fourth histamine receptor (H4) expressed in bone marrow. *Molecular pharmacology*, Vol. 59, No. 3, (03/01), pp. (420-6), ISSN 0026-895X

Lovenberg, T.W., Roland, B.I., Wilson, S.J., Jiang, X., Pyati, J., Huvar, A., Jackson, M.R., & Erlander, M.G. (1999). Cloning and functional expression of the human histamine H3 receptor. *Molecular pharmacology*, Vol. 55, No. 6, (06/99), pp. (1101-7), ISSN 0026-895X

Mah, L.J., Orlowski, C., Ververis, K., Vasireddy, R.S., El-Osta, A., & Karagiannis, T.C. (2011). Evaluation of the efficacy of radiation-modifying compounds using γH2AX as a molecular marker of DNA double-strand breaks. *Genome integrity*, Vol., 2, No.1, (06/11), pp. (3), ISSN 2041-9414

Malaviya, R., Morrison, A.R. & Pentland, A.P. (1996). Histamine in human epidermal cells is induced by ultraviolet light injury. *The Journal of investigative dermatology*, Vol. 106, No. 4, (04/96), pp. 785-9, ISSN 0022-202X

Malinski, C., Kierska, D., Fogel, W., Kinnunum, A., & Panula, P. (1993). Histamine: its metabolism and localization in mammary gland. *Comparative biochemistry and physiology. C: Comparative pharmacology*, Vol. 105, No. 2, (06/93), pp. (269-73), ISSN 0306-4492

Martner, A., Thorén, F.B., Aurelius, J., Söderholm, J., Brune, M. & Hellstrand, K. (2010). Immunotherapy with histamine dihydrochloride for the prevention of relapse in acute myeloid leukemia. *Expert review of hematology*, Vol 3, No. 4, (08/10) pp. 381-91, ISSN 1747-4086

Massari, N.A., Medina, V.A., Martinel Lamas, D.J., Cricco, G.P., Croci, M., Sambuco, L., Bergoc, R.M., & Rivera, E.S. Role of H4 receptor in histamine-mediated responses in human melanoma. *Melanoma research*, in press, ISSN 0960-8931

Masini, E., Fabbroni, V., Giannini, L., Vannacci, A., Messerini, L., Perna, F., Cortesini, C., Cianchi, F. (2005). Histamine and histidine decarboxylase up-regulation in colorectal cancer: correlation with tumor stage. 2. *Inflammation research : official journal of the European Histamine Research Society*, Vol. 54, No. Suppl 1, (40/05), pp. 80-1, ISSN 1023-3830

Medina, V., Cricco, G., Nuñez, M., Martín, G., Mohamad, N., Correa-Fiz, F., Sanchez-Jimenez, F., Bergoc, R., & Rivera, E. (2006). Histamine-mediated signaling processes in human malignant mammary cells. *Cancer biology & therapy*, Vol. 5, No. 11, (11/06), pp. (1462-71), ISSN 1538-4047

Medina, V., Croci, M., Mohamad, N., Massari, N., Garbarino, G., Cricco, P., Núñez, M., Martín, G., Crescenti, E., Bergoc, R., & Rivera, E. (2007). Mechanisms underlying the radioprotective effect of histamine on small intestine. *International journal of radiation biology*, Vol., 83, No. 10, (10/07), pp. (653-63), ISSN 0955-3002

Medina, V., Croci, M., Crescenti, E., Mohamad, N., Sanchez-Jiménez, F., Massari, N., Nuñez, M., Cricco, P., Martin, G., Bergoc, R., & Rivera, E. (2008). The Role of Histamine in Human Mammary Carcinogenesis. H3 and H4 Receptors as Potential Therapeutic Targets for Breast Cancer Treatment. *Cancer biology & therapy*, Vol. 7, No. 1, (06/08), pp. (27-35), ISSN 1538-4047

Medina, V.A., Massari, N.A., Cricco, G.P., Martín, G.A., Bergoc, R.M., & Rivera, E.S. (2009). Involvement of hydrogen peroxide in histamine-induced modulation of WM35 human malignant melanoma cell proliferation. *Free radical biology & medicine*, Vol. 46, No. 11, (06/09), pp. (1510-5), ISSN 0891-5849

Medina, V.A., Croci, C., Carabajal, E., Bergoc, R.M., & Rivera, E.S. (2010). Histamine protects bone marrow against cellular damage induced by ionizing radiation. *International journal of radiation biology*, Vol., 86, No. 4, (04/10), pp. (283-90), ISSN 0955-3002

Medina, V.A., & Rivera, E.S. (2010a). Histamine as a potential adjuvant to immuno and radiotherapy for cancer treatment. Discovering new functions for the oldest biogenic amine. *Current immunology reviews, special Issue; Advances in immunopathology*, Vol. 6, No. 4, (11/10), pp. (357-70), ISSN 1573-3955

Medina, V.A., & Rivera, E.S. (2010b). Histamine receptors and cancer Pharmacology. *British journal of pharmacology*, Vol. 161, No. 4, (10/10), pp. (755-67), ISSN 0007-1188

Medina, V., Prestifilippo, J.P., Croci, M., Carabajal, E., Bergoc, R.M., Elverdin, J.C., & Rivera, E.S. (2011a). Histamine prevents functional and morphological alterations of submandibular glands exerted by ionising radiation. *International journal of radiation biology*, Vol., 87, No. 3, (03/11), pp. (284-92), ISSN 0955-3002

Medina, V.A., Brenzoni, P.G., Martinel Lamas, D.J., Massari, N., Mondillo, C., Nuñez, M.A., Pignataro, O., & Rivera, E.S. (2011b). Role of histamine H4 receptor in breast cancer cell proliferation. *Frontiers in Bioscience (Elite Edition)*, Vol. 3, (06/11), pp. (1042-60), ISSN 1945-0494

Mizuguchi, H., Kitamura, Y., Kondo, Y., Kuroda, W., Yoshida, H., Miyamoto, Y., Hattori, M., Takeda, N., & Fukui, H. (2011). Histamine H_1 receptor gene as an allergic diseases-sensitive gene and its impact on therapeutics for allergic diseases. *Yakugaku Zasshi*, Vol. 131, No. 2, (02/11), pp. (171-8), ISSN 0031-6903

Morse, K.L., Behan, J., Laz, T.M., West, R.E., Greenfeder, S.A., Anthes, J.C., Umland, S., Wan, Y., Hipkin, R.W., Gonsiorek, W., Shin, N., Gustafson, E.L., Qiao, X., Wang, S., Hedrick, J.A., Greene, J., Bayne, M., & Monsma, F.J. (2001). Cloning and characterization of a novel human histamine receptor *The Journal of pharmacology and experimental therapeutics*, Vol. 296, No. 3, (03/01), pp. (1058-1066), ISSN 0022-3565

Muscoli, C., Cuzzocrea, S., Riley, D., Zweier, J., Thiemermann, C., Wang, Z., & Salvemini, D. (2003). On the selectivity of superoxide dismutase mimetics and its importance in pharmacological studies. *British journal of pharmacology*, Vol., 140, No. 3, (10/03), pp. (445-60), ISSN 0007-1188

Nagler, R.M. (2002). The enigmatic mechanism of irradiation-induced damage to the major salivary glands. *Oral diseases*, Vol. 8, No. 3, (05/02), pp. (141-6), ISSN 1354-523X

Nakamura, T., Itadani, H., Hidaka, Y., Ohta, M., & Tanaka, K. (2000). Molecular cloning and characterization of a new human histamine receptor, HH4R. *Biochemical and biophysical research communications*, Vol. 289, No. 2, (12/00), pp. (615-20), ISSN 0006-291X

Nakamura, Y., Smith, M., Krishna, A. & Terranova, P.F. (1987). Increased number of mast cells in the dominant follicle of the cow: relationships among luteal, stromal, and hilar regions. *Biology of reproduction*, Vol. 37, No. 3, (10/87), pp. 546-9, ISSN 0006-3363

Naredi, P. (2002). Histamine as an adjunct to immunotherapy. *Seminars in oncology*, No. 3, Suppl. 7, (06/02), pp. (31-4), ISNN 0093-7754

Nguyen, T., Shapiro, D.A., George, S.R., Setola, V., Lee, D.K., Cheng, R., Rauser, L., Lee, S.P., Lynch, K.R., Roth, B.L., & O'Dowd, B.F. (2001). Discovery of a novel member of the histamine receptor family. *Molecular pharmacology*, Vol. 59, No. 3, (03/01), pp. (427-33), ISSN 0026-895X

Nielsen, H.J., Christensen, I.J., Moesgaard, F., Kehlet, H. (2002). Ranitidine as adjuvant treatment in colorectal cancer. *The British journal of surgery*, Vol. 89, No. 1, (11/02), pp. (1416-22), ISSN 0007-1323

Nucifora, G., Smaller, B., Remko, R., & Avery, E.C. (1972) Transient Radicals of DNA Bases by Pulse Radiolysis. Effects of Cysteine and Cysteamine as Radioprotectors. Radiation Research, Vol. 49, No. 1, (06/72), pp. 96-111

Oda, T., Morikawa, N., Saito, Y., Masuho, Y., & Matsumoto, S. (2000). Molecular cloning and characterization of a novel type of histamine receptor preferentially expressed in leukocytes. *The Journal of biological chemistry*, Vol. 275, No. 47, (11/00), pp. (36781-6), ISSN 0021-9258

Parshad, R., Hazrah, P., Kumar, S., Gupta, S.D., Ray, R., & Bal, S. (2005). Effect of preoperative short course famotidine on TILs and survival in breast cancer. *Indian journal of cancer*, Vol. 42, no. 4, (10-12/05), pp. (185-190), ISSN 0019-509X

Pós, Z., Hegyesi, H., & Rivera, E. (2004). Histamine and cell proliferation, In: *Histamine Biology and Medical Aspects*, Falus A (editor), pp. (199-217), SpringMed Publishing, ISBN 963-9456-39X, Hungary

Pós, Z., Sáfrány, G., Müller, K., Tóth, S., Falus, A., & Hegyesi, H. (2005). Phenotypic profiling of engineered mouse melanomas with manipulated histamine production identifies histamine H2 receptor and rho-C as histamine-regulated melanoma progression markers. *Cancer research*, Vol. 65, No 10, (05/05), pp. (4458-66), ISSN:0008-5472

Potten, C.S., Owen, G., & Booth, D. (2002). Intestinal stem cells protect their genome by selective segregation of template DNA strands. *Journal of cell science*, Vol. 115, No. Pt 11, (06/02), pp. (2381-8), ISSN 0021-9533

Reynolds, J.L., Akhter, J., Adams, W.J., Morris, D.L. (1997). Histamine content in colorectal cancer. Are there sufficient levels of histamine to affect lymphocyte function? *European journal of surgical oncology*, Vol. 23, No. 3, (06/97), pp. (224-7), ISSN 0748-7983

Reynolds, J.L., Akhter, J.A., Magarey, C.J., Schwartz, P., Adams, W.J., & Morris, D.L. (1998). Histamine in human breast cancer. *The British journal of surgery*, Vol. 85, No. 4, (04/98), pp. (538-41), ISSN 0007-1323

Rivera, E.S., Cricco, G.P., Engel, N.I., Fitzimons, C.P., Martin, G.A., & Bergoc, R.M. (2000). Histamine as an autocrine growth factor: an unusual role for a widespread mediator. *Seminars in cancer biology*, Vol. 10, No. 1, (02/00), pp. (15-23), ISSN 1044-579X

Rudolph, M.I., Boza, Y., Yefi, R., Luza, S., Andrews, E., Penissi, A., Garrido, P. & Rojas, I.G. (2008). The influence of mast cell mediators on migration of SW756 cervical carcinoma cells. *Journal of pharmacological sciences*, Vol. 106, No. 2, (02/08), pp. 208-18, ISSN 1347-8613.

Sander, L.E., Lorentz, A., Sellge, G., Coëffier, M., Neipp, M., Veres, T., Frieling, T., Meier, P.N., Manns, M.P., Bischoff, S.C. (2006). Selective expression of histamine receptors H1R, H2R, and H4R, but not H3R, in the human intestinal tract. *British Medical Association*, Vol. 55, No. 4, (04/06), pp. (498-504), ISSN 0017-5749

Schwartz, J.C. (2011). The histamine H3 receptor: from discovery to clinical trials with pitolisant. *British journal of pharmacology*, Vol. 163, No. 4, (06/11), pp. (713-21), ISSN 0007-1188

Sieja, K., Stanosz, S., Von Mach-Szczypinski, J., Olewniezak, S., & Stanosz, M. (2005). Concentration of histamine in serum and tissues of the primary ductal breast cancer in women. *Breast*, Vol. 14, No. 3, (06/05), pp (236-41), ISSN 0960-9776

Smit, M.J., Hoffmann, M., Timmerman, H., & Leurs, R. (1999). Molecular properties and signaling pathways of the histamine H1 receptor. *Clinical and experimental allergy*, Vol. 29, No. Suppl. 3, (07/99), pp. (19-28), ISSN 0954-7894

Smuda, C., & Bryce, P.J. (2011). New developments in the use of histamine and histamine receptors. *Current allergy and asthma reports*, Vol. 11, No. 2, (04/11), pp. (94-100), ISSN 1529-7322

Soule, B.P., Simone, N.L., DeGraff, W.G., Choudhuri, R., Cook, J.A., Mitchell, J.B. (2010). Loratadine dysregulates cell cycle progression and enhances the effect of radiation in human tumor cell lines. *Radiation oncology*, Vol. 5, No. 8, (02/10), ISSN 1748-717X

Szincsák, N., Hegyesi, H., Hunyadi, J., Falus, A., & Juhász, I. (2002). Different h2 receptor antihistamines dissimilarly retard the growth of xenografted human melanoma cells in immunodeficient mice. *Cell biology international*, Vol 26, No 9, (02), pp. (833-6), ISSN:1065-6995

Szukiewicz, D., Klimkiewicz, J., Pyzlak, M., Szewczyk, G. & Maslinska, D. (2007). Locally secreted histamine may regulate the development of ovarian follicles by apoptosis. *Inflammation Research*, Vol. 56, Suppl 1, (04/07), pp. S33-4, ISSN 1023-3830

Takahashi, K., Tanaka, S., Ichikawa, A. (2001). Effect of cimetidine on intratumoral cytokine expression in an experimental tumor. *Biochemical and biophysical research communications*, Vol. 281, No. 5, (03/01), pp. (1113-9), ISSN 0006-291X

Tardivel-Lacombe, J., Morisset, S., Gbahou, F., Schwartz, J.C., & Arrang, J.M. (2001). Chromosomal mapping and organization of the human histamine H3 receptor gene. *Neuroreport*, Vol. 12, No. 2, (02/01), pp. (321-4), ISSN 0959-4965

Tomita, K., Izumi, K., & Okabe, S. (2003). Roxatidine- and cimetidine-induced angiogenesis inhibition suppresses growth of colon cancer implants in syngeneic mice. *Journal of pharmacological sciences*, Vol. 93, No. 3, (11/03), pp. (321-30), ISSN 1347-8613

Tomita, K., & Okabe, S. (2005). Exogenous histamine stimulates colorectal cancer implant growth via immunosuppression in mice. *Journal of pharmacological sciences*, Vol. 97, No. 1, (01/05), pp. (116-23), ISSN 1347-8613

Tomita, K., Nakamura, E., & Okabe, S. (2005). Histamine regulates growth of malignant melanoma implants via H2 receptors in mice. *Inflammopharmacology*, Vol. 13, No 1-3, (05), pp. (281-9), ISSN:0925-4692

Uçar, K. (1991). The effects of histamine H2 receptor antagonists on melanogenesis and cellular proliferation in melanoma cells in culture. *Biochemical and biophysical research communications*, Vol. 177, No 1, (05/91), pp. (545-50), ISSN:0006-291X

van Rijn, R.M., Chazot, P.L., Shenton, F.C., Sansuk, K., Bakker, R.A., & Leurs, R. (2006). Oligomerization of recombinant and endogenously expressed human histamine H(4) receptors. *Molecular pharmacology*, Vol. 70, No. 2, (08/06), pp. (604-15), ISSN 0026-895X

van Rijn, R.M., van Marle, A., Chazot, P.L., Langemeijer, E., Qin, Y., Shenton, F.C., Lim, H.D., Zuiderveld, O.P., Sansuk, K., Dy, M., Smit, M.J., Tensen, C.P., Bakker, R.A., & Leurs, R. (2008). Cloning and characterization of dominant negative splice variants of the human histamine H4 receptor. *The Biochemical journal*, Vol. 414, No. 1, (08/08), pp. (121-31), ISSN 0264-6021

von Mach-Szczypiński, J., Stanosz, S., Sieja, K., & Stanosz, M. (2009). Metabolism of histamine in tissues of primary ductal breast cancer. *Metabolism: clinical and experimental*, Vol. 58. No. 6, (06/09), pp. (867-70), ISSN 0026-0495

Wagner, W., Ichikawa, A., Tanaka, S., Panula, P., & Fogel, W.A. (2003). Mouse mammary epithelial histamine system. *Journal of physiology and pharmacology*, Vol. 54, No. 2, (06/03), pp. (211-23), ISSN 0867-5910

Wang, K.Y., Arima, N., Higuchi, S., Shimajiri, S., Tanimoto, A., Murata, Y., Hamada, T., & Sasaguri, Y. (2000). Switch of histamine receptor expression from H2 to H1 during differentiation of monocytes into macrophages. *FEBS letters*, Vol. 473, No. 3, (05/00), pp. (345-8), ISSN 0014-5793

Wasserman, T.H., & Brizel, D.M. (2001). The role of amifostine as a radioprotector. *Oncology (Williston Park, N.Y.)*, Vol., 15, No. 10, (10/01), pp. (1349-54), ISSN 0890-9091

Weigelt, C., Haas, R., & Kobbe, G. (2011). Parmacokinetic evaluation of palifermin for mucosal protection from chemotherapy and radiation. Expert opinion on drug metabolism & toxicology, Vol., 7, No. 4, (04/11), pp. (505-15505-15) ISSN 1742-5255

Wellendorph, P., Goodman, M.W., Burstein, E.S., Nash, N.R., Brann, M.R., & Weiner, D.M. (2002). Molecular cloning and pharmacology of functionally distinct isoforms of the human histamine H3 receptor. Neuropharmacology, Vol. 42, No. 7, (06/02), pp. (929-40), ISSN 0028-3908

Yang, L.P. & Perry, C.M. (2011). Histamine dihydrochloride: in the management of acute myeloid leukaemia. *Drugs*, Vol. 71, No. 1, (01/11), pp. 109-22, ISSN 0012-6667

Zampeli, E., & Tiligada, E. (2009). The role of histamine H4 receptor in immune and inflammatory disorders. *British journal of pharmacology*, Vol. 157, No. 1, (05/09), pp. (24-33), ISSN 0007-1188

4

Inhibitors of Proteinases as Potential Anti-Cancer Agents

Karolina Gluza and Paweł Kafarski
Department of Bioorganic Chemistry, Faculty of Chemistry
Wrocław University of Technology, Wrocław
Poland

1. Introduction

Cancer is a collection of over 100 devastating diseases that share a number of characteristics, a primary hallmark of which is out-of-control growth. However, in reality there are significant differences among these diseases, a fact that underlies the difficulties in the past few decades in their chemotherapeutic intervention. It is becoming evident that there are multiple routes to development of cancer, in part because so many distinct metabolic and biochemical steps can be altered to give rise to uncontrolled cell growth.

There is a positive correlation between the aggressiveness of a tumor and the secretion of various proteinases. Using bioinformatic analysis approximately 600 proteinases have been determined in human and mouse genomes (2-4% of the genome), many of which are orthologous (Puente et al., 2003). Only some of them are involved in tumor progression and growth, both at the primary and metastatic sites. As tumor progresses towards increased malignancy, it passes through several important stages that require the action of proteinases. First, the induction of angiogenesis requires degradation of the vascular basement membrane and the release of matrix-bound proangiogenic growth factors. Second, invasion of cancer cells into the surrounding tissue involves the dissolution of cell-cell junctions, degradation of the epithelial basement membrane and remodeling of extracellular matrix to allow cancer cells to be released from the primary tumor mass. Third, at least two key steps in metastasis require proteolysis: intravasation of cancer cells into the blood or lymphatic circulation at the primary site and then extravasation at the secondary site, where proteinases can play a part in promoting the colonization and growth of cancer. Proteinases may co-operatively mediate these steps with individual ones having distinct roles. Therefore, inhibition of their activity might be one of the means to combat the development of cancer. Despite of the described facts, recent findings have revealed that the functions of proteinases in tumors are significantly more complex and varied. For example, they are now seen as extremely important signaling molecules that are involved in numerous vital processes. Proteinase signaling pathways are strictly regulated, and the deregulation of their activities can lead to various pathologies, including cancer. Thus, construction of the inhibitor, which should have an impact on tumor progression and metastasis, cannot be done without placing certain proteinase in the proper metabolic context. Inhibitor therapy design is further complicated because different types of cancers utilize diverse proteinases at varying stages of cancer development.

Through the evolution, proteinases have adapted to the wide range of conditions found in human organism (variations in pH, reductive environment and so on) and they use several catalytic mechanisms for substrate hydrolysis. Basing on the chemical mechanism of their action human proteinases may be classified as: cysteine, serine, threonine, aspartic acid and metallo proteinases. In most cases specific inhibitors for each class of these enzymes are being designed.

A number of reviews on various aspects of the use of proteinase inhibitors as a mean to combat cancer have been published recently (Castro-Guillen et el., 2010; Lee et al., 2004; Magdolen et al., 2002; Pandey et al., 2007; Puxbaum & Mach, 2009; Turk, 2006). Therefore, in this review the current trends in designing of such inhibitors will be presented. Special emphasis will be put on rational design using the techniques which are based either on the knowledge of detailed mechanism of enzymatic catalysis or on three-dimensional structure of active sites of chosen enzymes. Indeed, several small-molecule drugs targeting proteinases obtained in that manner are already on the market and many more are in development.

2. Cysteine proteinases

Despite mounting evidence in the last 30 years showing that expression, localization and activation of lysosomal cysteine proteinases are aberrant in tumor cells, when compared to normal cells, this class of proteases has received little attention. Studies on increased expression, elevated activity and mislocalization of certain enzymes have indicated that members of the cysteine proteinases have been implicated in cancer progression. In mammalian cells, cysteine proteinases are localized mainly in the cytoplasm (calpain and caspase families) and lysosomal compartments (cathepsin and legumain families). Cathepsins are the most directly involved in tumor progression. There are 11 human cathepsins: B, C, F, H, K, L, O, S, W, V and X. These enzymes alongside with aspartic proteinases - cathepsins D and E are mainly involved in intracellular proteolysis within lysosomes. Their increased expression correlates with more aggressive tumors and poorer prognoses for patients (Berdowska, 2004). Cathepsins B and L expression is increased in many human cancers and these enzymes have been investigated most intensively (Bell-McGuinn, et al., 2007; Koblinski et al, 2000). In addition, the predominant expression of cathepsin K in osteoclasts has rendered this enzyme as a major target for the development of novel drugs against bone tumors (Lindeman et al., 2004).

The common belief is that cathepsin-mediated degradation of he extracellular matrix is primarily extracellular at the invasive front of tumor cells. This proteolytic process is associated both with early tumor development, affecting tumor cell proliferation and angiogenesis, and with dissemination of malignant cells from primary tumors (Turk et al 2004). Therefore inhibitors of cathepsins are most intensively studied.

Recent evidence reveals that tumor-promoting proteinases act as part of an extensive multidirectional network of proteolytic interactions. These networks involve various constituents of the tumor microenvironment, with cathepsin B being one of the best examples. An aspartic enzyme - cathepsin D converts pro-cathepsin B into cathepsin B. Cathepsin B can be also activated by a series of other proteinases with cathepsins C and G, urokinase-type plasminogen activator and tissue-type plasminogen activator being the most active ones. Finally, cathepsin B may undergo auto-activation under certain conditions. Activated cathepsin B cleaves a wide variety of targets depending on its subcellular localization in the tumor microenvironment. Some of its best-known substrates are proteins of extracellular matrix, as well as several important proteinases and their inhibitors (Skrzydlewska et al., 2005; Mason & Joyce, 2011). This complicated pattern of activity emphasizes the central role of cathepsin B in tumor progression simultaneously showing that design of its inhibitors as anticancer agents is a difficult task.

2.1 Cystatins

Cystatins are a superfamily of endogenous inhibitors of proteinases of papain family. So far, 25 representatives of these proteins have been determined. Their main function is to ensure protection of cells and tissue against the proteolytic activity of lysosomal peptidases that are released during normal cell death, or intentionally by proliferating cancer cells or by invading organisms, such as parasites. They exhibit low specificity towards their target proteases, meaning that one cystatin can inhibit several cathepsins. This is because they have apparently similar three-dimensional structure. In some types of cancers, the changes in cysteine cathepsin epression or activity have diagnostic or prognostic value with imbalance between cathepsins and cystatins being associated with tumor phenotype. Since the latter ones are able to inhibit cathepsins tumor-associated activity many studies have indicated their potential use in therapeutic approaches (Keppler, 2006; Kopitz et al, 2005; Palermo & Joyce, 2007). Indeed, one of these inhibitors, cystatin C (mostly the one isolated from egg white) has been used in preclinical research studies for more than 20 years, however, it has been introduced into clinical practice quite scarcely. Despite some isolated promising results (Saleh at al., 2006) this approach is also highly criticized (Keppler, 2006; Mussap & Plebani, 2004) with the greatest problems being high cost of the inhibitor (140 $ USA per milligram), its low bioavailability and short circulation time, and general skepticism amongst clinicians.

Despite the fact that cystatins of different families posses different biochemical properties their inhibitory properties are rather common. They are tight and reversible inhibitors of cathepsins and interact with the active sites of these proteinases via their inhibitory reactive site, made up of the juxtaposition of three regions of the molecule, which form a wedge-shaped edge that is highly complementary to the active site of papain family of proteinases (Fig. 1).

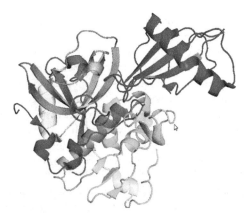

Fig. 1. Stefin A (violet) complexed with cathepsinB.

Thus, mimicking the segment of cystatin interacting with the cathepsin active site (Fig. 1) seems to be the method of choice. This approach is well represented by highly active inhibitor (N-1845, Fig. 2) of cathepsin B (K_i value of 0.088nM) containing an azaglycine residue in place of evolutionary conserved glycine residue in the N terminal part of cystatin (Wieczerzak et al., 2002). Further modification of this molecule, enforced by the use of molecular dynamic and NMR, afforded next potent and selective inhibitor of cathepsin B (K_i of 0.48 nM, Fig. 2) (Wieczerzak et al.; 2007).

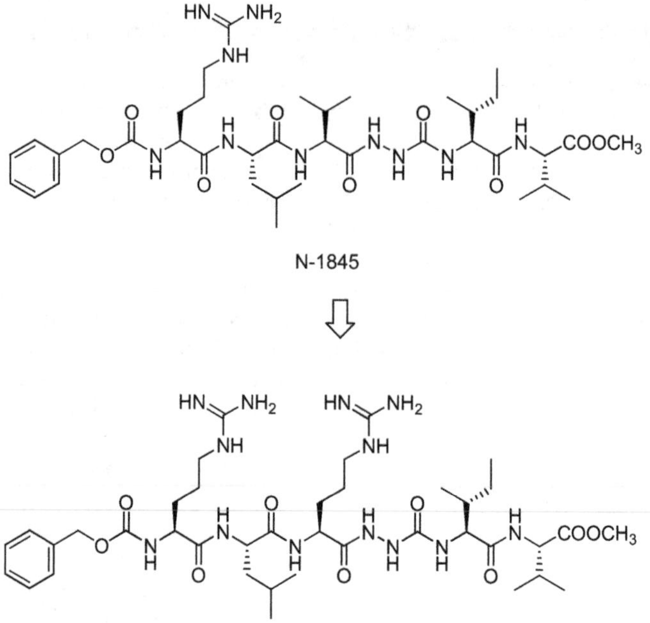

N-1845

Fig. 2. Two potent azapeptide inhibitors of cathepsin B.

2.2 Inhibitors from natural sources

General strategy employed for discovery of a new drug relays on random screening of libraries of newly available compounds and selection of these, which exhibit desired activity at micromolar range. The leads are then being modified in order to obtain significantly more potent and selective inhibitors, which might be further introduced as drugs. Nature is strongly exploited as a source of lead substances. Isolated in 1978 from *Aspergillus japonicus*, non-specific, irreversible inhibitor of cysteine proteinases, E-64 can serve as a good example (Hanada et al, 1978). The epoxysucciante fragment of this molecule reacts with active-site cysteine and binds covalently to the enzyme. By using this inhibitor as a frame and applying X-ray crystal structures of cathepsins B and L, specific inhibitors of these enzymes were designed (Fig. 3), prepared and shown to have promising anticancer activity in animal studies (Katunuma, 2011).

Traditionally, secondary metabolites from streptomyces show a wide range of diversity with respect to their biological activity and chemical nature. Therefore it is not surprising that their secondary metabolites appear to be interesting lead compounds. A mixture of two peptide metabolites from *Streptomyces* NCIM 2081 (Fig. 4) exhibited potent inhibitory action against papain and significantly inhibited tumor cell migration at subcytotoxic concentrations, indicating its remarkable potential to be developed as antimetastatic drug (Singh et al, 2010).

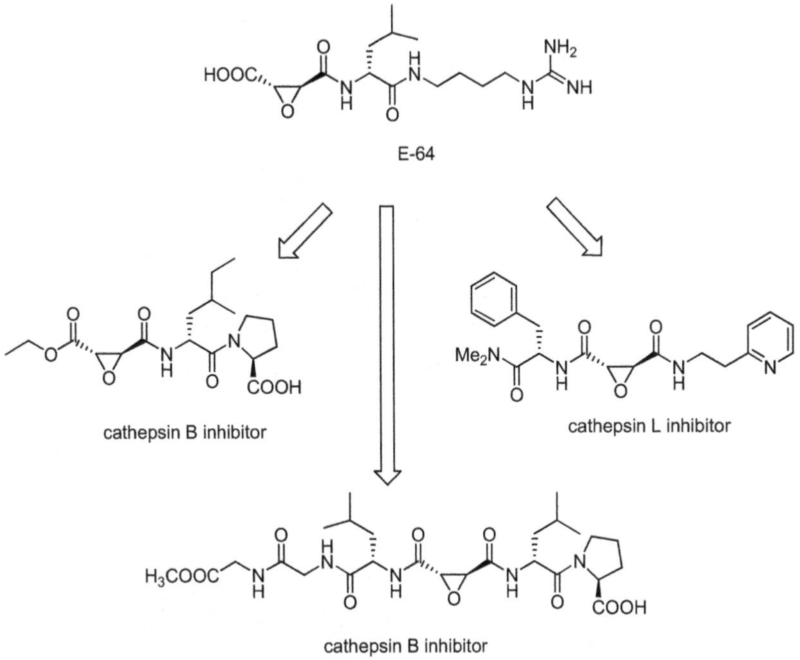

E-64

cathepsin B inhibitor

cathepsin L inhibitor

cathepsin B inhibitor

Fig. 3. Specific inhibitors of cathepsins B and L built up on the frame of E-64.

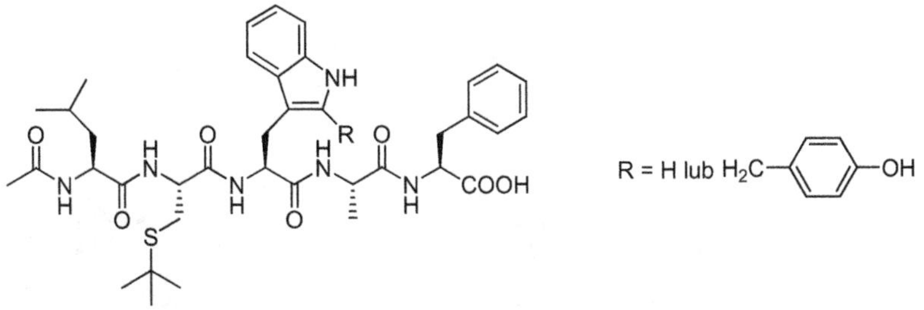

R = H lub H₂C—⟨⟩—OH

Fig. 4. Anticancer peptides produced by *Streptomyces* NCIM 2081.

2.3 Irreversible inhibitors

The majority of synthetic cysteine proteinase inhibitors contain a peptide segment for recognition by the chosen enzyme and an electrophilic functionality that is able to react with the thiolate moiety of active site cysteine. In most cases this results in covalent modification of the enzyme and irreversible inhibition. A wide variety of such reactive groups have been employed, including: azomethyl- or halomethyl ketone, acyloxymethyl ketone, acylhydroxamate, vinyl sulfone and chloromethyl sufoxide functions. It is also worth to mention that epoxysuccinates, described earlier, also fall within this class of inhibitors. Representative examples of structurally variable inhibitors are shown in Figure 5.

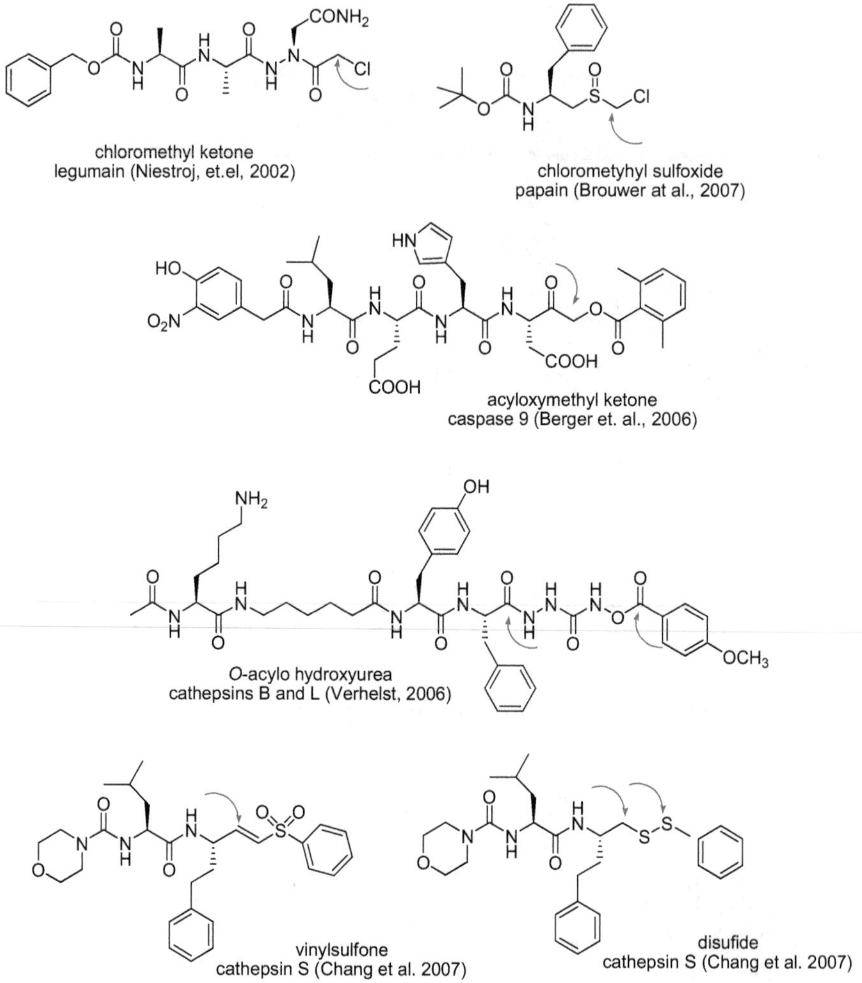

chloromethyl ketone
legumain (Niestroj, et.el, 2002)

chlorometyhyl sulfoxide
papain (Brouwer at al., 2007)

acyloxymethyl ketone
caspase 9 (Berger et. al., 2006)

O-acylo hydroxyurea
cathepsins B and L (Verhelst, 2006)

vinylsulfone
cathepsin S (Chang et al. 2007)

disufide
cathepsin S (Chang et al. 2007)

Fig. 5. Representative examples of irreversible inhibitors of cysteine proteinases. The curved arrows indicate possible sites of nucleophilic attack by the active site –SH of active site cysteine.

The reactivity of the electrophilic group greatly determines the selectivity and reaction rate of the formation of the covalent enzyme-inhibitor complex. With this respect halomethylketones are known to react not only with cysteine but also with serine proteinases, thus being non-selective. Although irreversible inhibitors possess high potency and selectivity, they are not considered to be viable drug candidates for treating diseases like cancer, osteoporosis or arthritis. This is because such inhibitors often react over time with other cysteine proteinases, thus causing toxic side effects or generating immunogenic adducts (Joyce et al., 2004).

Rational design of the peptidyl or peptidomimetic part of inhibitor requires X-ray determination of either cysteine proteinase alone or complexed with already known inhibitors. This provides the detailed insight into the active site and binding pockets of certain enzyme and makes the design process viable. The knowledge of the architecture of the active site of cathepsin B and molecular docking studies were used to design the mechanism-based inhibitor of this enzyme with dual action (Lim et el., 2004)). First, active site Cys-29 is acylated by the inhibitor, which is followed by transfer of acetyloxy moiety of the inhibitor catalyzed by His-199. Thus, two vital active site amino acids are blocked irreversibly (Fig. 6).

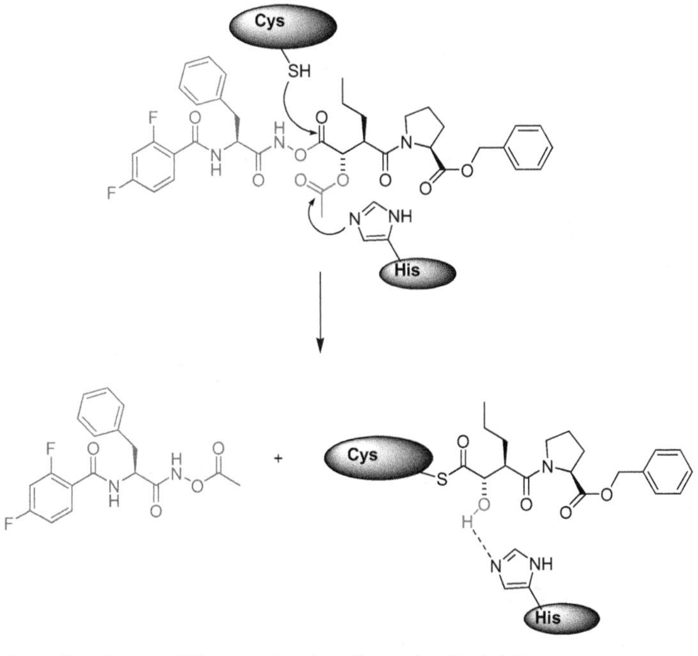

Fig. 6. Inhibition of cathepsin B by mechanism-base dual inhibitor.

2.4 Reversible inhibitors

The strategy in design of reversible inhibitors of cysteine proteinases is commonly the same as in the case of irreversible ones with the exception that the reaction between electrophilic warhead of the inhibitor and the enzyme is reversible. An aldehyde, a metyl ketone, a α-ketoamide or a nitrile groups usually act as the reactive electrophiles. Representative examples of such inhibitors are shown in Figure 7. Some of them are currently being profiled in animal models to further delineate the role of these enzymes in cancer disease processes.

A wide variety of these inhibitors were obtained using computer-aided design. For example, high-resolution X-ray crystallographic data and molecular modeling studies were used to find out one of the most potent inhibitors of cathepsin B (K_i=7nM) - dipeptide nitrile shown in Figure 8 (Greenspan et al., 2001). In the Figure 8 also the mechanism of reversible binding of this inhibitors was outlined.

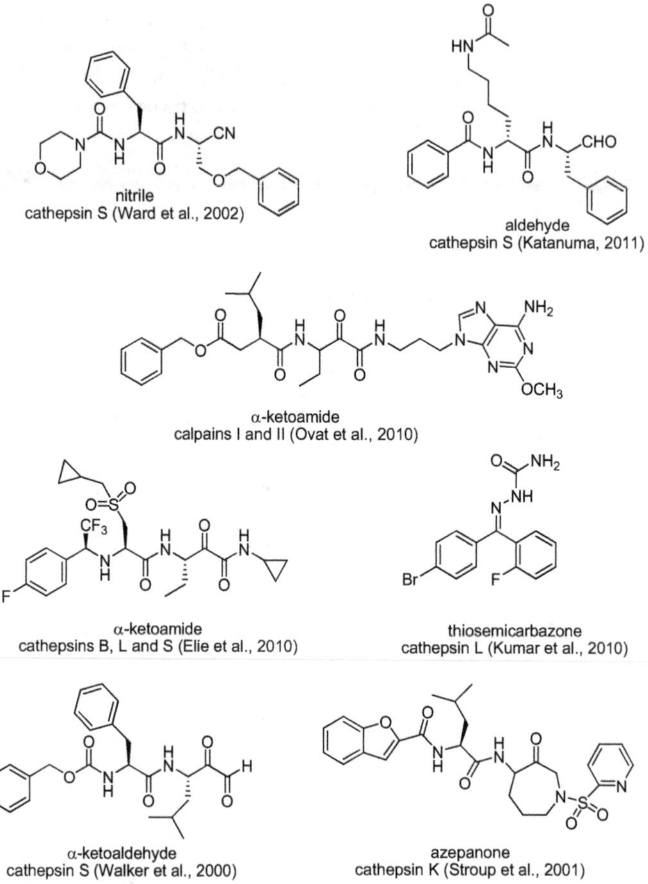
nitrile
cathepsin S (Ward et al., 2002)
aldehyde
cathepsin S (Katanuma, 2011)
α-ketoamide
calpains I and II (Ovat et al., 2010)
α-ketoamide
cathepsins B, L and S (Elie et al., 2010)
thiosemicarbazone
cathepsin L (Kumar et al., 2010)
α-ketoaldehyde
cathepsin S (Walker et al., 2000)
azepanone
cathepsin K (Stroup et al., 2001)

Fig. 7. Representative examples of reversible inhibitors of cysteine proteinases.

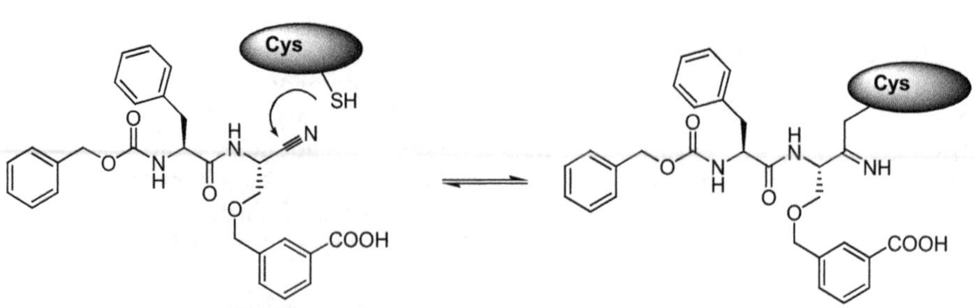
Cys
SH
COOH
Cys
NH
COOH

Fig. 8. Mechanism of inhibition of cathepsin B by dipeptidyl nitrile.

2.5 Metalloinhibitors

The field of metallodrugs is dominated by compounds, which interact with DNA and cause its direct damage. In recent years, however, it was well established that some of them exert cytotoxic activity affecting certain enzymes. Rhutenium (II)–arene derivatives exhibit remarkable selectivity towards solid tumors, most likely by inhibiting two vital enzymes for cancer development – thioredoxin reductase and cathepsin B. The most active inhibitor of cathepsin B is reversibly bound to the active site of the enzyme (Casini et al., 2008). Docking studies revealed that the most important interactions responsible for its activity are those with the residues flanking the active site (Fig. 9).

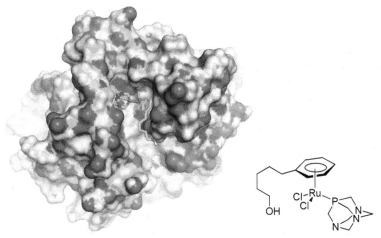

Fig. 9. The most active organorhutenium inhibitor of cathepsin B and its mode of binding in the active site of the enzyme as modeled by docking approach.

Quite contrary, newly synthesized series of organotelluranes appeared to be potent, irreversible inhibitors of cathepsins V and S (Piovan et al., 2011). Tellurium atom is an electrophilic center, which undergoes nucleophilic attack of cysteine thiol at the active site of the enzyme. In this reaction tellurium-halogen bond is broken and new tellurium sulfur bond is formed (Fig. 10). Considering the electrophilicity of the chalcogen, it is known that tellurium is less electronegative than selenium and, due to its greater capacity to stabilize the negative charge, bromide is a better leaving group than the chloride, we can explain the highest reactivity of the dibromo-organotelluranes toward cysteine cathepsins.

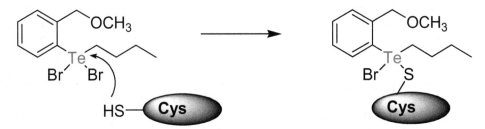

Fig. 10. Mechanism of irreversible inhibition of cathepsins by organotellurane.

3. Serine proteinases

Serine proteinases emerged during evolution as the most abundant and functionally diverse group of proteolytic enzymes - over one third of them belong to this class. They typically contain a catalytic triad of serine, histidine and aspartic acid residues in their catalytic active sites, which are commonly referred to as the charge relay system. This implies common mechanism of peptide bond hydrolysis. It goes through two-step hydrolytic process, which allows acylation of the serine residue by peptide substrate followed by hydrolysis of this adduct and regeneration of the enzyme.

Several serine proteinases have been implicated as important regulators of cancer development. This family includes enzymes involved in mediating of plasminogen (urokinase-type and tissue-type plasminogen activators), as well as serine proteinases stored in secretory lysosomes of various leukocytes, namely mast cell chymase, mast cell tryptase, and neutrophil elastase. Although most secreted serine proteinases emanate from host stromal cells, recent studies implicate a superfamily of cell-surface associated serine proteases, also known as Type II Transmembrane Serine Proteinases (TTSP), such as matriptase and hepsin, as important regulators of cancer development.

Plasmin proteolytic cascade is functionally contributing to neoplastic progression, including acquisition of a migratory and invasive phenotype by tumor cells, as well as remodeling of extracellular matrix components via activation of matrix metalloproteinases. Urokinase-type and tissue-type plasminogen activators (uPA and tPA respectively) regulate enzymatic activity of plasmin. uPA plays a crucial role in tissue remodeling, while tPA is important in vascular fibrinolysis (Naffara et al., 2009).

Mast cell-derived chymases and tryptases are stored in secretory granules. Their release into the extracellular milieu triggers a proinflammatory response as well as induces a cascade of protease activations, culminating in activation of matrix metalloproteinase 9. As a result neoplastic progression is observed (Fiorucci & Ascoli, 2004; Takai et el., 2004).

Neutrophil elastase, a serine protease abundantly present in neutrophil azurophilic (primary) granules, is transcriptionally activated during early myeloid development. Little is known about the role of this proteinase in cancer progression, however, it has the ability to cleave almost every protein contained within the extracellular matrix including, but not limited to: elastin, collagen, fibronectin, laminin, and proteoglycans. Interest in neutrophil elastase during neoplastic processes stems from recent clinical reports that correlate elevated expression of this enzyme with poor survival rates in patients with primary breast cancer and non-small cell lung cancer. It also has recently been found to initiate development of acute promyelocytic leukemia (Naffra et al., 2009; Sato et al., 2006)

Most serine proteinases are expressed by supporting tumor stromal cells, whereas membrane-anchored serine protease appear to be largely expressed by tumor cells at the cell surface and are thus ideally located to regulate cell–cell and cell–matrix interactions. Increasing evidence demonstrates that aberrant expression of enzymes such as matriptase and hepsin is a hallmark of several cancers and recent studies have defined molecular mechanisms underlying TTSP-promoted tumorigenesis, a processes causing carcinomas of skin, breast, and prostate (Choi et al., 2009). Similar association with cancer has led to great interest in kallikreins (Di Cera, 2009), a large family better known for its role in regulation of blood pressure through the kinin system. Prostate-specific antigen (PSA), a serine protease also belonging to the human kallikrein family, is best known as a prostate cancer biomarker since its expression is highly restricted to normal and malignant prostate epithelial cells.

3.1 Proteinous inhibitors

Typically serine proteinases have active site clefts that are relatively exposed to solvent. This permits the access to polypeptide loops of substrates and endogenous inhibitors. By forming strong proteinase-inhibitor complexes the latter ones regulate the activity of proteolytic enzymes and play important physiological roles in all organisms. Therefore, it is not surprising that they are considered as potential anticancer drugs and are already being tested in clinics.

Proteinous serine proteinase inhibitors were the first used against cancer and are so far the most intensively studied (Castro-Guillén et al., 2010; Otlewski et al., 2005). A small metalloprotein, Birk-Bowman inhibitor, isolated from soybeans as far as in 1946, is 8kDa polypeptide of the documented activity in a variety of tumors. Other members of this family have also proved their anti cancer activity, with field bean protease inhibitor being strongly active against skin and lung tumors, and tepary bean inhibitor affecting proliferation and metastasis of fibroblast (Castro-Guillén et al., 2010; Joanitti et al., 2010; Sakuhari et al., 2008). Another classes of similar inhibitors of serine proteinases also exhibit promising anti-cancer properties, to mention only: Kunitz-type inhibitors (Sierko et el., 2007; Wang et al., 2010), serpins (Catanzaro et al., 2011; Li et al., 2006), antileukoprotease (Xuan et el., 2008), nexin (Candia et el., 2006) and lunasin (Dia & de Meija, 2010; Hsieh et al., 2010).

Paradoxically, the action of proteinase inhibitors in some cases results in poorer prognosis and promotion of the cancer development (Fayard et al, 2009; Ozaki et al., 2009). This is contrary to what would be expected from proteinase inhibitor and shows that more detailed studies are required in order to understand their action. These observations also indicate the need for development of inhibitors of different types. Examination of crystal structures of inhibitors bound by various proteinases is a useful tool to study architecture and requirements of serine proteinase binding sites. This is because 3-5 amino acid residues of proteinaceus inhibitor, properly spatially located with respect to each other, interact with small binding region of the enzyme. The binding modes of Bowman-Birk inhibitor from *Vigna unguinocula* with β-chymotrypsin (Barbosa et. al., 2007), and structure of textilinin-1 from the venom of Australian *Pseudonaja textilis* snake complexed with trypsin (Millers et al., 2009) are shown in Figure 11 as representative examples.

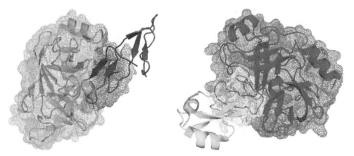

Fig. 11. The binding modes of Bowman-Birk inhibitor with β-chymotrypsin (left-hand side) and textilinin with trypsin

Mutation of the already known protein inhibitors is one of the means to construct highly specific inhibitors of chosen proteinase. Such strategy was applied to obtain specific and potent inhibitors of human kallikrein 14. A human serpin, named α-1-antichymotrypsin, was used to change its specificity by modifying five amino acids of its reactive center loop, a region involved in inhibitor–protease interaction. This region was replaced by two pentapeptides, previously selected by kallikrein 14 using phage-display technology. In this manner inhibitors with high reactivity towards the enzyme were generated (Fleber et al., 2006).

Sensing the binding site of chosen proteinase by studying structure of bound regions of its inhibitors and substrates is a classical tool for the design of new inhibitors of these enzymes. This concept is well illustrated by the discovery of cyclic peptides mimicking binding fragment of plasminogen activator (uPA) to its cell surface associated receptor (uPAR). The minimal portion of uPa able to bind effectively to uPAR was selected by systematic deletions of peptidyl fragments from the N- and C-terminus of the starting protein inhibitor. Cyclization of the minimal effective structure results in introduction of constrains that limit the conformational freedom of the molecule and ensure proper spatial arrangement of the amino acid residues interacting with the receptor. In that manner cyclic peptides, mimetics of uPA, (the most effective one is shown in Figure 12) were synthesized and found to effectively compete with uPA binding (Schmiedeberg et al., 2002).

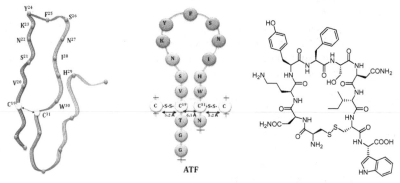

Fig. 12. Fragment of uPA selected as a scaffold for the preparation of cyclic peptidomimetics and the structure of the most effective of them

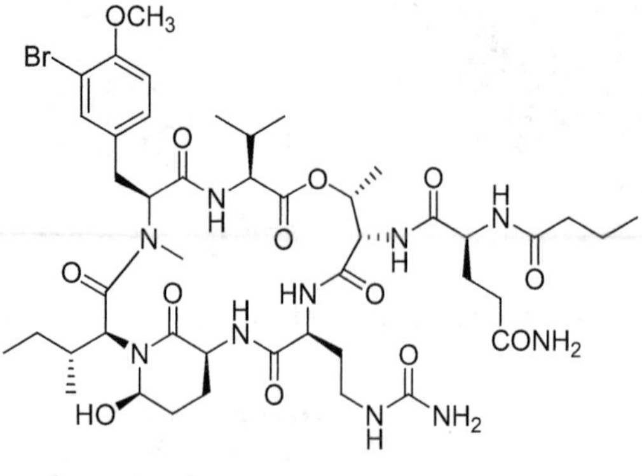

Fig. 13. Structure of Symplocamine A

Similar cyclic peptides, inhibitors of various proteinases, were also isolated from natural sources. For example, out of more than 100 compounds of this class isolated from cyanobacteria about half have been reported to inhibit trypsin or chymotrypsin. Recently isolated Symplocamine A (Figure 13), molecule of strong serine protease inhibitory activity, appeared to exert high level of cytotoxicity against variety of cancer cells *in vitro* thus being a potential agent against cancers (Linington et el., 2008).

3.2 Irreversible inhibitors

Similarly as in the case of cysteine proteinases irreversible inhibitors of serine proteinases are prominent class of their inactivators. They usually bind covalently to one of the nucleophilic moieties of amino acids present in an active site of the enzyme (most likely hydroxylic group of serine) using an electrophilic warhead. Although there are many classes of irreversible inhibitors of serine proteinases available today (Powers, et al., 2002) only limited examples entered clinical studies as anticancer agents. Therefore, new low-molecular inhibitors of enzymes involved in cancer development and metastasis are still strongly desirable. Recent studies are concentrated on the synthesis of inhibitors containing non-typical warheads (representative examples are shown in Figure 14).

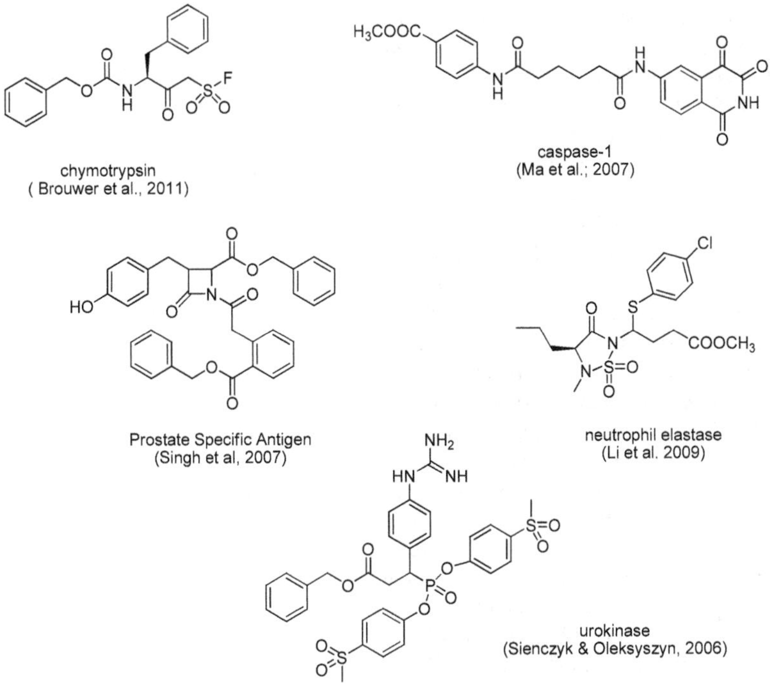

Fig. 14. Representative examples of irreversible inhibitors of serine proteinases.

Diphenyl phosphonates seem to be the most promising and general group of these inhibitors. They may be also classified as competitive transition-state analogues. On a molecular level they phosphonylate specifically active-site serine residue thus blocking the catalytic triad of serine, histidine and aspartic acids responsible for the formation of enzyme-substrate acyl intermediate and its further hydrolysis (Fig. 15). Anyway, the mode of action of phosphonates towards serine proteinases is not yet fully elucidated and minor variations were observed, depending on the targeted enzyme and conditions (Grzywa et al. 2007; Joossens et al., 2006; Sieńczyk et al., 2011; Sieńczyk & Oleksyszyn 2006; Sieńczyk & Oleksyszyn, 2009).

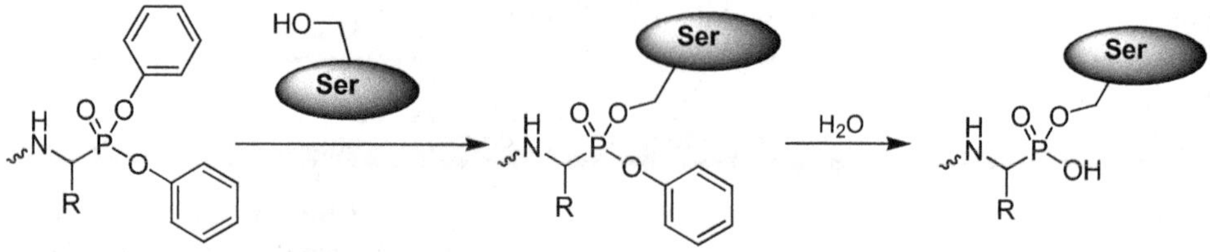

Fig. 15. Schematic illustration of the mechanism of action of the diphenyl α-aminophosphonate inhibitors of serine proteinases

3.3 Reversible inhibitors

Inhibitors of urokinase (also called urokinase-type plasminogen activator, uPA) are the biggest family of reversible serine protease inhibitors. Development of small molecule uPA inhibitors has began with aryl guanidines, aryl amidines, and acyl guanidines, molecules that contain positively charged guanidine, amidine, or simple amines as anchors able to interact with the negatively charged site chain of Asp189 (Lee et el., 2004). Although they exhibited moderate potency and poor selectivity they constituted a good starting point for the development of new effective generations of uPA inhibitors. Intensive studies using various approaches resulted in many inhibitors, which quite frequently revealed *in vitro* anticancer properties. Determination of three-dimensional structure of this enzyme either in native state or complexed with various inhibitors is vital for the design of new effectors of urokinase (Huai et al. 2008; Klinghofer et al. 2001; Sperl et. al. 2000).

For, example, an extremely simple inhibitor UK 122 (Fig. 16) was designed in a stepwise process. The first step was a selection of moderate inhibitors of uPA by screening a library of 16,000 synthetic compounds. This resulted in four promising inhibitors of the enzyme sharing very similar chemical structures. They were further optimized by using crystal structure of the enzyme-Amiloride complex and by applying molecular modeling methods. As a result UK 122 was found (Zhu et al., 2007). This compound significantly inhibited the migration and invasion of pancreatic cancer cell line.

Another example may be the use of three-dimensional quantitative structure-activity relationship (3D QSAR) studies to elucidate structural features required for uPA inhibition and to obtain predictive three-dimensional template for the design of new inhibitors. 3D QSAR was performed on five reported classes of the urokinase inhibitors by employing widely used CoMFA (Comparative Molecular Field Analysis) and CoMSIA (Comparative Molecular Shape Indices Analysis) methods (Bhongade & Gadad 2006). As a result the significance of various structural elements bound at different urokinase subsites was identified. These subsites may be combined to improve overall activity of newly designed inhibitors.

Inhibitors of other serine proteinases were studied as anticancer agents quite scarcely. Most of the obtained inhibitors were designed to affect with prostate specific antigen (PSA) and matriptase by adopting the procedures used for designing of other serine proteinase inhibitors. Some of them exhibit promising anticancer properties in cell culture systems. Representative examples of these inhibitors are shown in Figure 16.

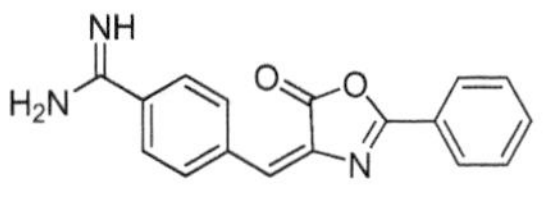

UK 122

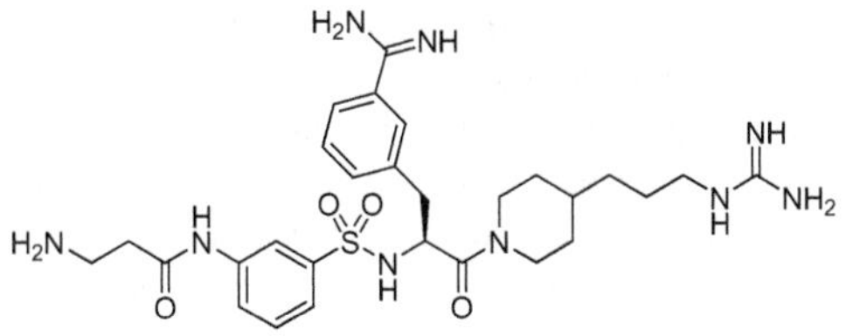

matriptase
(Steinmetzer et al., 2006)

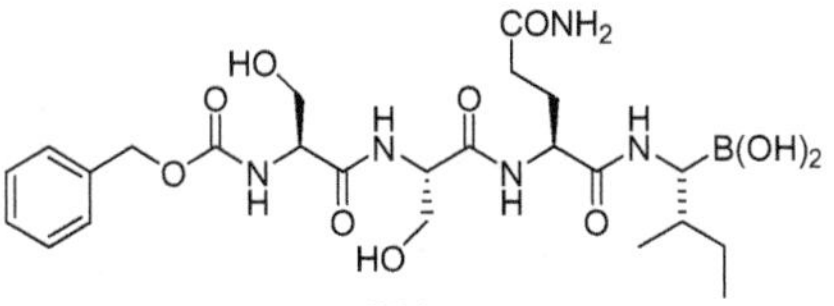

PSA
(LeBeauet.al. 2009)

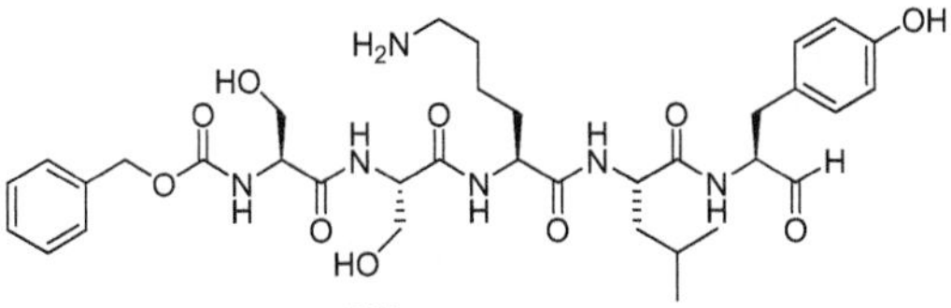

PSA
(LeBeauet.al. 2009)

Fig. 16. Representative examples of reversible inhibitors of serine proteinases.

4. Threonine proteinases

The sequencing of human genome revealed that threonine proteinases account only for about 5% of the whole pool of proteinases. From these proteinases, only proteasome is considered as a target for potential anticancer agents. Since tightly ordered proteasomal degradation of proteins plays crucial role in the cell cycle control potential of proteasome inhibitors is currently under intensive investigations.

The proteasome is a highly conserved intracellular nonlysosomal multicatalytic protease complex, degrading proteins usually tagged with a polyubiquitin chain. The 26S proteasome is a 2,000 kDa multisubunit cylindrical protein comprised of a 20S core catalytic component (the 20S proteasome) capped at one or both ends by 19S regulatory components (Figure 17). Proteasome 20S has three major sites of different activities designed as "chymotrypsin-like", "trypsin-like" and "caspase-like". These three activities are responsible for the cleavage of protein after hydrophobic, basic, and acidic amino acid residues, respectively. Analysis of the proteasome catalytic mechanism has revealed the importance of the N-terminal threonine as catalytic nucleophile. Thus, proteolytic machinery of the proteasome is an important target for the design of anticancer drugs (Abbenante & Fairlie, 2005; Delcros et al., 2003; Goldberg, 2007). A wide variety of inhibitors of proteasome were developed and evaluated (Delcros et al., 2003). This process culminated in discovery of bortezomib (*Velcade*, Figure 17), which decreases proliferation, induces apoptosis and enhances sensitivity of tumor cells to radiation or chemotherapy (Adams, 2002; Goldberg, 2007).

The most significant step in development of proteasome inhibitors was the decision by A. L. Goldberg and colleagues to create in 1993 the company *MyoGenics*. The goal was to synthesize proteasome inhibitors that could prevent muscle atrophy that occur in various disease states, such as cancer cachexia. This led to the production of a series of inhibitors that were freely distributed to academic laboratories and contributed to the enormous leap forward in understanding the multiple roles of the proteasome in cells.

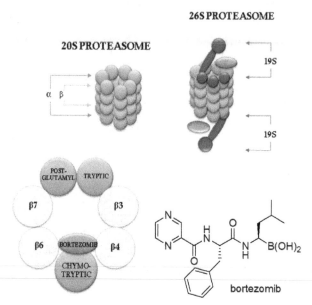

Fig. 17. Schematic structure of proteasome with indication of the binding site of bortezomib

4.1 Inhibitors from natural sources

The 20S proteasome is a tubular molecule with the proteolytic active sites on the inner surface. Thus, substrate molecules have to be translocated through the internal cavity to the catalytic sites. The X-ray crystallographic analysis has shown that the translocation channel is too narrow to allow passage of folded proteins. Protein substrates should be firstly unfolded and then degraded. Quite surprisingly, classical protein inhibitor of serine proteinases, bovine pancreatic trypsin inhibitor (BPTI) appeared to exert similar activity against proteaseome *in vitro* and *ex vivo* (Yabe & Koide, 2009). The molar ratio of BPTI to the proteasome 20S in the complex was estimated as approximately six to one, suggesting that two out of three proteinase activities of this complex were inhibited. This interesting finding has opened a new front in proteasome inhibition studies.

The majority of proteasome inhibitors have a structure of small cyclic and linear peptides built on scaffolds provided by natural substances. Lactacystin (Figure 18), produced by *Strepromyces* (Omura et. al., 1991), rearranges in neutral pH to highly reactive lactone-Omuralide, which irreversibly acylates proteasome active site threonine. Minute modification of the latter one led to the more potent inhibitor MNL-519 (Abbenante & Fairlie, 2005). Isolation of *Actinomycete* products – epoxomycin and eponemycin, and evaluation of their inhibitory activity (Hanada, et. al, 1992; Sugawara et al, 1990) has stimulated studies on their analogues (representative structure is shown in Fig. 18). This resulted in several potent inhibitors, which display non-typical mechanism of action (Elofsson et e., 1999; Zhou et el., 2009). A hemiacetal is first formed between the ketone portion of the inhibitor and threonine hydroxyl, followed by epoxide ring opening by the free amine of the N-terminal threonine to give a stable morpholino adduct.

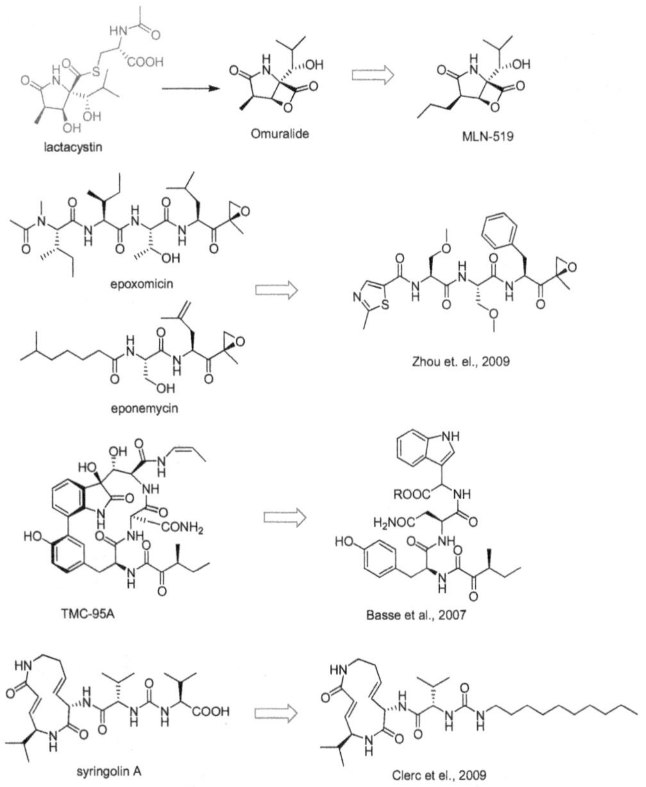

Fig. 18. Natural inhibitors of proteasome activity as scaffolds for synthesis improved ones.

Next example considers syringolines, reversible inhibitors of proteasome produced by *Pseudomonas siringae* (Coleman, et al. 2006). Elucidation of the crystal structure of syringolin B complexed with proteasome gave an insight into the structural requirements of good inhibitor. These findings were used successfully in the rational design and synthesis of a syringolin A-based lipophilic derivative, which proved to be one of the most potent proteasome inhibitors described so far (Clerc et el., 2009).

A limiting factor in the efficiency of peptidic inhibitors is that they are unstable in living organism because they are easily degraded by endogenous proteinases. This explains growing interest in non-peptidic inhibitors. Nature is an acknowledged source of such compounds and many inhibitors of proteasome were isolated and identified. These include such structurally diverse compounds as: ajoene isolated from garlic (Hassan, 2004), gliotoxin produced by *Aspergillus fumigatus* (Pahl et al., 1996), or triterpene-celastrol isolated from the root bark of medicinal plant *Tripterigium wolfordii* (Yang et al., 2006).

4.2 Synthetic inhibitors

The first inhibitors of proteasome were identified among the commercially available reversible tripeptide inhibitors of serine and cysteine proteinases. The easy access to the peptide aldehydes had lead to the development of a wide variety of inhibitors with an improved potency and selectivity. MG-132 (for its chemical structure see Figure 20) was one of the first synthetic inhibitors to be described and used in cell culture system (Adams & Stein, 1996). It exerts both, direct antiproliferative and cytotoxic effects towards tumor cells, and increases apoptosis induced by other agents. Recent studies have demonstrated the influence of absolute configuration of this tripeptide aldehyde on its cytotoxicity, with (L,D,L) isomer being the most active (Mroczkiewicz et al., 2010). Since a great number of tripeptide aldehydes contain side chains of non-coded amino acids but they usually correspond to natural L-amino acids this finding shed a new light on the importance of peptidyl absolute configuration.

Structurally related α-ketoaldehydes exert their action via mechanism similar to this described earlier for epoxyketones (Gräwert et al., 2011). This is a cyclization mechanism, which proceeds through formation of hemiketal with threonine hydroxyl followed by Schiff base formation between the nucleophilic N-terminal threonine and aldehyde moiety, which finally results in the reversible formation of a 5,6-dihydro-2H-1,4-oxazine ring (Figure 19). The examination of the binding mode of these inhibitors serves as a new lead for the development of anticancer drugs (Fig. 19).

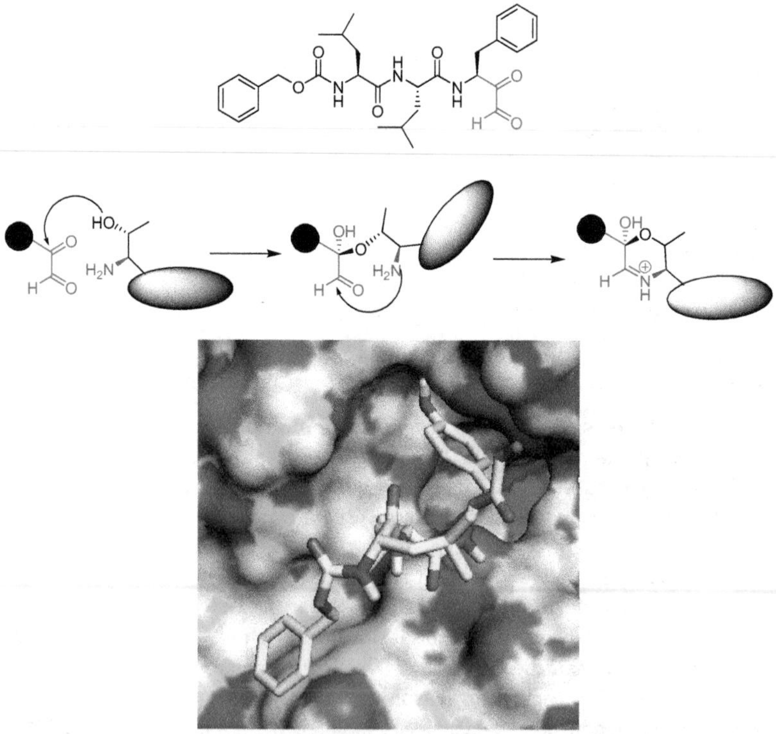

Fig. 19. Molecular mechanism of action of α–ketoaldehyde inhibitor of proteasome and the mode of its binding in the active site.

Searching for a new class of 20S proteasome inhibitors is a hot subject and to date a plethora of molecules that target the proteasome have been identified or designed (de Bettignies and Coux, 2010). Synthetic inhibitors possess a homogeneous structural profile - they are generally peptide-based compounds with a C-terminal pharmacophore function required for primary interaction with catalytic threonine of the enzyme. The peptide component seems to be important for determining specificity of the interactions with the enzymatic pockets. Essentially, most of these inhibitors act on the chymotrypsin-like activity of the proteasome although two remaining activities are also addressed.

Protection of the aldehyde moiety in a form of semicarbazone provides compounds that are more stable than counterpart aldehydes. They do not form adducts with cellular proteins and are irreversible inhibitors of proteasome requiring the action of this enzymatic complex to release inhibiting aldehyde. Thus, they may be classified as suicidal inhibitors. Recently two peptide semicarbazones, S-2209 and SC68896, were found to exert anti-melanoma and anti-glioma activities in preclinical studies (Baumann et el., 2009: Leban et al., 2008; Roth et el., 2009). For the latter one company was given an approval to start phase I/II clinical studies in 2011.

Structurally related N-acylpyrrole peptidyl derivatives were designed as irreversible inhibitors of proteasome. They appeared to possess unique biological profile and interact reversibly with β1 catalytic site of the proteasome also displaying good pharmacological properties (Baldisserotto et al., 2010). Molecular docking of the N-acylpyrrole molecule shown in Figure 20 enabled to rationalize the mode of their binding.

The vinyl sulfone group is less reactive than the aldehyde group but also binds irreversibly to the active sites. The advantage of vinylsulfone inhibitors is that they are easy to prepare. One of the most potent inhibitor - Ada(Ahx)$_3$-LLL-VFS, specifically and irreversibly inhibits both the constitutive and the induced proteasome by binding to their three active sites with approximately equal efficiencies (Kessler et al., 2001).

The screening of huge libraries of structurally variable compounds is a method for the identification of new cell-active inhibitors with novel chemical scaffolds. Such a procedure was also used in order to obtain new inhibitors of proteasome. Thus, a high-throughput screen of the Millennium Pharmaceuticals Inc. library (approximately 352,500 compounds) afforded 3015 hits, which were further optimized by applying X-ray crystallography and molecular modeling. In such manner 16 various structures were selected. They appear to exhibit high potency and selectivity towards β5 subunit of 20S proteasome. The crystal structures determined for the most active compounds (Fig. 20) enabled to determine the structural requirements of the inhibited subunit. Similar screening done on National Cancer Institute Diversity Set library composed of 1,992 compounds resulted in selection of four promising inhibitors of proteasome, with organocopper NCS 321206 (Fig.20) being the most active one (Lavelin et al., 2009).

Different approaches to the selection of new inhibitors of proteasome relayed on the use of computational tools, namely multistep structure-based virtual ligand screening strategy. First scoring engines were standardized using known inhibitors in order to obtain results similar to those found from crystallographic studies. It appeared that none of the presently developed scoring functions are fully reliable nor they fully correlate with experimental affinities. Therefore three protocols were used simultaneously - FRED, LigandFit and Surflex, to dock 300,000 compound collection (Chembridge). This enabled to select 200 molecules for further experimental testing, using MG-132 as a standard. Twenty of these molecules appeared to act as potent proteasome inhibitors showing variable profiles of activity. Thus six of them inhibited all three activities of proteasome, eleven of them inhibited two types of enzymatic activities, whereas three inhibited only one type of activity (Basse et al., 2010). The most active and selective inhibitors against chymotrypsin-like and trypsin-like activities are shown in Figure 20.

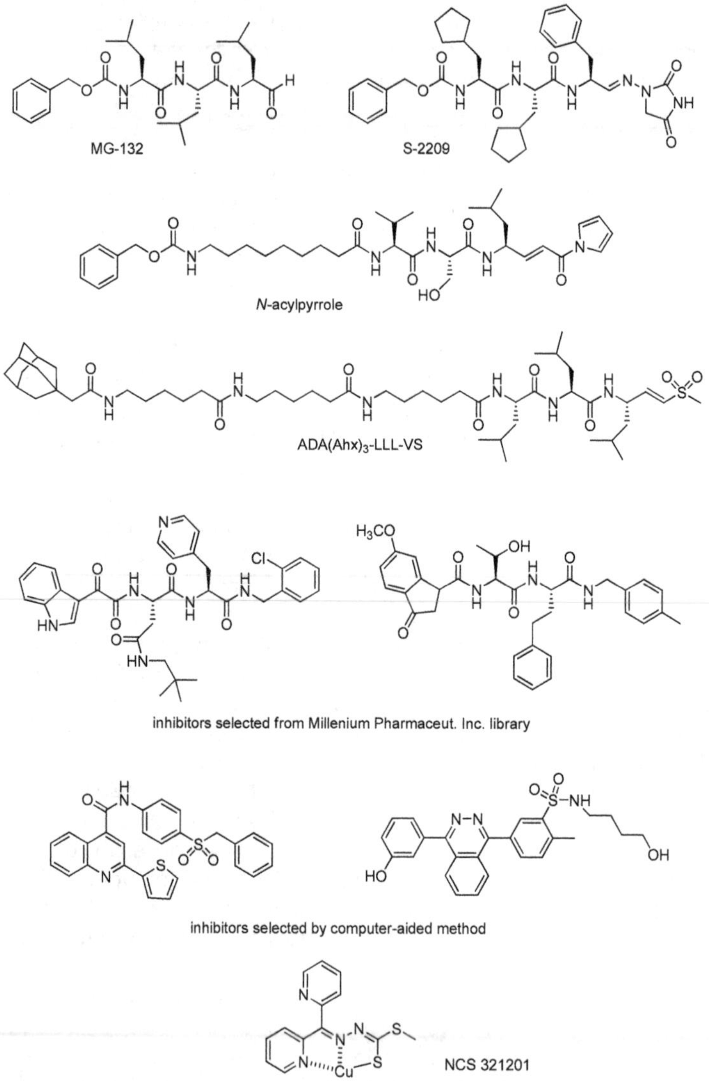

Fig. 20. Structurally diverse, synthetic inhibitors of proteasome.

The discovery of bortezomib was followed by intensive preclinical and clinical studies on many cancer models and cancer patients. This drug was approved in 2003 for treatment of multiple myeloma as a second line of the therapy. Today it is taken by approximately 50,000 patients worldwide (Goldberg, 2007) and is still being tested clinically against other forms of cancer. Interestingly, recent studies have indicated that this drug is a multiple inhibitor and affects also serine proteinases in cell lysates (Arastu-Kapur et al., 2011). This finding may explain better the clinical profile of this drug. Alongside with physiologic studies synthesis and evaluation of inhibitory activity of its analogues have been carried out. Although in some cases inhibitors of similar potency were obtained (Aubin et al., 2005; Vivier et al., 2005; Zhu et al, 2010) none of them was found to be better than bortezomib.

5. Aspartic proteinases

This is the smallest family of proteinases, which accounts for only 3% of them and includes several physiologically important enzymes such as pepsin, chymosin, renin, gastricsin, cathepsin D and cathepsin E. Some members of this family, in particular cathepsins D and E, have been implicated in cancer progression. High cathepsin D expression is associated with shorter disease-free and overall survival in patients with breast cancer, whereas in patients with ovarian or endometrial cancer, cathepsin E expression has been reported to be associated with tumor aggressiveness.

Quite surprisingly, the aspartic protease napsin A, expressed in lung cells, where it is involved in the processing of surfactant protein B, suppressed tumor growth in HEK293 cells in a manner independent of its catalytic activity (Ueno et al., 2008). Further insight into mechanism involved may help in producing new drugs for renal cancer.

The most extensively investigated aspartic proteinase in the context of cancer is cathepsin D, with a particular emphasis on its role in breast cancer (Benes et al, 2008). In these studies several inhibitors of this enzyme are most commonly used including peptidomimetic pepstatin (Umezawa et al., 1970) and protein inhibitors from potato and tomato (Carter et al., 2002). Search for new inhibitors of this enzyme is practically limited to peptides containing non-typical amino acid – statine. Inhibitors of this type were obtained from both natural sources as well as were synthesized basing on the crystal structure of pepstatin A (Fig. 21) complexed by this enzyme. Statine, which is a component of pepstatin A, may be considered as an analogue of tetrahedral intermediate (or transition-state) of the enzymatic hydrolysis of L-leucylglycine (Fig. 21). Therefore it is not surprising that most of cathepsin D inhibitors contain this amino acid or its analogue within peptidic chain (Bi et al., 2000; McConnell et al., 2003). Of special interest are grassystatins (Fig. 21) isolated from cyanobacterium *Lyngbya* cf. *confervoides*. These peptidomimetics are equally active against cathepsins D and E (Kwan et al., 2009).

The new approach to the identification of inhibitors is appropriate selection of DNA aptamers strongly interacting with chosen enzyme. This methodology was used to identify the aptamer SF-6-3, which selectively and very strongly binds cathepsin E (Naimuddin et al., 2007).

6. Metalloproteinases

Metalloproteinases are the largest class of proteinases in human genome. They are a range of enzymes possessing metal ions in their active sites. Most of them are dependent on zinc ions, which play catalytic functions. Understanding their mechanism of action is of key importance to rational design of potent and specific inhibitors of these enzymes and, consequently, to obtain drugs of improved properties. Therefore, a substantial effort has been made to study the mode of binding of their substrates and inhibitors, as well as to elucidate the three dimensional structure of these enzymes and to define the detailed mechanisms of catalyzed reactions. Despite extensive experimental and theoretical studies the mechanism by which the catalytic center of metalloproteinases functions is still the subject of debate and several mechanism have been proposed (Mucha et al., 2010).

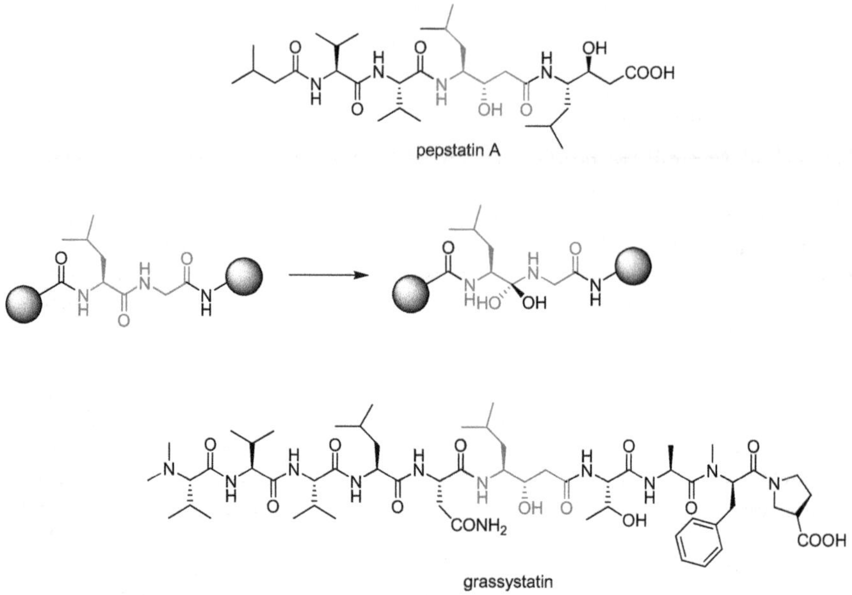

pepstatin A

grassystatin

Fig. 21. Pepstatin A and grassystatin as transition-state analogues of peptide hydrolysis.

Matrix metalloproteinases (MMPs), a disintegrin and metalloproteinases (ADAMs, adamalysins) and tissue inhibitors of metalloproteinases (TIMPs) together comprise an important set of proteins that are regulatory in matrix turnover and regulate growth factor bioavailability. There are 23 MMP, 32 ADAM and 4 TIMP proteins present in humans. This shows how complex system is involved in tumorigenesis and its regulation. For example, four tissue inhibitors of metalloproteinases (TIMP1, TIMP2, TIMP3 and TIMP4) are the main endogenous inhibitors for all the metallo-endopeptidases, of which there are more than 180.

6.1 Matrix metalloproteinases

Matrix metalloproteinases (MMPs) consist of a multigene family of zinc dependent extracellular endopeptidases implicated in tumor growth and the multistep processes of invasion and metastasis, including proteolytic degradation of extracellular matrix, alteration of the cell–cell and cell–matrix interactions, cell migration and angiogenesis (Gialeli et al., 2011). These structurally and functionally related endoproteinases share common functional domains and activation mechanisms. The MMPs were the first proteinase targets seriously considered for combating cancer. After encouraging preclinical results in various cancer models several of the MMP inhibitors were tested in advanced clinical trials but all failed because of severe side effects or no major clinical benefit (Turk et el., 2006). These include: hydroxamate inhibitors batimastat, marimastat, and prinomastat and the non-hydroxamate ones such as neovastat (an extract from shark cartilage of a molecular mass up to 500kDa introduced by Aeterna) rebimastat and tanomastat (Fig. 22).

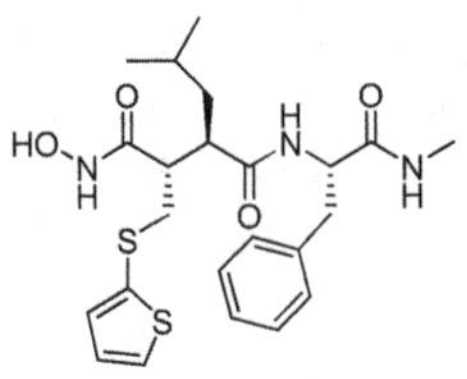

batimastat (*British Biotech*)

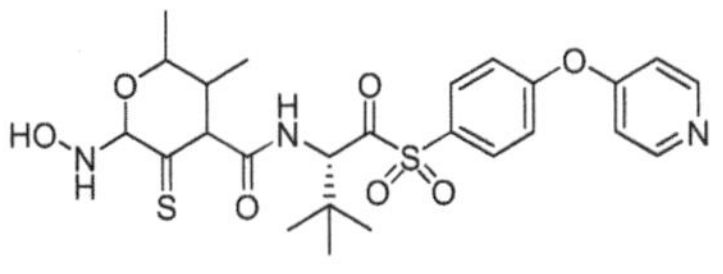

prinomastat (*Aguron*)

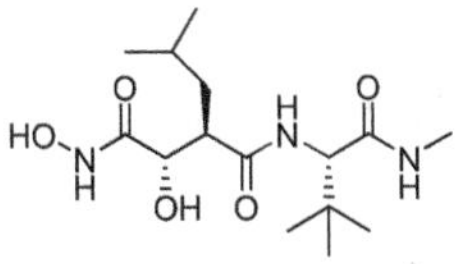

marimastat (*British Biotech*)

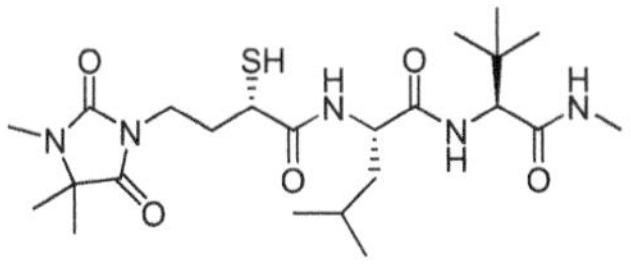

rebimastat (*Bristol-Meyers Squibb*)

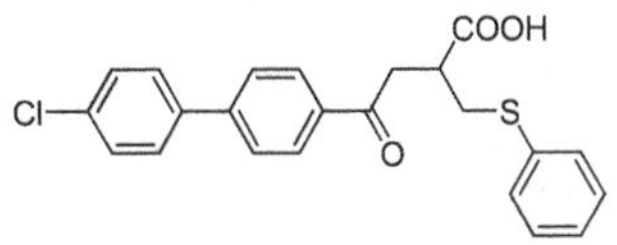

tanomastat (*Bayer*)

Fig. 22. Matrix metalloproteinase inhibitors, which failed in clinical studies. In parentheses companies, which introduced these compounds are given.

Clinical studies indicated that timeframe of targeting MMPs differs, depending on the stage of cancer, because the expression profile, as well as the activity of these enzymes, is not the same in the early stage compared to advanced cancer disease. As a consequence, the use of broad-spectrum inhibitors raises concerns that certain MMPs that exert anticancer effects are inhibited, which in turn may result in promotion of the disease (Gialeli et al., 2011). Thus, pharmacological targeting of cancer by the development of a new generation of effective and selective inhibitors to individual matrix metalloproteinases is an emerging and promising area of research (Devel et al., 2010; Manello, 2006). However, despite intense efforts, very few highly selective inhibitors of these metalloproteinases have been discovered up to now. This is because MMPs have catalytic domains composed of 160–170 amino acid residues that share a marked sequence similarity, with the percentage of identical residues being in the range of 33% to 90%. The three dimensional structure of the catalytic domains of 12 out of 23 human MMPs has been solved either by X-ray crystallography or NMR (Maskos, 2005), and the results supported that they are of significant similarity. The other cause of low specificity of most of MMP inhibitors is that their action relays on strong complexation of zinc ion present in the active sites of these enzymes. This is especially true in the case of hydoxamic acid-based inhibitors (Yiotakis & Dive, 2008), which are the most intensively studied so far (Attolino et al., 2010; Fisher & Mobashery, 2006; Nuti et al., 2010).

Among different zinc-binding groups, the phosphoryl moiety was thought to be the weakest binder. Indeed, it turns out that numerous peptide analogues with a phosphorus-containing moiety replacing the scissile amide bond have been found to regulate the activity of metalloproteinases (Collinsová & Jiraček, 2000). The intense optimization of the phosphinic inhibitor structures, using parallel or combinatorial chemistry, is generally required to identify nanomolar inhibitors and to get selectivity (Dive et al., 2004). Without selective inhibitors, which are indispensable tools for studying the structure and the role of individual enzymes at different stages of complex tumorigenesis, anticancer strategies based on MMP inhibition are unlikely to provide important therapeutic benefits. Two representative inhibitors of this class of inhibitors are shown in Figure 23.

High-throughput screening of chemical libraries has also led to the discovery of unusual MMP inhibitors, selective against MMP-13. Among these, a new class of MMP inhibitors that do not possess a zinc-binding group and thus do not interact directly with the zinc active site ion is of special interest (Fig. 23) (Chen et al., 2000).

6.2 Aminopeptidases

Aminopeptidases are proteolytic enzymes that hydrolyze peptide bonds from the amino termini of polypeptide chains with the release of a single amino acid residue from polypeptide substrates. Although their involvement in tumorigenesis was well established the studies on their anticancer properties are far less developed than studies on MMPs. This may also result from the fact that physiologic role of these enzymes is far more complex.

A plethora of inhibitors of aminopeptidases have been synthesized and tested clinically against various pathological disorders, including cancers (Bauvois & Dauzonne, 2006; Mucha et al., 2010; Selvakumar et al., 2006; Wickström et al., 2011). Bestatin, a general inhibitor of aminopeptidases and aspartyl proteinases, has been the most intensively studied (Fig. 24). It was originally isolated from *Streptomyces olivoreticuli* more than 30 years ago (Umezawa et al., 1976). Bestatin studies in biological systems both *in vitro* and *in vivo*, resulted in discovery of several interesting properties of this compound such as ability to induce apoptosis in cancer cells, and anti-angiogenic, anti-malarial or immunomodulatory effects. Presently, bestatin (Ubenimex®) is on Japanese market where it is applied for treatment of cancer and bacterial infections. Examples of successful inhibition of aminopeptidases by bestatin include aminopeptidase N (CD13), leucine aminopeptidase (LAP) and aminopeptidase B. These aminopeptidases, as well as methionine aminopeptidase 2 are the most exploited targets to obtain new anticancer agents.

In contrast to MMPs selectivity of the inhibitor is not a required feature and in most cases general inhibitors of aminopeptidases are used in clinical studies. Such an example is tosedostat (Fig. 24) (Krige et. al, 2008; Moore et al., 2009), a hydroxamic acid inhibitor of M1 family of aminopeptidases (especially leucine aminopeptidase), which is now being introduced to the market by Chroma Therapeutics. In clinical studies tosedostat was well tolerated, given orally once a day, and it has produced encouraging response rates in difficult to treat patients with acute leukemia and a variety of blood related cancers. Tosedostat (CHR-2797) is a prodrug and exposure of cancer cells to this drug results in the generation of the active metabolite CHR-79888 (Fig. 24), which is poorly membrane-permeable, what limits its pharmacological activity. The use of prodrug results in intracellular accumulation of CHR-79888 and desirable physiological effect.

6.3 Carboxypeptidases

Carboxypeptidases cleave the peptide bond of amino acid residue at the carboxylic terminus of protein or peptide. Humans contain several types of carboxypeptidases, which have diverse functions ranging from catabolism to protein maturation. There is practically lack of information about the role of carboxypeptidases in tumorigenesis. However, some of them were proposed as markers of individual tumors (Kemik et al., 2011; Lee et al., 2011). This indicates that they also might be considered as targets in anticancer therapy. Indeed, there are two reports on antitumor activity of two endogenous protein inhibitors of carboxypeptidases – latexin (Pallares et al., 2005) and retinoic acid-induced tumor suppressor retinoic acid receptor responder 1 (RARRES 1) (Sahab et al., 2011).

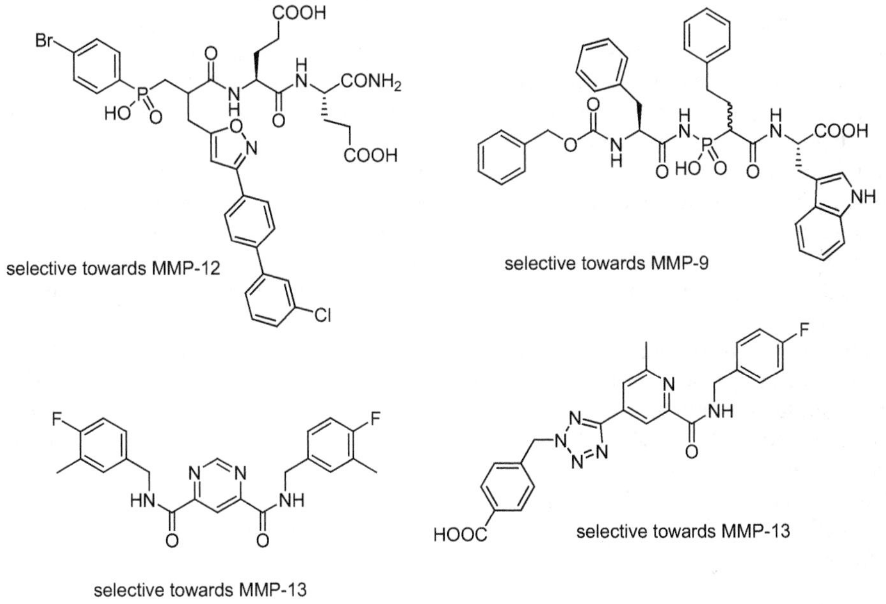

selective towards MMP-12

selective towards MMP-9

selective towards MMP-13

selective towards MMP-13

Fig. 23. Selective MMP inhibitors.

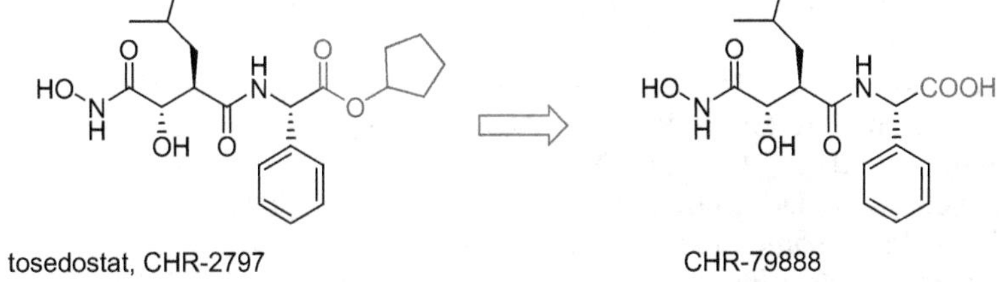

bestatin

tosedostat, CHR-2797

CHR-79888

Fig. 24. Bestatin and tosedostat – general inhibitors of aminopeptidases and promising anticancer drugs.

7. Conclusion

Looking back at the progress made with anticancer therapies using inhibitors of various proteinases it is hard to consider it as particularly successful. Today the major successful areas in protease-targeted therapies are the cardiovascular, inflammatory and infectious diseases (mostly anti-HIV), however, the intensive studies on therapies of cancer and neurodegradative disorders are predicted. This is a good prognosis if taking into account that the annual spending for protease-directed drugs amounts close to US$ 10 billion annually (Turk, et al., 2006).

It is worth to note that past drug failures are not worthless. They provide not only invaluable lessons but are also a useful resource of data, which could still be used.

In order to achieve more satisfactory results, better understanding of the proteolytic network in tumor envinroment and increased knowledge in protease biology based on comprehensive analysis of protease activity in physiologically relevant conditions are required. The fact that tumor cells are only one part of the tumor environment and that extracellular matrix components and stromal cells are important contributors to the proteolytic activity of tumors should also be taken into consideration. For example, the use of transgenic animals may help in elucidation of the role of individual components of this complex networks.

Also the techniques of inhibitor design are developing significantly with *in silico* structure-based ligand design and various types of high-throughput screening being the major ones. Today's strategy in inhibitor design is to provide compounds complementary to active sites of the inhibited proteins, while the other concepts are used scarcely. One of the solutions is to design allosteric inhibitors altering proteinase activity by binding outside the enzyme active site, most likely in the cavity lacking any physiological role. The development of computer-aided methods for drug design (especially docking procedures) might be very helpful in this respect.

8. Acknowledgment

This work is dedicated to Professor Francisco Palacios from University of Basque Country at Vitoria on the occasion of his 60th birthday.
Authors thank Polish Ministry of Science and Higher Education for financial support.

9. References

Abbenante, G.; Fairlie, D. P. (2005) Protease Inhibitors in the Clinic. *Medicinal Chemistry* Vol. 1 (No. 1): 71-104

Adams, J. (2002) Development of the Proteasome Inhibitor PS-341. *Oncologist* Vol. 7 (No. 1): 9-16.

Adams, J. & Stein, R. (1996) Novel Inhibitors of the Proteasome and Their Therepeutic Use in Inflammation. *Annual Reports in Medicinal Chemistry* Vol. 31: 279-288.

Arastu-Kapur, S.; Anderl, J. L.; Karus, M.; Parlati, F.; Shenk, K. D.; Lee, S. J.; Muchamuel, T.; Bennett, M. K.; Driessen, C.; Ball, A. J. & Kirk, C. J. (2011) Non-proteasomal Targets of the Proteasome Inhibitors Bortezomib and Carfilzomib: a Link to Clinical Adverse Effects. *Clinical Cancer Research* Vol. 17 (No. 9): 2734-2743.

Attolino, E.; Calderone, V.; Dragoni, E.; Fragai, M.; Richichi, B.; Luchinat, C. & Nativi, C. (2010) Structure-based Approach to Nanomolar, Water Soluble Matrix Metalloproteinases Inhibitors (MMPIs). *European Journal of Medicinal Chemistry* Vol. 45 (No. 12): 5919-5925.

Aubin, S.; Martin, B.; Delcros, J.-G.; Arlot-Bonnemains, J & Baudy-Floc'h, M. (2005) Retro Hydrazino-azapeptoids as Peptidomimetics of Proteasome Inhibitors. *Journal of Medicinal Chemistry* Vol. 48 (No. 1): 330-334.

Baldisserotto, A.; Ferretta, V.; Destro, F.; Franceschini, C.; Marastoni, M.; Gavioli, R. & Tomatis, R. (2010) α,β-Unstaurated N-Acylpyrrole Peptidyl Derivatives: New Proteasome Inhibitors. *Journal of Medicinal Chemistry* Vol. 53 (No. 17): 6511-6515.

Barbosa, J. A. R. G.; Silva, R. P.; Teles, R. C. L.; Esteves, G. F.; Azevedo, R. B.; Ventura, M. M. & de Freitas, S. M. (2007) Crystal Structure of tyhe Bowman-Birk Inhibitor from *Vigna unguiculata* Seeds in Complex with β-Chymotripsin at 1,55 Å Resolution and Its Structural Properties in Association with Proteinases. *Biophysical Journal* Vol. 92 (No. 5): 1638-1650.

Basse, N.; Piguel, S.; Papapostolu, D.; Ferrier-Berthelot, A.; Richy, N.; Pagano, M.; Sarthou, P.; Sobczak-Thépot, J.; Reboud-Ravaux, M. & Vidal, J. (2007) Linear TMC-95 Based Proteasome Inhibitors. *Journal of Medicinal Chemistry* Vol. 50 (No. 12): 2842-2850.

Basse, N.; Montes, M.; Maréchal, X.; Qin, L.; Bouvier-Durand, M.; Genin, E.; Vidal, J. ; Villoutreix, B. O. & Reboud-Ravaux, M. (2010) Novel Organic Proteasome Inhibitors Idnetified by Virtual and in Vitro Screening. *Journal of Medicinal Chemistry* Vol. 53 (No. 1): 509-513

Baumann, P.; Müller, K.; Mandl-Weber, S.; Leban, J.; Doblhofer, R.; Ammendola, A.; Baumgartner, R.; Oduncu, F. & Schmidmaier, R. (2009) The Peptide-semicarbazone S-2209, a Representative of New Class of Proteasome Inhibitors, Induces Apoptosis and Cell Growth Arrest in Multiple Myeloma Cells. *British Journal of Haemathology* Vol. 144 (No. 6): 875-886.

Bauvois, B. & Dauzonne, D. (2006) Aminopeptidase N/CD13 (EC 3.4.11.2) Inhibitors: Chemistry, Biological Evaluations and Therapeutic Prospects. *Medicinal Research Reviews* Vol. 26 (No. 1): 88-130.

Bell-McGuinn, K. M.; Garfall, A. M.; Bogyo, M.; Hanahan, D. & Joyce, J. A. (2007) Inhibition of Cysteine Cathepsin Protease Activity Enhances Chemotherapy Regimens by Decreasing Tumor Growth and Invasiveness in a Mouse Model of Multistage Cancer. *Cancer Research* Vol. 67 (No. 15): 7378-7385.

Benes, P.; Vetwicka, V.& Fusek, M. (2008) Cathepsin D – Many Functions of One Aspartic Protease. *Critical Reviews in Oncology/Hematology* Vol. 68 (No. 1): 12-28.

Berdowska, I. (2004) Proteases as Disease Markers. *Clinica Chimica Acta* Vol. 342 (No. 1-2): 41-69.

Bhongade, B. A. & Gadad, A. K. (2006) Insight into the Structural Requirements of Urokinase-Type; Plasminogen Activator Inhibitors Based on 3D QSAR CoMFA/CoMSIA Models, *Journal of Medicinal Chemistry* Vol. 49 (No. 2): 475-489.

Blackburn, C.; Gigstad, K. M.; Hales, P.; Garcia, K.; Jones, M.; Bruzzese, M. J.; Barrett, C.; Liu, J. X.; Soucy, T. A.; Sappal, D. S.; Bump, N.; Olhava, E. J.; Fleming, P.; Dick, L. R.; Tsu, C.; Sintchak, M. D. & Blank J. L. (2010) Characterization of a New Series of Non-Covalent Proteasome Inhibitors with Exquisite Potency and Selectivity for the 20S β5-Subunit, *Biochemical Journal* Vol. 430 (No. 3): 461-476.

Brouwer, A. J.; Bunschoten, A. & Liskamp, R. M. J. (2007) Synthesis and Evaluation of Chloromethyl Sulfoxides as a New Class of Selective Irreversible Cysteine Protease Inhibitors. *Bioorganic & Medicinal Chemistry* Vol. 15 (No. 22): 6985-6993.

Brouwer, A. J.; Ceylan, T.; Jonker, A. M.; van der Linden, T & Liskamp R. M. J. (2011) Synthesis and Biological Evaluation of Novel Irreversible Serine Protease Inhibitors Using Amino Acid Based Sulfonyl Fluorides as an Electrophilic Trap. *Bioorganic & Medicinal Chemistry* Vol. 19 (No. 7): 2397-2406.

Candia, B. J.; Hines, W. C.; Heaphy, C. N.; Griffith, J. K. & Orlando, R. A. (2006) Protease Nexin I Expression Is Altered in Human Breast Cancer. *Cancer Cell International* Vol. 16 (31 May 2006): 16.

Carter, S. A.; Lees, W. A.; Hill, J.; Brzin, J.; Kay, J. & Phylip, L. H. (2002) Aspartic Protease Inhibitors from Tomato and Potato are More Potent Against yeast Proteinase A than Cathepsin D. *Biochimica and Biophysica Acta (BBA) – Protein Structure anhd Molecular Enzymology* Vol. 1596 (No. 1): 76-82.

Casini, A.; Gabbiani, C.; Sorrentino, S.; Rigobello, M. P.; Bindoli, A.; Geldbach, T. J.; Marrone, A.; Re, N.; Hartinger, C. G.; Dyson, P. J. &Messori, L. (2008) Emerging Protein Targets for Anticancer Metallodrugs: Inhibition of Thioredoxin Reductase and Cathepsin B by Antitumor Ruthenium (II) – Arene Compounds. *Journal of Medicinal Chemistry* Vol. 51 (No. 21): 6773-6781.

Castro-Guillén, J. L.; Garcia-Gasca, T & Blanco-Labra, A. (2010) Chapter V. Protease Inhibitors as Anticancer Agents. In: *New Approaches in the Treatment of Cancer.* V. C. Mejia Vazquez & S. Navarro (Eds.), 91-124, Nova Science Publishers, ISBN 978-1-61728-304-9

Catanzaro, J. M.; Guierriero, J. L.;Liu, J.; Ullman, E.; Sheshadri, N.; Chen, J. J. & Zong, W.-X. (2011) Elevated Expression of Squamus Cell Carcinoma Antigen (SCAA) Is Associated with Human Breast Carcinoma. *PloS ONE* Vol. 6 (No. 4): 1-8, e19096

Chang, W.-S. W.; Wu, H.-R.; Wu, C.-W. & Chang, J.-Y. (2007) Lysosomal Cysteine Protease Cathepsin S as a Potential Target for Anti-cancer Therapy. *Journal of Cancer Molecules* Vol. 3 (No. 1): 5-14.

Chen, J. W.; Nelson, F. C.; Levin, J. I.; Mobilio, D.; Moy, F. J.; Nilakantan, R.; Zask, A. & Powers, A. (2000) Structure-based Design of a Novel, Potent and Selective Inhibitor for MMP-13Utilizing NMR Spectroscopy and Computer-Aided Molecular Design. *Journal of American Chemical Society* Vol. 122 (No. 40): 9648-9654.

Choi, S.-Y.; Bertram, S.; Głowacka, I. ; Park, Y. W. & Pöhlmann, S. (2009) Type II Transmembrane Serine Proteases in Cancer and Viral Infections. *Trends in Molecular Medicine* Vol. 15 (No. 7): 303-312.

Clerc, J.; Groll, M.; Illich, D. J.; Bachmann, A. S.; Huber, R.; Schellenberg, B.; Dudler, R. & Kaiser, M. (2009) Synthetic and Structural Studies on Syringolins A and B Reveal Critical Determinants of Selectivity and Potency of Proteasome Inhibition. *Proceedings of the National Academy of Sciences of the United States of America* Vol.106 (No. 16): 6507-6512.

Coleman, C. S.; Rocetes, J. D., Park, D. J.; Wallick, C. J.; Warn-Cramer, B. J.; Michael, K.; Dudler, R. & Bachmann, A. S. (2006) Syringolin A, a new plant elicitor from the phytopathogenic bacterium Pseudomonas syringae pv. syringae, inhibits the proliferation of neuroblastoma and ovarian cancer cells and induces apoptosis. *Cell Proliferation* Vol. 39 (No. 6) 599-609.

Collinsová, M. & Jiraček, J. (2000) Phosphinic Acid Compounds in Biochemistry, Biology and Medicine. *Current Medicinal Chemistry* Vol. 7 (No. 6): 629-647.

De Bettignies, G. & Coux, O. (2010) Proteasome Inhibitors: Dozens of Molecules and Still Counting. *Biochimie* Vol. 92 (No. 11): 1530-1545.

Decros, J. G.; Baudy Floc'h, M.; Prignet, C. & Arlot-Bonnemais, Y. (2003) Proteasome Inhibitors as Therapeutic Agents: *Current Medicinal Chemistry* Vol. 10 (No.6): 479-503.

Devel, L.; Czarny, B.; Beau, F.; Georgiadis, D.; Stura, E. & Dive, V. (2010) Third Generation of Matrix Matalliproteinase Inhibitors: Gain in Selectivity by Targeting the Depth of S' Cavity. *Biochemie* Vol. 92 (No. 11): 1501-1508.

Dia, V. P. & de Mejia, E. G. (2010) Lunasin Promotes Apoptosis in Human Colon Cancer Cells by Mitochondrial Pathway Activation and Induction of Nuclear Clusterin Expression. *Cancer Letters* Vol. 295 (No. 1): 44-53.

Di Cera, E. (2009) Serine Proteases. *IUBMB Life* Vol. 15 (No. 5): 510-515.

Dive, V.; Georgiadis, D.; Matziari, M.; Makaritis, A.; Beau, F.; Cuniasse, P. & Yiotakis, A. (2004) Phosphinic Peptides as Zinc Metalloproteinase Inhibitors. *Cellular and Molecular Life Science* Vol. 16 (August 2004): 2010–2019.

Elie, B. T.; Gocheva, V.; Shree, T.; Dalrymple, S. A. Holsinger, L. J. & Joyce, J. A. (2010) Identification and Pre-Clinical Testing of a Reversible Cathepsin Protease Inhibitor Reveals Anti-Tumor Efficacy in a Pancreatic Cancer Model. *Biochimie* Vol. 92 (No.11): 1618-1624.

Elofsson, G.; Splittgerber, U.; Myung, J.; Mohan, R. & Crews, C. M. (1999) Towards Subunit-Specific Proteasome Inhibitors: Synthesis and Evaluation of Peptide α',β'-Epoxyketones. *Chemistry & Biology* Vol. 6 (No. 11): 811-822.

Fayard, B.; Bianchi, F.; Dey, J.; Moreno, E.; Djaffer, S.; Hynes, N. E. & Monard, D. (2009) The Serine Protease Inhibitor Protease Nexin-1 Controls Mammary Cancer Metastasis through LPR-1-Mediated MMP9 Expression. *Cancer Research* Vol. 69 (No. 14): 5690-5698.

Fleber, L. M.; Kündig, C.; Borgoño, C. A.; Chagas, J. R.; Tasinato, A.; Jichlinski, P.; Gygi, C. M.; Leisinger, H.-J.; Diamandis, E. P.; Deperthes, D. & Cloutier, S. M. (2006)Mutant Recombinant Serpins as Highly Specific Inhibitors of Human Kallikrein 14. *FASEB Journal* Vol. 273 (No. 11): 2505-2514.

Fiorucci, L. & Ascoli, F. (2004) Mast Cell Tryptase, a Still Enigmatic Enzyme. *Cellular and Molecular Life Sciences* Vol. 61 (No.11): 1278-1295.

Fisher, J. J. & Mobashery, S. (2006) Recent Advances in MMP Inhibitor Design. *Cancer Metastasis Review* Vol. 25 (No. 1): 115-136.

Gialeli, C.; Theocharis, A. D. & Karamanos, N. K. (2011) Roles of Matrix Metalloproteinases in Cancer Progression and Their Pharmacological Targeting. *FEBS Journal* Vol. 276 (No. 1): 16-27.

Goldberg, A. (2007) Functions of the Proteasome: from Protein Degradation to Immune Surveillance to Cancer Therapy. *Biochemical Society Transactions* Vol. 35 (No. 1): 12-17.

Gräwert, M. A.; Gallastegui, N.; Stein, M.; Schmidt, B.; Kloetzel, P.-M.; Huber, R. & Groll, M. (2010) Elucidation of the α-Keto Aldehyde Binding Mechanism: A Lead Structure Motif for Proteasome Inhibition. *Angewandte Chemie International Edition* Vol. 50 (No. 2): 542-544

Greenspan, P. D.; Clark, P. N.; Tommasi, R. A.; Cowen, S. D.; McQuire, L.W. Farley D. L.; van Dauzer, J. H.; Goldber, R. L.; Zhou, H.; Du, Z.; Fitt, J. J.; Coppa, D.E.; Fang, Z.; Macchia, W.; Zhu, L.; Capparelli, M. P.; Goldstein, R.; Wigg, A. M.; Doughty, J. R.; Bohacek, R. S. & Knap.A. K. (2001) Identification of Dipeptidyl Nitriles as Potent and Selective Inhibitors of Cathepsin B through Structure-based Drug Design. *Journal of Medicinal Chemistry* Vol. 44 (No. 26): 4524-4534.

Grzywa, R.; Dyguda-Kazimierowicz, E.; Sieńczyk, M.; Feliks, M.; Sokalski, W. A. & Oleksyszyn, J. (2007) The Molecular Basis of Urokinase Inhibition: from the Nonempirical Analysis of Instramolecular Interactions to the Prediction of Binding Affinity. *Journal of Molecular Modeling* Vol. 13 (No. 6-7): 677-683.

Hanada, M.; Sugawara, K.; Kaneta, K.; Toda, S.; Nishiyama, Y.; Tomita, K.; Yamamoto, H.; Konishi, M. & Oki, T. (1992) Epoxomycin, a New Antitumor Agent of Microbial Origin. *Journal of Antibiotics (Tokyo)* Vol. 45 (No. 11): 1746-1752.

Hanada, K.; Tamai, N.; Yamagishi, N.; Ohmura, S. Sawada, J. & Tanaka, I. (1978) Isolation and Identification of E-64, A New Thiol Protease Inhibitor. *Agricultural and Biological Chemistry Tokyo* Vol. 42 (No. 3): 523-528.

Hassan, H. T. (2004) Ajoene (Natural Garlic Compound): A New Anti-Leukaemia Agent for AML Therapy. *Leukemia Research* Vol. 28 (No. 7): 667-671.

Hsieh, C. C.; Hernández-Ledesma, B.; Jeong, H. J.; Park, J. H. & de Lumen, B. O. (2010) Complementary Roles in Cancer Prevention: Protease Inhibitor Makes the Cancer Preventive Lunasin Bioavailable. *Plos ONE* Vol. 5 (No.1): 1-9, e8890.

Huai, Q.; Zhou, A.; Lin, L.; Mazar, A. P.; Parry, G. C.; Callahan, J.; Shaw, D. E.; Furie, B.; Furie, B. C. & Huang, M. (2008) Crystal Structures of Two Human Vironectin, Urokinase and UrokinaseReceptor Complexes. *Nature Structural and Molecular Biology* Vol. 15 (No. 4): 422-423.

Joanitti, G. A.; Azevedo, R. B. & Freitas, S. M. (2010) Apoptosis and Lysosome Membrane Permeabilization Induction on Breast Cancer Cells by Anticancerogenic Bowman-Birk Protease Inhibitor from *Vigna unguiculata* Seeds. *Cancer Letters* Vol. 293 (No. 1): 73-81.

Joossens, J.; Van der Veken, P.; Surpetanu, G.; LAmbeit, A.-M.; El-Sayed, I.; Ali, O. M.; Augustyns, K. & Haemers, A. (2006) Diphenyl Phosphonate Inhibibtors for the Urokinase-Type Plasminogen Activator: Optimization of the P4 Position. *Journal of Medicinal Chemistry* Vol. 49 (No. 19): 5785-5793.

Joyce, J. A.; Baruch, A.; Chehade, K.; Meyer-Morse, N.; Giraudo, E.; Tsai, F. Y.; Greenbaum, D. C.; Harger, J. H.; Bogyo, M. & Hanahan, D. (2004) Cathepsin Cysteine Proteases are Effectors of Invasive Growth and Angiogenesis During Multistage Tumorigenesis. *Cancer Cell* Vol. 5 (No. 5): 443-453.

Katunuma, N. (2011) Structure-based Development of Specific Inhibitors for Individual Cathepsins and Their Medical Applications. *Proceedings of Japan Academy of Sciences, Series B, Physical and Biological Sciences* Vol. 87 (No.2): 29-38.

Kemik, O.; Kemik, A. S.; Sumer, A.; Beğenik, H.; Dügler, A. C.; Purisa, S. & Tuzun, S. (2011) The Relationship Among Acute-phase Response Proteins, Cytokines, and Hormones in Various Gastrointestinal Cancer Types Patients with Cachectic. *Human & Experimental Toxicology* Vol. 30: doi: 10.1177/0960327111405864, first published on April 18, 2011.

Keppler, D. (2006) Mini Review. Towards Novel Anti-Cancer Strategies Based on Cystatin Function. *Cancer Letters* Vol. 235 (No. 2): 159-175.

Kessler, B. M.; Tortorella, D.; Altun. M.; Kisselev, A. M.; Fiebiger, E.; Hekking, B. G.; Ploegh, H. L. & Overkleeft, H. S. (2001) Extended Peptide-based Inhibitors Efficiently Target the Proteasome an Reveal Overlapping Specificities of the Catalytic β-Subunits. *Chemistry & Biology* Vol. 8 (No. 9): 913-929.

Klinghofer, V.; Steward, K.; McGonigal, T.; Smith, R.; Sarthy, A.; Nienaber, V.; Butler, C.; Dorwin, S.; Richardson, P.; Weitzberg, M.; Wendt, M.; Rockway, T.; Zhao, Z.; Hulkower, K. L. & Giranda, V. L. (2001) Species Specificity of Aminidine-Based Urokinase Inhibitors. *Biochemistry* Vol. 40 (No. 31): 9125-9131.

Koblinski, J. E.; Abram, M. & Sloane, B. F. (2000) Unraveling the Role of Proteases In Cancer. *Clinica Chimica Acta* Vol. 291 (No. 2): 113-135.

Koguchi, Y.; Kohno, J.; Nishio, M.; Takahashi, A.; Okuda, T.; Ohnuki, T. & Komatsubara, S. (2000) TMC-95A, B, C and D, Novel Proteasome Inhibitors Produced by *Apiospora montagnei* Sacc. TC 1093. Taxonomy, Production, Isolation, and Biological Activities. *Journal of Antibiotics (Tokyo)* Vol. 53 (No. 2): 105-109.

Kopitz, C.; Anton, M. Gansbacher, B. & Krüger, A. (2005) Reduction of Experimental Human Fibrosarcoma Lung Metastasis in Mice by Adenovirus-mediated Cystatin C Overexpression in the Host. *Cancer Research* Vol. 65 (no. 19): 8608-8612.

Krige, D.; Needham, L. A.; Bawden, L. J.; Flores, N.; Farmer, H.; Miles, L. E. C.; Stone, E.; Callaghan, J.; Chandler, S.; Clark, V. L.; Kirwin-Jones, P.; Legris, V.; Owen, J.; Patel, T.; Wood, S.; Box, G.; Laber, D.; Odedra, R.; Wright, A.; Wood, L. M.; Eccles, S. A.; Bone, E. A.; Ayscough, A. & Drummond, A. H. (2008) CHR-2797: An Antiproliferative Aminopeptidase Inhibitor that Leads to Amino Acid Deprivation in Human Leukemic Cells. *Cancer Research* Vol. 68 (No. 16): 6669-6679.

Kumar, G. D. K.; Chavarria, G. E.; Charlton-Sevcik, A.; Arispe, W. M.; MacDonough, M. T.; Strecker, T. E.; Chen, S.-E.; Siim, B. G.; Chaplin, D. J.; Trawick, M. L. & Pinney, K. G. (2010) Design, Synthesis and Biological Evaluation of potent Thiosemicarbazone Based Cathepsin L Inhibitors. *Bioorganic & Medicinal Chemistry Letters* Vol.20 (No. 4): 1415-1419.

Kwan, J. C.; Eksioglu, E. A.; Liu, C.; Paul, V. J. & Leusch, H. (2009) Grassystatins A-C from Marine Cyanobacteria, Potent Cathepsin E Inhibitors That Reduce Antigen Presentation. *Journal of Medicinal Chemistry* Vol. 52 (No. 18): 5732-5747.

Lavelin, I.; Beer, A.; Kam, Z.; Rotter, V.; Oren, M.; Navon, A. & Geiger, B. (2009) Discovery of Novel Proteasome Inhibitors Using a High Content Cell Base Screening System. *PloS ONE* Vol. 4 (No. 12): e8503.

Leban, J.; Blisse, M.; Krauss, B.; Rath, S.; Baumgartner, R. & Seifert, M. H. J. (2008) Proteasome Inhibition by Peptide Semicarbazones. *Bioorganic & Medicinal Chemistry* Vol. 16 (No. 18): 4579-4588.

Lee, M.; Fridman, R. & Mobashery, S. (2004) Extracellular Proteases as Targets for Treatment of Cancer Metastases. *Chemical Society Reviews* Vol. 33 (No. 7): 401-409.

Lee, T. K.; Murthy, S. R. K.; Cawley, N. X.; Dhanvantari, S.; Hewitt, S. M.; Lou, H.; Lau, T.; Ma, S.; Huynh, T.; Wesley, R. A.; Ng, I. O.; Pacak, K.; Poon, R. T. & Loh, Y. P. (2011) An N-Terminal Truncated Carboxypeptidase E Splice Isoform Induces Tumor Growth and Is a Biomarker for Predicting Future Metastasis in Human Cancers, *The Journal of Clinical Investigation* Vol. 121 (No. 3): 880-892.

Li, X.; Yin, S.; Meng, Y.; Sakr, W. & Sheng, S (2006) Endogenous Inhibition of Histone Deacylase 1 by Tumor-Suppressive Maspin. *Cancer Research* Vol. 66 (No. 18): 9323-9329.

Li, Y.; Dou, D.; He, G.; Lushington, G. H. & Groutas, W. C. (2009) Mechanism-Based Inhibitors of Serine Proteases with High Selectivity Through Optimization of S′ Subsite Binding. *Bioorganic & Medicinal Chemistry* Vol. 17 (No. 10): 5336-5342.

Lim, I. T.; Meroueh, S. O.; Lee, M.; Heeg, M. J. & Mobashery, S. (2004) Strategy in Inhibition of Cathepsin B, A Target in Tumor Invasion and Metastasis. *Journal of American Chemical Society* Vol. 126 (No. 33): 10271-10277.

Lindeman, J.H.; Hanemaaijer, R.; Mulder, A.; Dijkstra, P. D.; Szuhai, K.; Bromme, D.; Verheijen, J. H. & Hogendoorn P. C. (2004) Cathepsin K is Principal Protease in Giant Cell Tumor of Bone. *American Journal of Pathology* Vol. 165 (No.2): 593-600.

Linington, R. G.; Edwards, D. J.; Shuman, C. F.; McPhail, K. L.; Matainaho, T. & Gerwick, W. H. (2008) Symploxacine A, a Potent Cytotoxin and Chymotrypsin Inhibitor from the Marine Cyanobacterium *Symploca* sp. *Journal of Natural Products* Vol. 71 (No. 1): 22-27.

Ma, X.-Q.; Zhang, H.-J.; Hang, Y.-H.; Chen, Y.-H.; Wu, F.; Du, J.-Q.; Yu, H.-P.; Zhou, Z.-L.; Li, J.-Y.; Nan, F.-J. & Li. J. (2007) Novel Irreversible Caspase-1 Inhibitor Attenuates the Maturation of Intracellular Interleukin -1β. *Biochemistry & Cell Biology* Vol. 85 (No. 1): 56-65.

Magdolen, U.; Krol, J.; Sato, S.; Mueller, M. M.; Sperl, S.; Krüger, A.; Schmidtt, M. & Magdolen, V. (2002) Natural Inhibitors of Tumor-Associated Proteases. *Radiology and Oncology* Vol. 36 (No. 2): 131-143.

Manello, F. (2006) Natural Bio-Drugs as Natural Matrix Metalloprotreinase Inhibitors: New Perspectives on The Horison? *Recent Patents on Anti-cancer Drug Discovery* Vol. 1 (No. 1):91-103

Maskos, K. (2005) Crystal Structures of MMPs in Complex with Physiological and Pharmacological Inhibitors. *Biochimie* Vol. 87 (No. 3-4): 249-263.

Mason, S. D. & Joyce, J. A (2011) Proteolytic Networks in Cancer. *Trends in Cell Biology* Vol. 21 (No. 4): 228-237.

McConnell, R. M.; Godwil, W. E.; Stefan, A.; Newton, C.; Myers, N. & Hatfield, S. E. (2003). Synthesis an Cathepsin D Inhibition of Peptide-hydroxyethyl Amine Isosteres with Cyclic Tertiary Amines. *Letters in Peptide Science* Vol. 10 (No. 2): 69-78.

Miller, E. K.-I.; Trabi, M.; Masci, P.P.; Lavin, M. F.; de Jersey, J. & Guddast, L. W. Crystal Structure of Textinilin-1, a Kunitz-Type Serine Protease Inhibitor from the Venom of the Australian Common Brown Snake (*Pseudonaja textilis*). *FEBS Journal* Vol. 276 (No. 11): 3162-3175.

Moore, H. E.; Davenport, E. L.; Smith E. M.; Mularikrishnan, S.; Dunlop, A. S.; Walker, B. A.; Krige, D.; Drummond, A. H.; Hooftman, L.; Morgan, G. J. & Davies, F. E. (2009) Aminopeptidase Inhibition as a Targeted Treatment Strategy in Myeloma. *Molecular Cancer Therapeutics* Vol.8 (No. 4): 762-770.

Mroczkiewicz, M.; Winkler, K.; Nowis, D.; Placha, G.; Golob, J. & Ostaszewski, R. (2010) Studies on the Synthesis of All Stereoisomers of MG-132 Proteasome Inhibitors in the Tumor Targeting Approach. *Journal of Medicinal Chemistry* Vol. 53 (No. 4): 1509-1518.

Mucha, A.; Drąg, M.; Dalton, J. & Kafarski. P. Metallo-peptidase Inhibitors. *Biochimie* Vol. 92 (No. 11): 1509-1529.

Mussap, M & Plebani, M. (2004) Biochemistry and Clinical Role of Human Cystatin C. *Critical Reviews in Clinical Laboratory Sciences* Vol. 41 (No. 5-6): 467-550.

Naffara, N. I.; Andreu, P. & Coussens, L. M. (2009) Delineating Protease Functions During Cancer Development. In: *Proteases and Cancer. Methods and Protocols*. T. M. Antalis & T. H. Bugge (Eds.) 1-33, Humana Press, New York.

Naimuddin, M.; Kitamura, K.; Kinoshita, Y.; Honda-Takahashi, Y.; Murakami, M.; Ito, M.; Yamamoto, K.; Hanada, K.; Husimi, Y. & Nishigaki, K. (2007) Selection-by-function: Efficient Enrichement of Cathepsin E Inhibitors from a DNA Library. *Journal of Molecular Recognition* Vol. 20 (No. 1): 58-69.

Niestroj, A. J.; Feuβner, K.; Heiser, U.; Dando, P. M.; Barrett, A.; Gerhardtz, B. & Demuth, H. U. (2002) Inhibition of Mammalian Legumain by Michaels Acceptors and AzaAsn-Halomethylketones *Biological Chemistry* Vol. 383 (No. 7-8): 1205-1214.

Nuti, E.; Casalini, F.; Avramova, S. I.; Santamaria, S.; Fabbi, M.; Ferrini, S.; Marinelli, L.; La Pietra, V.; Limongelli, V.; Novellino, E.; Cercignani, G.; Orlandini, E.; Nencetti, S. & Rosello, A. (2010) Potent Arylsulfonamide Inhibitora of Tumor Necrosis Factor-α Converting Enzyme Able to Reduce Activated Leucocyte Cell Adhesion Molecule Shedding in Cancer Cell Models. *Journal of Medicinal Chemistry* Vol. 53 (No. 6): 2622-2635.

Omura S.; Fujimoto, T.; Matsuzaki, K.; Moriguchi, R.; Tanaka, H. & Sasaki, Y. (1991) Lactacystin, a Novel Microbial Metabolite, Induces Neuritogenesis of Neuroblastoma Cells. *Journal of Antibiotics* Vol. 44 (No.1): 113-116.

Otlewski, J.; Jeleń, F.; Zakrzewska, M. & Oleksy. A (2005) The Many Faces of Protease-Protein Inhibitor Interaction. *The EMBO Journal* Vol. 24 (No. 7): 1303-1310.

Ovat, A.; Li, Z. Z.; Hampton, C. Y.; Asress, S. A.; Fernández, F. M.; Glass, J. D. & Powers, J. C. (2010) Peptidyl α–Ketoamides with Nucleobases, Methylpiperazine and Dimethylaminoalkyl Substituents as Calpain Inhibitors. *Journal of Medicinal Chemistry* Vol.53 (No.17): 6326-6336.

Ozaki, N.; Ohmuraya, N.; Hirota, M.; Ida, S.; Wang, J.; Takamori, H.; Higashiyama, S.; Baba, H. & Yamamura, K.-I. (2009) Serine Protease Inhibitor Kazal Type 1 Promotes Proliferation of Pancreatic Cancer Cells through the Epidermal Growth Factor Receptor. *Molecular Cancer Research* Vol. 7 (No. 9): 1572-1581.

Pahl, H. L.; Krauss, B.; Schulze-Osthoff, B.; Decker, T.; Traenckner, E. B.; Vogt, M.; Myers, C.; Parks, T.; Warring, P.; Mühlbacher, A.; Czernilofsky, A. P. & Baeuerle, P. A (1996) The Immosuppresive Fungal Metabolite Gliotoxin Specifically Inhibits Transcription Factor NF-κB. *Journal of Experimental Medicine* Vol. 183 (No. 4): 1829-1840.

Palermo, C. & Joyce, J. A. (2007) Cysteine Cathepsin Proteases as Pharmacological Targets in Cancer. *Trends in Pharmacological Sciences* Vol. 29 (No. 1): 22-28

Pallares, I.; Bonet, R.; Garcia-Castellanos, R.; Ventura, S.; Avilés, F. X.; Vendrell, J. & Gomis-Rüth, F. X. (2005) Structure of Human Carboxypeptidase A4 with Its Endogenous Protein Inhibitor, Latexin. *Proceedings of the National Academy of Sciences of the United States of America* Vol. 102 (No. 11): 3978-3983.

Pandey, R.; Patilo, N. & Rao, M. (2007) Proteases and Protease Inhibitors: Implications in Antitumorigenesis and drug Development. *International Journal of Human Genetics* Vol.17, (No. 1): 67-82.

Piovan, L.; Alves, M. F. M.; Juliano, L.; Brömme, D.; Cunha R. L. O. R. & Andrade, L. H. (2011) Structure-Activity Relationship of Hypervalent Organochalcogenanes as Inhibitors of Cysteine Cathepsins V and S. *Bioorganic & Medicinal Chemistry* Vol. 19 (No. 6): 2009-2014.

Powers, J. C.; Asqian, J. L.; Ekici, O. D. & James, K. E. (2002) Irreversible Inhibitors of Serine, Cysteine and Thereonine Proteases. *Chemical Reviews* Vol.102 (No. 12): 4639-4650.

Puente, X. S.; Sanchez,L. M.; Overall, C. M. & Lopez-Otin, C. (2003). Human and Mouse Proteases: A Comparative Genomic Approach. *Nature Reviews: Genetics* Vol. 4 (No. 7): 544-558.

Puxbaum, V & Mach, L. (2009) Proteinases and Their Inhibitors in Liver Cancer. *World Journal of Hepatology* Vol. 31 (No. 1): 28-34.

Roth, P.; Kissel, M.; Herrmann, C.; Eisele, G.; Leban, J.; Weller, M. & Schmidt, F. (2009) SC68896, a Novel Small Molecule Proteasome Inhibitor, Exerts Antiglioma Activity *In vitro* and *In vivo*. *Clinical Cancer Research* Vol. 15 (No. 21): 6609-6618.

Sahab, Z. J.; Hall, M. D.; Me Sung, Y.; Dakshanamurthy, S.; Ji, Y.; Kumar, D. & Byers, S. W. (2011) Tumor Suppressor RARRES 1 Interacts with Cytoplasmic Carboxypeptidase AGBL2 to Regulate α–Tubulin Tyrosination Cycle. *Cancer Research* Vol. 71 (No. 4): 1219-1228.

Sakuhari, N.; Suzuki, K.; Sano, Y.; Saito, T.; Yoshimura, H.; Nishimura, Y.; Yano, T.; Sadzuka, Y. & Asano, R. (2008) Effect of a Single Dose Administration of Bowman-Birk Inhibitor Concentrate on Anti-Proliferation and Inhabitation of Metastasis in M5076 Ovarian Sacroma-Bearing Mice. *Molecular Medicine Reports* Vol. 1 (No. 5): 903-907.

Saleh, Y.; Wnukiewicz, J.; Andrzejak, R. Trziszka, T. Siewiński, M. Ziolkowski, P. & Kopeć, W. (2006) Cathepsin B and Cysteine Protease Inhibitors In Human Tongue Cancer: Correlation with Tumor Staging and In Vitro Inhibition of Cathepsin B by Chicken Cystatin. *Journal of Cancer Molecules* Vol. 2 (No. 2): 67-72.

Sato, T.; Takahashi, S.; Mizumoto, T.; Harao, M.; Akizuki, M.; Takasugi, M.; Fukutomi, T. & Yamashita, J.-I. (2006) Nautrophil Elastase and Cancer. *Surological Oncology* Vol. 15 (No. 4): 217-222.

Schmideberg, N.; Schmitt, M.; Rölz, C.; Truffault, V.; Sukopp, M.; Bürgle, M.; Wilhelm, O. G.; Schmalix, W.; Magdolen, V & Kessler, H. (2002) Synthesis, Solution Structure, and Biological Evaluation of Urokinase Type Plasminogen Activator (uPA)-Derived Receptor Binding Domain Mimetics. *Journal of Medicinal Chemistry* Vol. 45 (No. 23): 4894-4994.

Selvakumar, P.; Lakshmikuttayamma, A.; Dimmock, J. R. & Sharma, R. K. (2006) Methionine Aminopeptise 2 and Cancer. *Biochimica et Biophysica Acta – Reviews on Cancer* Vol. 1765 (No. 2): 148-154.

Sieńczyk, M & Oleksyszyn, J. (2006) Inhibition of Trypsin and Urokinase by Cbz-Amino(4-guanidinophenyl)methanephosphonate Aromatic Ester Derivatives: The Influence of the Ester Group on Their Biological Activity. *Bioorganic & Medicinal Chemistry Letters* Vol. 16 (No. 11): 2886-2890

Sieńczyk, M. & Oleksyszyn, J. (2009) Irreversible Inhibition of Serine Proteases – Design and in Vivo Activity of Diaryl α–Aminophosphonate Derivatives. *Current Medicinal Chemistry* Vol. 16 (No. 13): 1673-1687.

Sieńczyk M.; Winiarski, Ł.; Kasperkiewicz, P.; Psurski, M.; Wietrzyk, J. & Oleksyszyn, J. (2011) Simple Phosphonic Inhibitors of Human Neutrophil Elastase. *Bioorganic & Medicinal Chemistry Letters* Vol. 21 (No. 5): 1310-1314.

Sierko, E.; Wojtukiewicz, M. Z. & Kisiel, W. (2007) The Role of Tissue Factor Pathway Inhibitor-2 in Cancer Biology. *Seminars in Thrombosis and Homeostasis* Vol. 33 (No. 7): 653-659.

Singh, J. P.; Tamang, S.; Rajamohanan, P. R.; Jima, N. C.; Chakraborty, G.; Kundu, G. C.; Gaikwad, S. M. & Khan, M. I. (2010) Isolation, Structure and Functional Elucidation of Modified Pentapeptide, Cysteine Protease Inhibitor (CPI-2081) from *Streptomyces Species* 2081 that Exhibit Inhibitory Effect on Cancer Cell Migration. *Journal of Medicinal Chemistry* Vol. 53 (No. 14): 5121-5128.

Skillman, A. G.; Lin, B.; Lee, C. E.; Kunz, I. D.; Ellman, J. A. & Lynch, G. (2000) Plasminogen Activator Inhibitors Based on 3D QSAR CoMFA/CoMSIA Models; Journal of Medicinal Chemistry Vol. 49 (no. 2) 457-489. Novel Cathepsin D Inhibitors Block the Formation of Hyperphosphorylated Tau Fragments in Hippocampus. *Journal of Neurochemistry* Vol. 74 (No. 4): 1459-1477.

Skrzydlewska, E.; Sulkowska, M.; Koda, M. & Sulkowski S. (2005) Proteolytic-antiproteolytic Balance and Its Regulation in Carcinogenesis. *World Journal of Gastroenterology* Vol. 11 (No. 9): 1251-1266.

Sperl, S.; Jacob, U.; Arroya de Parad, N.; Stürzerbecher, J.; Wilhelm, O. G.; Bode W.; Magdolen, V.; Huber, R. & Moroder, L. (2000) 4-(Amidomethyl)phenylguanidine Derivatives as Non Peptidic Highly Selective Inhibitors of Human Urokinase. *Proceedings of the National Academy of Sciences of the United States of America* Vol. 97 (No. 10): 5113-5118.

Stroup, G. B.; Lark, M. W.; Veber, D. F.; Battacharyya, A.; Blake, S.; Dare, L. C.; Erhard, K. F.; Hoffman, S. J.; James, I. E.; Marquis, R. W.; Ru, Y.; Vasco-Moser, J. A.; Smith, B. R.; Tomaszek, T. & Gowen, M. (2001) Potent and Selective Inhibition of Human Cathepsin K Lead to Inhibition of Bone Resorption in Vivo in a Non-Human Primate. *Journal of Bone and Mineral Research* Vol.16 (No. 10): 1739-1746.

Sugawara,K.; Hatori, M.; Nishiyama, Y.; Tomita, K.; Kamei, H.; Konishi, M. & Oki, T. (1990) Eponemycin, a New Antibiotic Active Against B16 Melanoma. I. Production, Isolation, Structure and Biological Activity. *Journal of Antibiotics (Tokyo)* Vol. 43 (No. 1): 8-18.

Takai, S.; Jin, D.; Muramatsu, M. & Miyazaki, M. (2004) Cymase as a Novel Target for the Prevention of Vascular Diseases. *Trends in Pharmacological Science.* Vol. 25 (No. 10): 518-522.

Turk, B. (2006) Targeting Proteases: Successes, Failures and Future Prospects. *Nature Reviews: Drug Discovery* Vol. 5 (September 2006): 785-799.

Turk, V.; Kos, J. & Turk, B. (2004) Cysteine Cathepsins (Proteases) - on The Main Stage of Cancer? *Cancer Cell* Vol. 5 (No. 5): 409-410.

Umezawa, H.; Aoyagi, T.; Morishima, H.; Matsuzaki, H. & Hamada, M. (1970) Pepstatin a New Pepsin Inhibitor Produced by Actinomycetes. *Journal of Antibiotics (Tokyo)* Vol. 23 (No. 5): 259-262.

Umezawa, H.; Aoyagi, T.; Suda, H.; Hamada, M. & Takeuchi, T. (1976) Bestatin, an Inhibitor of Aminopeptidase B, Produced by Actinomycetes. *Journal of Antibiotics (Tokyo)* Vol. 29 (No. 1): 97-99.

Ueno, T.; Elmberger, G.; Weaver, T. E.; Toi, M & Linder, S. (2008) The Aspartic Protease Napsin A Suppresses Tumor Growth Independent on its Catalytic Activity. *Laboratory Investigation* Vol. 88 (No. 3): 256-263.

Velhelst, S. H. L.; Witte, M. D.; Arastu-Kapur, S.; Fonovic, M. & Bogyo, M. (2006) Novel Aza Peptide Inhibitors of and Active Site Probes of Papain Family Cysteine Proteases. *ChemBioChem* Vol. 7 (No. 5): 824-827

Vivier, M.; Jarrousse, A.-S.; Bouchon, B.; Galmier, M.-J.; Auzeloux, P.; Sauzieres, J. & Madelmont, J. C. (2005) Preliminary studies of New Proteasome Inhibitors in the

Tumor Targeting Approach: Synthesis and in Vitro Toxicity. *Journal of Medicinal Chemistry* Vol. 48 (No. 21): 6731-6740.

Ward, Y. D.; Thomson, D. S.; Frye, L. L.; Cywin, C. L.; Morwick, T.; Emmanuel, M. J.; Zindell, L.; McNell, D.; Bekkall, Y.; Girardot, M.; Hrapchak, M.; De Turi, M.; Crane, K.; White, D.; Pav, S.; Wang, Y.; Hao, M. H.; Grygon, C. A.; Labadia, M. E.; Freeman, D. M.; Davidson, W.; Hopkins, J. L.; Brown, M. L. & Spero, D. M. (2002) Design and Synthesis of Dipeptide Nitriles as Reversible and Potent Cathepsin S Inhibitors. *Journal of Medicinal Chemistry* Vol. 45 (No. 25): 5471-5482.

Wickström, M.; Larsson, R.; Nygren, P. & Gullbo, J. (2011) Aminopeptidase N (CD13) as a Target for Cancer Chemotherapy. *Cancer Science* Vol. 102 (No. 3): 501-508.

Wieczerzak, E.; Drabik, P.; Łankiewicz, L.; Ołdziej, S.; Grzonka, Z.; Abrahamson, M.; Grubb, A. & Brömme, D. (2002) Azapeptides Structurally Based upon Inhibitory Sites of Cystatins as Potent and Selective Inhibitors of Cysteine Proteases. *Journal of Medicinal Chemistry* Vol. 45 (No. 19): 4202-4211.

Wieczerzak, E.; Rodziewicz-Motowidło, S.; Jankowska, E.; Giełdoń, A. & Ciarkowski, J. (2007) An Enormously Active and Selective Azapeptide Inhibitors of Cathepsin B. *Journal of Peptide Science* Vol. 13 (No. 8): 536-543.

Xuan, Q.; Yang, X.; Mo, L.; Huang, F.; Pang, Y.; Qin, M.; Chen, Z.; He, M.; Wang, Q. & Mo, Z.-N (2008) Expression of Serine Protease Kallikrein 7 and Its Inhibitor Antileukoprotease is Decreased in Prostate Cancer. *Archives of Pathology and Laboratory Medicine* Vol. 132 (No. 11): 1796-1801.

Yabe, K. & Koide, T. (2009) Inhibition of the 20S Proteosome by a Protein Proteinase Inhibitor: Evidence that Natural Serine Proteinase Inhibitor Can Inhibit a Threonine Proteinase. *Journal of Biochemistry* Vol. 145 (No. 2): 217-227.

Yang, H.; Chen, D.; Cui, Q. C.; Yuan, X. & Dou, Q. P. (2006) Celastrol, a Triterpene Extracted from the Cinese "Thunder of God Vine", Is a Potent Proteasome Inhibitor and Suppresses Human Prostate Cancer Growth in Nude Mice. *Cancer Research* Vol. 66 (No. 9): 4758-4765.

Yang, Z.-Q.; Kwok, B. H. B.; Lin, S.; Koldobskiy, M. A.; Crews, C. M. & Danishefsky, S. J. (2003) Simplified Synthetic TMC-95A/B Analogues Retain the Potency of Proteasome Inhibitory Activity. *ChemBioChem* Vol. 4 (No. 6); 508-513

Yotaklis, A.; & Dive, V. (2008) Synthesis and Site Directed Inhibitors of Metzicind: Achievement and Perspectives. *Molecular Ascpects of Medicine* Vol. 29 (No. 2): 329-338.

Zhou, H.-J.; Aujay, M. A. ; Bennett, M.K. ; Dajee, M. ; Demo, S. D.; Fang, Y.; Ho, M. N.; Jiang. J.; Kirk, C. J.; Laiding, G. J.; Lewis. E. R.; Lu, Y.; Muchamuel, T.; Parlati, F.; Ring, E.; Shenk, K. D.; Shields, J.; Showonek, P. J.; Stanton, T.; Sun, C. M.; Sylvain, C.; Woo, T. M. & Yang, J. (2009) Design and Synthesis of Orally Bioavailable and Selective Epoxyketone Proteasome Inhibitor (PR-047). *Journal of Medicinal Chemistry* Vol. 52 (No. 9): 3028-3028.

Zhu, M.; Gokhale, V. M.; Szabo, L.; Munoz, R. M.; Baek, H.; Bashyam, S.; Hurley, L. H.; Von Hoff, D. D. & Han, H. (2007) Identification of Novel Inhibitor of Urokinase-Type Plasminogen Activator. *Molecular Cancer Therapeutics* Vol. 6 (No. 4): 1348-1356.

Zhu, Y.; Zhu, XC.; Wu, G.; Ma, Y.; Li, Y.; Zhao, X.; Yuan, Y.; Yang, J.; Yu, S.; Shao, F.; Li, R.; Ke. Y.; Lu, A.; Liu, Z. & Zhang, L. (2010) Synthesis in Vitro and in Vivo Biologial Evaluation, Docking Studies and Structure – Activity Relationship (SAR) Discussion of Dipeptidyl Boronic Acid Proteasome Inhibitors Composed of β–Amino Acids. *Journal of Medicinal Chemistry* Vol. 53 (No. 5): 1990-1999.

5

Histone Deacetylase Inhibitors as Therapeutic Agents for Cancer Therapy: Drug Metabolism and Pharmacokinetic Properties

Ethirajulu Kantharaj and Ramesh Jayaraman
S*BIO Pte Ltd
Singapore

1. Introduction

The processes of absorption (A), distribution (D), metabolism (M) and excretion (E) (collectively referred as ADME) determine the pharmacokinetics (PK) of a compound. Lack of optimum PK is one of the major reasons for compounds to fail in the clinic resulting in high attrition rates. In the beginning of 1990, 39% of the drugs failed in the clinic due to poor PK emphasizing its importance in drug development (Waterbeemd and Gifford, 2003). In 1988, a study of the pharmaceutical companies in UK showed that non-optimal PK was one of the major reasons (~40%) for termination of drugs in development (Prentis et al., 1988). In the last two decades this number dropped to ~ 10% (Yengi et al., 2007). The main reasons for this significant drop in the number of compounds failing for PK reasons can be attributed to the following: a) application of concepts of drug metabolism and PK to design compounds in medicinal chemistry programs (Smith et al., 1996); b) development of *in vitro* ADME assays that are predictive of *in vivo* behavior (PK) of drugs (Obach et al., 1997; Venkatakrishnan et al.,2003; Pelkonen and Raunio, 2005; Thompson,2000; Fagerholm, 2007); c) use of the Lipinski rule of 5 to design oral drugs (Lipinski, 2000); d) development of computer programs to predict the human PK parameters and profiles based on *in vitro* ADME properties of drugs (Jamei et al., 2009); e) PK/PD correlation studies in preclinical setting and f) high throughput screening of ADME properties in *in vitro* and *in vivo* assays for hundreds of compounds in the lead identification to lead optimization stages of drug discovery. The consequence of all the above mentioned developments in ADME have resulted in the frontloading of non-drug like compounds early in drug discovery and ultimately reducing the attrition rates of compounds in the clinic.

Histone acetylases (HATs) and Histone deacetylases (HDACs) are enzymes that carry out acetylation and deacetylation, respectively, of histone proteins (Minucci and Pelicci, 2006). Histone proteins form a complex with DNA called as nucleosomes, which are the structural units of chromatin. The interplay of HATs and HDACs activities regulate the structure of chromatin and control gene expression. The aberrant expression of HDACs has been linked to the pathogenesis of cancer (Minucci and Pelicci, 2006). Histone deacetylase inhibitors

(HDACi) are an emerging class of therapeutic agents that induce tumor cell cytostasis, differentiation and apoptosis in various hematologic and solid malignancies (Mercurio et al., 2010; Stimson et al., 2009). They are known to exert their anti-tumor activity by inhibiting the HDACs, which play an important role in controlling gene expression by chromatin remodeling, that affect cell cycle and survival pathways (Stimson et al., 2009). Inhibitors of histone deacetylases (HDACi) also show promising anti-inflammatory properties as demonstrated in a number of animal and cellular models of inflammatory diseases and for diabetes (Christensen et al., 2011). The HDACi Zolinza (Vorinostat/ Suberolyanilide hydroxamic acid [SAHA]) and Romidepsin (FK228) have been approved by the FDA (United States Food and Drug Administration) for the treatment of cutaneous T cell Lymphoma (CTCL) (Mann et al., 2007, Grant et al.,2010) and for peripheral T cell lymphoma (PTCL)(http://www.accessdata.fda.gov/drugsatfda_docs/appletter/2011/022393s004ltr.p df) as such demonstrating clinical "proof-of-principle" for this class of compounds.

Four groups of HDAC inhibitors have been characterized: (i) short chain fatty acids (e.g., Sodium butyrate and phenylbutyrate), (ii) cyclic tetrapeptides (e.g., Depsipeptide and Trapoxin), (iii) benzamides (e.g. MGCD0103 (Mocetinostat), CI-994 and MS-275 (Entinostat)), and (iv) hydroxamic acids (e.g., SAHA [Vorinostat/Zolinza]), LBH589 (Panabinostat), SB939 (Pracinostat), ITF2357 (Givinostat), PXD101 etc). Table 1 shows compounds that are currently in different stages of clinical development.

The clinical progress that has been made by hydroxamic acid derivatives as HDAC inhibitors is of particular interest because they are usually considered as non-druggable and are down-prioritized in lead identification campaigns attributing to their poor physicochemical and ADME properties. SB939 (Pracinostat) is a potent HDACi that was discovered and developed at S*BIO (Wang et al., 2011; Novotny-Diermayr et al, 2011) to overcome some of the ADME and PK/PD (Pharmacokinetic/Pharmacodynamic) limitations of the current HDACi. The pharmacokinetics and drug metabolism aspects of the four classes of HDACi have not been reviewed extensively. In this article, we review the pharmacokinetic and drug metabolism properties of SB939 and the preclinical and clinical ADME aspects of other HDAC inhibitors in the clinic.

2. Short chain fatty acids

2.1 Sodium butyrate (SB)

Sodium butyrate is a short chain fatty acid inhibitor of HDAC enzymes that is in phase 2 clinical trials. The PK of SB in preclinical species was characterized by poor bioavailability, short $t_{1/2}$ (< 5 min in mice and rabbits), leading to challenges in oral administration (Coradini et al, 1999; Daniel P et al, 1989). Butyrate was found to be transported by via a carrier mediated transport system MCT1 in Caco-2 cells suggesting that the absorption of SB might be saturable (Stein et al., 2000). SB has been reported to significantly increase the cytochrome P450 3A4 (CYP3A4) activity in Caco-2 cells transfected with CYP3A4 (Cummins et al; 2001) and induce P glycoprotein (PgP) *in vivo* (Machavaram et al., 2000). Due to its low potency very high doses were required to achieve pharmacological concentrations in animals and humans (Kim and Bae, 2011). In PK studies in mice and rats, SB showed rapid clearance (CL) with non-linear PK resulting from the high doses (up to 5 g/kg in mice), based on which the authors indicated that high doses would be problematic in humans (Egorin et al., 1999). In a clinical pharmacology study in leukemia patients, where SB was administered as continuous intravenous (IV) infusions (at a dose of 500 mg/kg/day) over a

Compound name	Structure	Class	Stage of clinical development*
Vorinostat (ZOLINZA™)		Hydroxamic Acid	Approved (2006)
Romidepsin (Istodax)		Cyclic peptide	Approved (2009)
MGCD0103 (Mocetinostat)		Benzamide	Phase 2
LBH589 (Panabinostat)		Hydroxamic Acid	Phase 2
SB939 (Pracinostat)		Hydroxamic Acid	Phase 2
ITF2357 (Givinostat)		Hydroxamic Acid	Phase 2
PXD101 (Belinostat)		Hydroxamic Acid	Phase 2

Compound name	Structure	Class	Stage of clinical development[*]
CI994 (Tacedinaline)		Benzamide	Phase 2
MS-275 (Entinostat)		Benzamide	Phase 2
Sodium Butyrate		Short chain fatty acid	Phase 2
Sodium Phenylbutyrate		Short chain fatty acid	Phase 2
CUDC-101		Hydroxamic acid	Phase 1
JNJ-26481585		Hydroxamic acid	Phase 1
CRA 24781 (PCI-24781)		Hydroxamic acid	Phase 1
Sodium Valproate		Short chain fatty acid	Phase 2

[*]Reference from http://www.fda.gov

Table 1. HDAC inhibitors in clinical development

10 day period, SB declined rapidly post infusion with a very short $t_{1/2}$ (~ 6 min), with high systemic clearance (CL~5 L/h/kg) and low volume of distribution (V_d =0.74 L/kg) (Miller et al., 1987). The amount of unchanged SB in urine was minimal suggesting that SB's clearance was primarily by metabolism. The authors concluded that the lack of efficacy of SB in the leukemic patients was due to its low plasma levels and very short $t_{1/2}$ (Miller et al., 1987).

2.2 Sodium phenyl butyrate (PB)

Sodium phenyl butyrate (PB) is an aromatic fatty acid HDACi, with low potency of 0.5 mM that is in phase 2 trials for cancer. PB (Buphenyl) has already been approved by the FDA for patients with hyperammonemia (Gilbert et al., 2001).

In a phase 1 study in patients with solid tumors, the PK of PB was characterized by rapid absorption (time of peak concentration [t_{max}] ~1.8 h), dose proportional increase in oral exposures between doses of 9 and 36 g/day, a short $t_{1/2}$ of 1 h, with mean absolute oral bioavailability (F) of 78% (Gilbert et al., 2001). In the same study, the major circulating metabolites of PB were phenylacetate (PA) and phenyacetylglutamine (PG), the exposures of which were 46-66% and 70-100% respectively of PB, suggesting extensive metabolic clearance of PB in humans. The highest percentage of patients that showed stable disease was from the 36 g/day cohort, in which the time above 0.5 mM was ~ 4.0 h (Gilbert et al., 2001). In another phase 1 study in patients with myelodysplastic syndrome (MDS) and acute myelogenous leukemia (AML), where PB was dosed as IV infusions, PB showed non-linear PK between 125 and 500 mg/kg/day, with PA and PG being formed as major metabolites (Gore et al., 2001). The low potency of PB requires very high doses in humans, leading to non-linear kinetics, thus making it a less attractive chemotherapeutic agent. In another phase 1 study, where PB was evaluated as continuous IV infusions (120 h) in solid tumors, the PK of PB was best described by saturable elimination, and PG was the major metabolite found in urine which was indicative of extensive metabolic clearance of PB in humans (Carducci et al., 2001). In the same study the plasma clearance (CL) of PB increased during the infusion period in some patients at higher dose levels. In a dose escalation oral study of PB in patients with glioma, who also received anticonvulsants concomitantly, the mean CL of PB was significantly higher than in solid tumor patients, and the possible reason was attributed to the induction of cytochrome P450 (CYP450) enzymes by anticonvulsants (Phuphanich et al., 2005). Thus it appears that the CYP450 metabolism might play a significant role in clearance of PB in humans.

2.3 Sodium valproate

Sodium valproate is a short chain fatty acid that is currently in phase 1 and 2 clinical trials in patients with solid tumors and hematological malignancies (Federico and Bagella, 2011). Sodium valproate (Depakote) has been previously approved for use in epilepsy patients and is in medical use for the last 3 decades (Federico and Bagella, 2011). It is a moderately potent inhibitor of class 1 HDAC enzymes with promising antitumor effects *in vitro* and *in vivo*. The human ADME of sodium valproate is characterized by a) high plasma protein binding (PPB) of 90 % with concentration dependent PPB; b) weak inhibitor of some CYP450, epoxide hydrolase and glucoronosyl transferases; c) entirely metabolized by the liver via glucoronidation and β-oxidation pathways with less than 3% of unchanged parent drug found in the urine; d) minimum drug-drug interaction (DDI) potential with CYP450 inhibitors as CYP450 mediated oxidation is a minor pathway ; e) high absolute oral bioavailability (90%); f) mean terminal half-life of 9-16 h (Depakote prescribing information, http://www.accessdata.fda.gov/drugsatfda_docs/label).

3. Cyclic tetrapeptides

3.1 Romidepsin (FK228, depsipeptide, ISTODAX™)

Romidepsin is a bicyclic peptide that was isolated as a secondary metabolite from a naturally occurring soil bacterium, and found to be a potent anti-tumor agent *in vitro* and *in vivo* (Ueda et al., 1994) and subsequently found to be a potent HDACi. It was approved by the FDA for treatment of patients with refractory CTCL (Mercurio et al., 2010). Romidepsin is a high molecular weight drug (Mw ~ 541), highly lipophilic, and insoluble in water, necessitating intraperitoneal and subcutaneous administrations in pharmacology studies (Ueda et al., 1994). The *in vitro* PPB of Romidepsin to human plasma was 92-94 % over a concentration of 50-1000 ng/mL, indicating high binding (http://www.accessdata.fda). Romidepsin is a substrate of PgP and MRP1 (Xiao et al., 2005). Depsipeptide was extensively metabolized by human liver microsomes, leading to the formation of at least 10 different metabolites, and was found to be primarily metabolized by CYP3A4 *in vitro* (Shiraga et al., 2005). Among the metabolites formed, mono-oxidation, di-oxidation, reduction of disulfide metabolites and two unidentified metabolites were the major metabolites in humans (http://www.accessdata.fda). It did not seem to inhibit any of the major human CYP450 enzymes *in vitro*, and there are no reports on its effect on the induction of human CYP450s (http://www.accessdata.fda). The preclinical PK of depsipeptide was characterized by high systemic CL and long $t_{1/2}$ (~ 6.0 h) in mice (Graham et al., 2006). In rats, the volume of distribution at steady state (V_{ss}) was very high (100 L/kg) and systemic CL was high (~ 49 L/h/kg), $t_{1/2}$ was short (18 min), and had poor oral bioavailability (F= ~ 2-11%) (Li and Chan, 2000). The low F in rats may be could be due to high first-pass effect, poor solubility and PgP efflux. Systemic CL (~1.8 L/h/kg) and $t_{1/2}$ (205 min) were moderate in nonhuman primates (Berg et al., 2004). In a radiolabelled mass-balance study in rats with FK228, approximately 98% of the dose was recovered in excreta with ~ 79% of the dose in the feces, and biliary clearance appeared to be the main clearance mechanism (http://www.accessdata.fda; Shiraga et al., 2005). Unchanged FK228 accounted for 3% of the dose, with > 30 metabolites detected in bile, indicating extensive metabolism of FK228 (Shiraga et al., 2005). The clinical PK of Romidepsin was characterized by low V_{ss} (54 L), low CL (20 L/h), and a short $t_{1/2}$ (~ 3.5 h) (http://www.accessdata.fda; Woo et al., 2009). The intra-patient variability was moderate to high (30-80%) and the inter-patient variability was high (50-70%) (http://www.accessdata.fda;). Despite the high inter-patient variability the AUC and C_{max} increased dose proportionally (http://www.accessdata.fda).

Romidepsin is the only HDACi that seems to be a PgP substrate. Romidepsin induced PgP expression in the HCT15 tumor cell line and conferred resistance to its action (Xiao et al., 2005). A possibility of correlation between PgP induction and the poor response rate of Romidepsin in cancer patients has been proposed (Xiao et al., 2005).

4. Benzamides

4.1 Mocetinostat (MGCD0103)

Mocetinostat (MGCD0103), an aminophenyl benzamide, is a potent inhibitor of HDAC 1, 2, and 3 enzymes and has recently completed Phase 2 clinical trials (Mercurio et al., 2010). It is a small molecule (Mw~396) and moderately lipophilic (LogP=2.6). There is no information available on its permeability, microsomal stability, metabolism, plasma protein binding, CYP450 inhibition and induction. In preclinical PK studies in mice, rat and dog,

Mocetinostat showed moderate V_{ss} (0.35 -0.91 L/kg), moderate to high CL (1.7 to 4.3 L/h/kg), short $t_{1/2}$ (0.6-1.3 h), with F ranging between low (mice =12%), moderate (rat=47%) and low-high (dogs=1-92%) (Zhou et al., 2008). In preclinical PK and PD studies, where the dihydrobromo salt of Mocetinostat was used, the dosing formulations required acidification and cosolvent addition indicating solubility issues (Zhou et al, 2008). In a phase 1 study in patients with leukemia, the oral PK of Mocetinostat was characterized by rapid absorption (t_{max} = 0.5-1.2 h), mean elimination $t_{1/2}$ of 7-11 h, and a dose related increase in peak plasma concentration (C_{max}) and area under the concentration-time curve (AUC) between 20 and 60 mg/m^2 and tended to plateau at higher doses (Garcia-Manero et al., 2011). Based on the lack of accumulation upon repeated dosing, it was suggested that induction or inhibition of drug elimination was unlikely in humans (Le Tourneau and Siu, 2008).

4.2 CI994 (N-acetyldinaline)
CI994 (N-acetydinaline), belonging to the benzamide class, is a HDACi with promising antitumor activities in preclinical xenograft models, and subsequently progressed to phase 1 2 clinical trials (Richards et al., 2006). CI994, a small molecule (MW=269.3) and with poor aqueous solubility, was developed as an acetylated analogue of Dinaline (GOE-1734), which, also showed equivalent antitumor activity (LoRusso et al., 1996). CI994 was eventually identified as an active metabolite of Dinaline (LoRusso et al., 1996). Limited data is available on its *in vitro* ADME. It showed low PPB in mice (20%) (Foster et al., 1997). In an oral PK and metabolism study in mice, where CI-994 was dosed once daily at 50 mg/kg for 14 days, it showed moderately rapid absorption (t_{max}= 30-45 min), 2 compartment disposition with a terminal $t_{1/2}$ on day 1 (9.4 h) being longer than on day 14 (3.4 h), and oral CL ranging between 0.42 (Day 1) -0.52 (day 14) ml/min (Foster et al., 1997). High amounts of unchanged drug (42-58% of dose) were found in the urine with minimal amounts in fecal samples, suggesting that renal clearance was a major clearance pathway for CI-994. Low amounts of Dinaline were found in urine and feces indicating that *in vivo* conversion of CI-994 to Dinaline were not significant. In rhesus monkeys, the PK of CI-994 was characterized by low volume of distribution (V_d) (0.3 L/kg) and CL (0.05 L/h/kg), a moderate $t_{1/2}$ (7.4 h), and high brain penetration (Riva et al., 2000). The oral bioavailability of CI-994 in preclinical species was 100% (Riva et al., 2000). In a phase 1 study in cancer patients following oral dosing (5-15 mg/m^2), CI-994 showed rapid absorption (t_{max} 0.7-1.6 h), oral CL ranging between ~30-48 ml/min/m^2), dose proportional increases in C_{max} and AUC, and moderately long $t_{1/2}$ (7.4-14 h) (Prakash et al., 2001). In the same study, no food effects were observed on the oral PK of CI-994.

4.3 Entinostat (MS-275)
Entinostat (MS-275) is a small molecule, synthetic benzamide that is currently in phase 2 trials (Mercurio et al., 2010). It is moderately lipophilic (LogD= 1.79), with moderate plasma protein binding (fraction unbound [f_u] ranged between 0.375 to 0.439 in preclinical species, and 0.188 in humans) (Hooker et al., 2010; Acharya et al., 2006). In preclinical pharmacology studies, the t_{max} of Entinostat ranged between 30-40 minutes with a $t_{1/2}$ of ~ 1 h in rats, mice and dogs, and the oral bioavailability was high (F~ 85%) (Ryan et al., 2005). In a radiolabeled tissue distribution and brain penetration study in baboons, radioactivity was cleared both by renal and biliary systems, and showed poor brain penetration (Hooker et al,

2010). The authors concluded that PgP mediated efflux was probably not the main mechanism for the poor brain penetration.

The clinical PK of Entinostat, in cancer patients, was characterized by variable absorption rates (t_{max} ranged between 0.5 to 60 h), a mean terminal elimination half-life of ~ 52 h, low oral clearance (CL/F=17.4 L/h/m^2), nearly dose proportional increase in exposures with dose (range 2-12 mg/m^2), and with substantial interpatient variability (Ryan et al., 2005). The nearly 50 fold longer $t_{1/2}$ in humans was not predicted based on the preclinical PK (Ryan et al., 2005). The possible reasons for the extended $t_{1/2}$ in humans were attributed to entero-hepatic recirculation and higher binding to human plasma proteins to some extent (Ryan et al., 2005). In an *in vitro* study, no metabolites could be detected after incubation of MS-275 in human liver microsomes, indicating that hepatic metabolism was a minor pathway of elimination in humans (Acharya et al., 2006).

5. Hydroxamic acids

5.1 Vorinostat (suberoylanilide hydroxamic acid [SAHA], ZOLINZA^{TM})

Vorinostat (SAHA, ZOLINZA™), belonging to the hydroxamic acid class, was the first HDACi to be clinically approved for the treatment of refractory cutaneous T-cell lymphoma (Mann et al., 2007). Vorinostat (M_w=264) is poorly soluble in aqueous solutions ~ 191 µg/mL [~0.7 mM] (Cai et al., 2010), has a pKa of 9.2 and a LogP ~1.0 (http://www.accessdata.fda). It was moderately permeable in Caco-2 cell permeability assays (~ 2 X 10^{-6} cm/sec), based on which, and its poor solubility, it was classified as a Biopharmaceutical Classification System (BCS) class 4 drug (http://www.accessdata.fda). It displayed low to moderate binding to plasma proteins, with mean PPB of 71.3, 62.5, 43.6, 32.4, and 31.1 % in human, rabbit, dog, rat and mouse plasma, respectively (http://www.accessdata.fda). The mean blood-to-plasma partition ratio was 1.2, 0.7, and 2.0 in rat, dog and human blood, respectively (http://www.accessdata.fda). In *in vitro* metabolism studies, using S9 and liver microsomal fractions from rat, dog and humans, the major metabolic pathway was O-glucoronidation of Vorinostat in all the 3 species, and a minor pathway was the hydrolysis of parent to 8-anilino-8-oxooctanoic acid (8-AOO) (http://www.accessdata.fda). In metabolism studies with hepatocytes from rat, dog and humans, the major metabolites formed in all the 3 species were 4-anilino-4-oxobutanoic acid (4-AOB, β-oxidation product) and 8-AOO (hydrolysis). In dog hepatocytes, the O-glucoronide was also a major metabolite, with human hepatocytes generating small amounts of it (http://www.accessdata.fda). The CYP450 enzymes were not responsible for the biotransformation of Vorinostat (http://www.accessdata.fda).

In preclinical studies in rats and dogs (Sandhu et al., 2007), the PK of Vorinostat was characterized by high systemic CL (7.8 and 3.3 L/h/kg in dog (> liver blood flow of ~ 1.9 L/h/kg) and rat (=liver blood flow of 3.3 L/h/kg), respectively), low to moderate V_{ss} (1.6 and 0.6 L/kg in dog and rat respectively), short half-lives (12 min in dog and rat), and poor oral bioavailability (11 % and ~ 2% in dog and rat, respectively). The O-glucoronide and 4-AOB metabolites of Vorinostat were detected in significant levels in both the species following oral dosing (AUC ratio of O-glucoronide to Vorinostat was ~ 1.0 and 2.3 in dog and rat, respectively; and the AUC ratio of 4-AOB to Vorinostat was 10 and 23 in dog and rat, respectively). In excretion studies with radiolabeled Vorinostat, 89-91% and 68-81% of the total dose was recovered in urine of rat and dog, respectively. The major metabolites in rat urine (over a period of 24 h) were acetaminophen-O-sulfate (~16-19%), 4-AOB (47-48%),

6-anilino-oxohexanoic acid (6-AOB) (~10-14%), O-glucoronide in trace amounts, and the parent accounting for 0.7- 5%. In dog urine, the major metabolites found were 4-AOB (31-34%), ortho-hydroxyaniline O-sulfate (17-21%), with minor amounts of the O-glucoronide and carnitine esters of 6-AOH and 8-AOO. Thus, Vorinostat was primarily cleared by metabolism and renally excreted in rat and dog. The data suggest that the low bioavailability of Vorinostat in rat and dog was due to a high first-pass effect and not due to absorption since the > 90% of the dose was recovered in urine, indicative of high intestinal absorption (fraction of dose absorbed [F_a]=0.8-1.0) (Sandhu et al., 2007). Vorinostat did not inhibit any of the major human CYP450 enzymes (http://www.accessdata.fda). It did not significantly induce CYP1A2, 2B6, 2C9, 2C19 and 3A4 in freshly cultured human hepatocytes, although the induction activity of 2C9 and 2C19 were suppressed at the highest concentration (http://www.accessdata.fda). In the first clinical trial in cancer patients Vorinostat was administered intravenously as a 2 h infusion (Kelly et al., 2003). The intravenous route was chosen due to predictions of poor oral bioavailability based on its preclinical ADME properties (Kelly et al., 2003). In a subsequent phase 1 trial, Vorinostat was dosed orally in patients with advanced cancer in which the oral PK was also characterized (Kelly et al., 2005). Vorinostat showed dose proportional increase in C_{max} and AUC following single oral doses of 100, 400 and 600 mg, with the average terminal $t_{1/2}$ ranging between ~ 92 to 127 minutes, median t_{max} ranging between 53 to 150 minutes, and an absolute oral bioavailability of 43%. No apparent changes were observed in PK following multiple oral dosing. The $t_{1/2}$ following oral dosing was longer than the $t_{1/2}$ observed after i.v. dosing (range of ~35-42 min), suggesting that the elimination of Vorinostat was absorption rate limited (Kelly et al., 2005). In another study investigating the PK of Vorinostat, at 400 mg, and its major metabolites in cancer patients, the mean serum exposures of the O-glucoronide and 4-AOB were 3-4 fold and 10-to-13 fold higher, respectively, than that of Vorinostat (Rubin et al., 2006). In the same study, up to 18% and 36% of the O-glucoronide and 4-AOB, respectively, were recovered in urine, with the parent accounting for < 1 % of the total dose, clearly indicating that Vorinostat was cleared primarily by metabolism in humans, and that the O-glucoronide and 4-AOB were the major metabolites. The main enzymes responsible for the formation of the O-glucoronide were identified as the UDP-glucoronosyltransferases (UGTs), such as the UGTs 2B17 and 1A9, which are expressed in the liver, and the extrahepatic UGTs 1A8 and 1A10 (Balliet et al.,2009). UGT2B17 was one of the major enzymes contributing to the formation of the O-glucoronide of Vorinostat in humans (Balliet et al., 2009). Since UGTs are known to show extensive polymorphism, including UGT2B17, they have been associated with the variable PK and response of Vorinostat in patients (Balliet et al., 2009).

There have been no reports on allometric scaling or the predictions of human PK based on preclinical ADME data so far.

5.2 Panabinostat (LBH589)

Panabinostat (LBH589) is a cinnamic hydroxamic acid and a potent pan HDAC inhibitor that is currently in phase 2 clinical trials (Mercurio et al., 2010). Very little information is available on its preclinical ADME characteristics. It showed poor oral bioavailability in rodents (F=6% in rats) and moderate F in dogs (33-50%) (Konsoula et al, 2009).

Like SAHA, Panabinostat was first tried as an intravenous formulation in the phase 1 clinical trials (Giles et al., 2006). In that study, LBH589 showed dose proportional increase in

C_{max} and AUC between 4.8 and 14 mg/m^2, with the terminal half-life ranging between 8-16 h. The V_{ss} and CL were not reported. The oral PK of Panabinostat was characterized by rapid absorption (t_{max} =1-1.5 h), linear increase in dose between 20 and 80 mg and the terminal $t_{1/2}$ ranged between 16-17 h (Prince et al, 2009). In an oral mass-balance study in patients with advanced cancer, following a single oral dose of 20 mg of ^{14}C radioactively labeled Panabinostat, 87% of the administered dose was recovered in the excreta, with unchanged drug accounting for <3% of the administered dose in the feces, suggesting good oral absorption and extensive metabolism (Clive et al, 2006). The major circulating metabolites were glucoronidation products of Panabinostat, in addition to hydrolysis and reduction products. Thus, it appears that there is no single major metabolic pathway for the elimination of Panabinostat in humans. CYP3A4 does not significantly contribute to the elimination of Panabinostat in humans (DeJonge et al, 2009). Human PK data suggest that Panabinostat is a permeable drug and the poor bioavailability in preclinical rodents could be due high first-pass and poor solubility.

5.3 Givinostat (ITF2357)

Givinostat (ITF2357) is a pan HDAC inhibitor, belonging to the hydroxamic acid class that is currently in phase 2 trials for many hematological malignancies (Mercurio et al., 2010). Preclinical ADME information is either limited or qualitative for Givinostat. Metabolism was the primary clearance mechanism in preclinical species like rats, dogs, rabbits and monkeys, with excretion being biliary or renal (Furlan et al, 2011). In a phase 1 study in healthy volunteers, the oral PK of Givinostat was characterized by rapid absorption, dose proportional increases in C_{max} and AUC upon single and multiple oral dosing, and the terminal half-life ranged between 5-7 h (Furlan et al, 2011). Two major circulating metabolites of Givinostat, a carboxylate and an amide formed due to oxidation and reduction of the hydroxamic acid group, were detected at significant levels in plasma.

5.4 Belinostat (PXD101)

Belinostat (PXD101) is a hydroxamic acid class potent pan HDAC inhibitor that is currently in phase 2 clinical trials (Mercurio et al., 2010). It is a small molecule (Mw 318) and sparingly soluble in aqueous solutions (Urbinati et al., 2010). Preclinical ADME information on Belinostat is limited. Preclinical pharmacodynamic studies in mice (Plumb et al., 2003) and PK studies in non-human primates (Warren et al 2008) have been performed using IV administrations, suggesting that Belinostat may have poor solubility and bioavailability issues. However, in dogs an oral bioavailability of 30-35% was reported (Steele et al, 2011). In rhesus monkeys, clearance was rapid (425 $mL/min/m^2$) with a $t_{1/2}$ of 1.0 h (Warren et al 2008). In a PK/PD study in mice following IV dosing at 200 mg/kg, Belinostat declined rapidly in plasma (ca $t_{1/2}$ ~ 0.4 h), suggesting high systemic clearance (Marquard et al 2008). In the same study a correlation was observed between tumor concentrations and histone 4 acetylation levels indicating that Belinostat penetrated solid tumors.

In a phase 1 clinical study in patients with solid tumors, where Belinostat was administered as a 30 min IV infusion, its PK was characterized by dose proportional increase in AUC and C_{max}, and a short $t_{1/2}$ (0.45 to 0.79 h) (Steele et al., 2008). The oral PK of Belinostat following a 1000 mg/m^2 dose in patients with solid tumors, was characterized by mean t_{max} of 1.9 h (although the oral concentration-time profile showed a flat absorption phase), with a mean

$t_{1/2}$ of 1.5 h (Steele et al, 2011). High variability was observed in oral clearance (39-71%) due to which dose proportionality analysis was not attempted. The oral $t_{1/2}$ was longer than that of the IV, which was attributed to a slow absorption rate (Steele et al., 2011). Oral bioavailability ranged between low to moderate (20-50%) in patients with advanced solid tumors (Kelly et al., 2007). Although a correlation between H4 acetylation and concentrations was observed following oral dosing at 1000 mg/m^2 (Steele et al., 2011), recent phase 2 trials have employed IV dosing of Belinostat (Cashen et al., 2011). In another Phase 1 study, where the metabolism of Belinostat was studied in patients with hepatocellular carcinoma, five metabolites were identified (Wang et al, 2010). Glucoronidation was the most significant pathway of metabolism, and the methylated and amide (reduction of hydroxamic acid) products were also detected. The acid and N-glucoside forms of Belinostat were found as minor metabolites. In an *in vitro* assay using 12 isoforms forms of human UGTs, Belinostat was mainly cleared by UGT1A1 (Wang et al., 2010). The data taken together suggest that Belinostat was primarily cleared by phase 2 metabolism, involving UGT1A1, in humans.

5.5 CUDC-101

CUDC-101 is a small molecule (Mw 434.5) hydroxamic acid HDACi, synthesized by incorporating the hydroxamic acid group into the epidermal growth factor receptor (EGFR) pharmacophore, that exhibited antiproliferative effects *in vitro* and *in vivo* (Cai et al., 2010; Lai et al, 2010). The preclinical ADME of CUDC-101 is not available (Cai et al., 2010). The fact that CUDC-101 was dosed IV in the preclinical efficacy studies suggests that it may have had poor oral bioavailability (Cai et al., 2010). CUDC-101 is currently in phase 1 trials (Cai et al., 2010)

5.6 JNJ-26481585

JNJ-26481585 is a second-generation, small molecule hydroxamic acid based potent pan-HDACi that is currently in phase 1 trials (Mercurio et al., 2010). The preclinical ADME information for this compound is minimal. JNJ-26481585 has been shown to undergo extensive first-pass metabolism resulting in poor oral bioavailability in rodents, due to which it had to be dosed intraperitoneally (IP) in xenograft models (Arts et al., 2009). In a phase 1 oral PK/PD study in solid tumor patients, the exposures of JNJ-26481585 (dosed *q.d.* in 3 weekly cycles) increased dose proportionally between 2 and 12 mg (Postel-Vinay et al., 2009). In the same study promising antitumor activity was observed indicating orally active exposures were achieved in humans.

5.7 CRA-024781(PCI-24781)

CRA-024781(PCI-24781) is a small molecule, hydroxamic based pan HDACi that is currently in phase 1 trials (Mercurio et al., 2010). In preclinical murine models of efficacy, its PK was characterized by a very short $t_{1/2}$ (~ 7 min), very high CL (~ 18 L/h/kg) and high V_{ss} (~ 9 l/kg) (Buggy et al., 2006). It was administered intravenously at high doses of up to 200 mg/kg in the efficacy models, most probably owing to poor oral bioavailability and high CL (Buggy et al, 2006). In a phase 1 study in patients with solid tumors, where PCI-24781 was dosed as a 2 h IV infusion, the mean elimination $t_{1/2}$ was ~ 6 h, high CL and moderately high V_{ss}, low oral bioavailability of 28%, with the carboxylic acid and amide metabolites formed at ~ 60 % of the parent (Undevia et al., 2008).

5.8 Pracinostat (SB939)

Pracinostat (SB939) is a hydroxamic acid based potent HDACi that is in multiple phase 2 clinical trials (http://clinicaltrials.gov/ct2/results?term=Sb939) in patients with solid tumors and hematological malignancies. Since the clinically advanced hydroxamic acid HDACi (Zolinza, Panabinostat and Belinostat) had ADME liabilities, such as poor solubility and oral bioavailability, we sought to identify a candidate that would achieve pharmacologically active exposures in humans when dosed orally. Pracinostat is a small molecule (Mw 359) moderately lipophilic base (LogD$_{7.4}$ =2.1) with high aqueous solubility (>100 mg/mL in water for the HCl salt of SB939) and high permeability with low efflux which indicated that Pracinostat would show high intestinal absorption *in vivo* (Wang et al., 2011). Based on its solubility and permeability Pracinostat was categorized as a BCS class 1 compound (S*BIO Data files). In preclinical PK studies Pracinostat showed higher oral bioavailability in mice (F=34%) and dogs (F=65%), than Zolinza, Panabinostat and Belinostat (table 2). The superior efficacy of Pracinostat, over Zolinza and Belinostat, when dosed orally in murine xenograft models was consistent its improved PK profile (Novotny-Diermayr et al., 2011). Pracinostat was found to selectively accumulate in tumors which correlated well with increased and prolonged acetylation levels in tumor which, in turn correlated with high tumor growth inhibition in mice (Novotny-Diermayr et al., 2011).

Preclinical ADME of Pracinostat was characterized by: a) in *in vitro* liver microsomal stability studies, Pracinostat was most stable in human and dog, moderate in mouse, and least stable in rat; b) uniform PPB of 84-94% in preclinical species and humans; c) was metabolized mainly by human CYP3A4 and 1A2; d) did not inhibit the major human CYPs except moderate inhibition of 2C19 (~ 6 µM); e) lack of significant induction of human CYP3A4 and 1A2 *in vitro*; f) metabolite identification studies using liver microsomes showed the formation of N-deethylation and bis-N-deethylation as major metabolites in addition to minor oxidative products; g) a glucoronidation product of SB939 was found as the major metabolite in rat urine following oral dosing; h) PK: high systemic clearance of 9.2, 4.5 and 1.5 L/h/kg in mice, rat and dog, respectively and high volume of distribution (V$_{ss}$ ranged between 1.7 to 4.2 L/kg) in preclinical species; i) moderate F in mice and dogs and poor in rats (Jayaraman et al., 2011). In PK/PD studies in HCT116 xenograft models, studying the relationship between tumor growth inhibition and the PK/PD indices such as AUC/IC$_{50,HCT116}$, C$_{max}$/ IC$_{50,HCT116}$, and time above IC$_{50,HCT116}$, Pracinostat was found to have the highest PK/PD ratios for all the three PK/PD parameters when compared to Vorinostat, Panabinostat and Belinostat (figure 1) (Jayaraman et al., 2009).

Pracinostat showed linear allometric relationships for V$_{ss}$ and CL in preclinical species. Prediction of human PK parameters using allometry indicated oral exposures would be achieved in humans with an acceptable t$_{1/2}$ which, was subsequently found to be consistent with the observed data from cancer patients (Jayaraman et al., 2011). The human PK of Pracinostat was simulated with the Simcyp ADME simulator (Jamei et al., 2009) using the physico-chemical and *in vitro* ADME data. The simulated PK profiles were in good agreement with the observed mean data, and the mean oral clearance and AUCs were predicted reasonably well (within 2 fold of observed data) (Jayaraman et al., 2011). Furthermore, simulations of drug-drug interactions (DDI) of Pracinostat in humans with the potent CYP3A inhibitor and inducers, ketoconazole and rifampicin, respectively, and with omeprazole (substrate of 2C19) showed lack of potential DDI at the clinically relevant dose of 60 mg (Jayaraman et al., 2011).

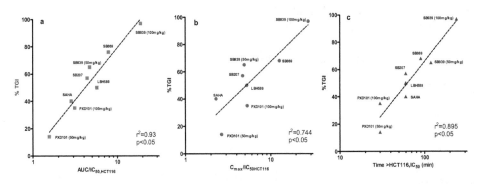

Fig. 1. The relationship between tumor growth inhibition (%TGI) and PK/PD parameters for
HDACi in the murine HCT116 xenograft model (Jayaraman et al., 2009). a) AUC/$IC_{50, HCT116}$;
b) C_{max}/ $IC_{50, HCT116}$; c) time above $IC_{50, HCT116}$.

Parameter	mice				dog	
	Pracinostat (SB939)	Vorinostat (SAHA)	Belinostat (PXD101)	Panabinostat (LBH589)	Pracinostat (SB939)	Vorinostat (SAHA)
C_{max}(ng/mL)	2632	501	489	116	1537	35
t_{max}(h)	0.17	0.5	0.17	0.17	0.8	0.7
$t_{1/2}$(h)	2.4	0.75	1.3	2.9	4.1	0.2
AUC_{0-inf} (ng.h/mL)	1841	619	287	126	4481	55
F (%)	34	8.3	6.7	4.6	65	2

Table 2. Comparison of preclinical pharmacokinetics of Pracinostat with that of other
advanced hydroxamic acid HDACi.

In the first phase 1 study in patients with solid tumors, Pracinostat showed rapid absorption
($t_{max} = 0.9$-2 h), dose proportional increase in C_{max} and AUC between 10 and 60 mg doses, a
mean terminal $t_{1/2}$ of ~ 7 h, and lack of significant accumulation on repeated dosing (Yong et
al, 2011). In the same study, pharmacologically active concentrations were achieved at the
starting dose of 10 mg, and a dose dependent increase in histone acetylation was observed.
At the 60 mg dose high acetylation levels was observed in all patients indicating sustained
target inhibition, and two of the patients experienced prolonged disease stabilization. The
clinical PK of Pracinostat was superior to the other hydroxamic acid HDACi in the clinic
(table 3). The high aqueous solubility, permeability, good oral bioavailability and
predictable human PK of Pracinostat contributed to obtaining active exposures in the clinic
when dosed orally, which was in contrast to the intravenous dosing of Zolinza, Panabinostat
and Belinostat in the initial clinical trials. The terminal $t_{1/2}$ of Pracinostat was longer than
that of Zolinza and Belinostat, and shorter than Panabinostat.

In summary, the superior preclinical ADME of Pracinostat over Zolinza, Panabinostat and Belinostat was translated into the clinic.

Parameter	Pracinostat (SB939)[*]	Vorinostat (SAHA)[#]	Panabinostat (LBH589)[%]	Belinostat (PXD101)[$]
Dosage regimen	thrice weekly	once daily	thrice weekly	once daily
Recommended Dose (mg)	60	400	20	250
$t_{1/2}$(h)	7-9	0.8-3.9	16	1.5
AUC_{0-inf}(ng.h/mL)	1226(3.4µM)	1716 (6.5 µM)	183(0.54 µM)	2767 (8.7 µM)
Remarks	Orally active exposures achieved at FTIM[&]. Best-in-class profile.	FTIM dose was given IV due to poor F in preclinical species.	FTIM dose was given IV due to poor F in preclinical species. Limited exposure.	FTIM dose was given IV due to poor F in preclinical species. Poor PK/PD

* Yong et al., 2011
\# Rubin et al., 2006
% Prince et al., 2009
$ Steele et al., 2011
& first time in Man

Table 3. Comparison of oral clinical pharmacokinetics of Pracinostat with hydroxamic acid HDAC inhibitors

6. Conclusions

The clinical use of the less potent short chain fatty acid HDACi (PB, SP and sodium valproate) in cancer patients was limited by the requirement of high doses and short half-life. The cyclic peptide drug Depsipeptide had to be administered intravenously because of poor solubility and oral bioavailability. The most clinically advanced hydroxamic acid HDACi such as Zolinza, Belinostat and Panabinostat were initially administered IV in patients owing to their poor solubility and oral bioavailability in preclinical species. Formulations were subsequently developed for oral administration. We succeeded in designing the hydroxamic acid pan HDACi Pracinostat (SB939) which had high solubility and permeability, with superior preclinical ADME and PK/PD properties when compared to the other hydroxamic acid HDACi, which subsequently helped to achieve pharmacologically active exposures upon oral dosing in cancer patients.

7. References

[1] van de Waterbeemd H and Gifford E. 2003. ADMET IN SILICO MODELLING: TOWARDS PREDICTION PARADISE? *Nat Rev Drug Disc* 2:192-204

[2] Prentis RA, Lis Y and Walker SR. 1988 Pharmaceutical innovation by the seven UK-owned pharmaceutical companies (1964-1985). *Br. J. Clin. Pharmacol.* 25: 387-396

[3] Yengi LG, Leung L, and Kao J. 2007. The evolving role of drug metabolism in drug discovery and development. *Pharm Res.* 24(5): 842-858

[4] Smith DA., Jones BC, and Walker DK.1996. Design of drugs involving the concepts and theories of drug metabolism and pharmacokinetics. *Med Res Rev.* 16(3):243-266

[5] Obach RS, Baxter JG, Liston TE, Silber BM, Jones BC, MacIntyre F, Rance DJ, Wastall P.1997. The prediction of human pharmacokinetic parameters from preclinical and in vitro metabolism data. *J Pharmacol Exp Ther* 283(1):46-58.

[6] Venkatakrishnan K, von Moltke LL, Obach RS, Greenblatt DJ. 2003. Drug metabolism and drug interactions: application and clinical value of in vitro models. *Curr Drug Metab.* 4(5):423-59.

[7] Pelkonen O and Raunio H. 2005. In vitro screening of drug metabolism during drug development: can we trust the predictions? *Expert Opin Drug Metab Toxicol* 1(1):49-59

[8] Thompson TN. 2000. Early ADME in support of drug discovery: the role of metabolic stability studies. *Curr Drug Metab* 1(3): 215-241

[9] Fagerholm U .2007. Prediction of human pharmacokinetics-gastrointestinal absorption. *J Pharm Pharmacol* 59:905-916

[10] Lipinski CA. 2000. Drug-like properties and the causes of poor solubility and poor permeability. *J Pharmacol and Toxicol Meth* 44: 235- 249

[11] Jamei M, Marciniak S, Feng K, Barnett A, Tucker G, Rostami-Hodjegan A.2009. The Simcyp population-based ADME simulator. *Expert Opin Drug Metab Toxicol* 5(2):211-223

[12] Minucci S and Pelicci PG. 2006. Histone deacetylase inhibitors and the promise of epigenetic (and more) treatments for cancer. *Nat. Rev. Cancer* 6(1):38-51

[13] Mercurio C, Minucci S, and Pelicci PG. 2010. Histone deacetylases and epigenetic therapies of hematological malignancies. *Pharmacol Res.* 62(1):18-34.

[14] Stimson L, Wood V, Khan O, Fotheringham S, and La Thangue NB. 2009. HDAC inhibitor-based therapies and haematological malignancy. *Ann Oncol.* 20(8):1293-302.

[15] Christensen DP, Dahllöf M, Lundh M, Rasmussen DN, Nielsen MD, Billestrup N, Grunnet LG, Mandrup-Poulsen T. 2011. HDAC inhibition as a novel treatment for diabetes mellitus. *Mol Med.* doi: 10.2119/molmed.2011.00021

[16] Mann BS, Johnson JR, Cohen MH, Justice R, Pazdur R. 2007. FDA approval summary: vorinostat for treatment of advanced primary cutaneous T-cell lymphoma. *Oncologist.* 12(10):1247-52.

[17] Grant C, Rahman F, Piekarz R, Peer C, Frye R, Robey RW, Gardner ER, Figg WD, Bates SE. 2010. Romidepsin: a new therapy for cutaneous T-cell lymphoma and a potential therapy for solid tumors. *Expert Rev Anticancer Ther.* 10(7):997-1008.

[18] Wang H, Yu N, Chen D, Lee KC, Lye PL, Chang JW, Deng W, Ng MC, Lu T, Khoo ML, Poulsen A, Sangthongpitag K, Wu X, Hu C, Goh KC, Wang X, Fang L, Goh KL, Khng HH, Goh SK, Yeo P, Liu X, Bonday Z, Wood JM, Dymock BW, Kantharaj E, Sun ET. 2011. Discovery of (2E)-3-{2-Butyl-1-[2- (diethylamino)ethyl]-1H-benzimidazol-5-yl}-Nhydroxyacrylamide (SB939), an Orally Active Histone Deacetylase Inhibitor with a Superior Preclinical Profile. *J Med Chem* in press.

[19] Novotny-Diermayr V, Sangthongpitag K, Hu CY, Wu X, Sausgruber N, Yeo P, Greicius G, Pettersson S, Liang AL, Loh YK, Bonday Z, Goh KC, Hentze H, Hart S, Wang H,

Ethirajulu K, Wood JM. 2010. SB939, a novel potent and orally active histone deacetylase inhibitor with high tumor exposure and efficacy in mouse models of colorectal cancer. *Mol Cancer Ther.* 9(3):642-52.

[20] Coradini D, Pellizzaro C, Miglierini G, Daidone MG, Perbellini A. 1999. Hyaluronic acid as drug delivery for sodium butyrate: improvement of the anti-proliferative activity on a breast-cancer cell line. *Int J Cancer.*81(3):411-6.

[21] Daniel P, Brazier M, Cerutti I, Pieri F, Tardivel I, Desmet G, Baillet J, Chany C. 1989. Pharmacokinetic study of butyric acid administered in vivo as sodium and arginine butyrate salts. *Clin Chim Acta.* 181(3):255-63.

[22] Stein J, Zores M, Schröder O. 2000. Short-chain fatty acid (SCFA) uptake into Caco-2 cells by a pH-dependent and carrier mediated transport mechanism. *Eur J Nutr.* 39(3):121-5.

[23] Cummins CL, Mangravite LM, Benet LZ. 2000. Characterizing the expression of CYP3A4 and efflux transporters (P-gp, MRP1, and MRP2) in CYP3A4-transfected Caco-2 cells after induction with sodium butyrate and the phorbol ester 12-O-tetradecanoylphorbol-13-acetate. *Pharm Res.* 18(8):1102-9.

[24] Machavaram KK, Gundu J, Yamsani MR. 2000. Effect of various cytochrome P450 3A and P-glycoprotein modulators on the biliary clearance of bromosulphaphthalein in male wistar rats. *Pharmazie.* 59(12):957-60.

[25] Hyun-Jung Kim and Suk-Chul Bae. 2011. Histone deacetylase inhibitors: molecular mechanisms of action and clinical trials as anti-cancer drugs. *Am J Transl Res* 3(2): 166-179

[26] Egorin MJ, Yuan ZM, Sentz DL, Plaisance K, Eiseman JL. 1999. Plasma pharmacokinetics of butyrate after intravenous administration of sodium butyrate or oral administration of tributyrin or sodium butyrate to mice and rats. *Cancer Chemother Pharmacol.*43(6):445-53.

[27] Miller AA, Kurschel E, Osieka R, Schmidt CG. 1987. Clinical pharmacology of sodium butyrate in patients with acute leukemia. *Eur J Cancer Clin Oncol.* 23(9):1283-7

[28] Gilbert J, Baker SD, Bowling MK, Grochow L, Figg WD, Zabelina Y, Donehower RC, Carducci MA. 2001. A phase I dose escalation and bioavailability study of oral sodium phenylbutyrate in patients with refractory solid tumor malignancies. *Clin Cancer Res.* 7(8):2292-300.

[29] Gore SD, Weng LJ, Zhai S, Figg WD, Donehower RC, Dover GJ, Grever M, Griffin CA, Grochow LB, Rowinsky EK, Zabalena Y, Hawkins AL, Burks K, Miller CB. 2001. Impact of the putative differentiating agent sodium phenylbutyrate on myelodysplastic syndromes and acute myeloid leukemia. *Clin Cancer Res.* 7(8):2330-9.

[30] Carducci MA, Gilbert J, Bowling MK, Noe D, Eisenberger MA, Sinibaldi V, Zabelina Y, Chen TL, Grochow LB, Donehower RC. 2001. A Phase I clinical and pharmacological evaluation of sodium phenylbutyrate on an 120-h infusion schedule. *Clin Cancer Res.* 7(10):3047-55.

[31] Phuphanich S, Baker SD, Grossman SA, Carson KA, Gilbert MR, Fisher JD, Carducci MA. 2005. Oral sodium phenylbutyrate in patients with recurrent malignant gliomas: a dose escalation and pharmacologic study. *Neuro Oncol.* 7(2):177-82.

[32] Federico M and Bagella L. 2011. Histone deacetylase inhibitors in the treatment of hematological malignancies and solid tumors. *J Biomed Biotechnol.* 2011:475641

[33] http://www.accessdata.fda.gov/drugsatfda_docs/label/2009/018723s039lbl.pdf

[34] Ueda H, Nakajima H, Hori Y, Fujita T, Nishimura M, Goto T, and Okuhara M. 1994. FR901228, a novel antitumor bicyclic depsipeptide produced by Chromobacterium

violaceum No. 968. I. Taxonomy, fermentation, isolation, physico-chemical and biological properties, and antitumor activity. *J Antibiot (Tokyo)*. 47(3):301-10.

[35] Xiao JJ, Foraker AB, Swaan PW, Liu S, Huang Y, Dai Z, Chen J, Sadée W, Byrd J, Marcucci G, and Chan KK. 2005. Efflux of depsipeptide FK228 (FR901228, NSC-630176) is mediated by P-glycoprotein and multidrug resistance-associated protein 1. *J Pharmacol Exp Ther*. 313(1):268-76

[36] Shiraga T, Tozuka Z, Ishimura R, Kawamura A, and Kagayama A. 2005. Identification of cytochrome P450 enzymes involved in the metabolism of FK228, a potent histone deacetylase inhibitor, in human liver microsomes. *Biol Pharm Bull*. 28(1):124-9.

[37] Graham C, Tucker C, Creech J, Favours E, Billups CA, Liu T, Fouladi M, Freeman BB 3rd, Stewart CF, and Houghton PJ. 2006. Evaluation of the antitumor efficacy, pharmacokinetics, and pharmacodynamics of the histone deacetylase inhibitor depsipeptide in childhood cancer models in vivo. *Clin Cancer Res*. 12(1):223-34.

[38] Li Z, and Chan KK. C.2000. A subnanogram API LC/MS/MS quantitation method for depsipeptide FR901228 and its preclinical pharmacokinetics. *J Pharm Biomed Anal*. 22(1):33-44.

[39] Berg SL, Stone J, Xiao JJ, Chan KK, Nuchtern J, Dauser R, McGuffey L, Thompson P, and Blaney SM. 2004. Plasma and cerebrospinal fluid pharmacokinetics of depsipeptide (FR901228) in nonhuman primates. *Cancer Chemother Pharmacol*. 54(1):85-8.

[40] Woo S, Gardner ER, Chen X, Ockers SB, Baum CE, Sissung TM, Price DK, Frye R, Piekarz RL, Bates SE, Figg WD. 2009. Population pharmacokinetics of romidepsin in patients with cutaneous T-cell lymphoma and relapsed peripheral T-cell lymphoma. *Clin Cancer Res*. 15(4):1496-503.

[41] Zhou N, Moradei O, Raeppel S, Leit S, Frechette S, Gaudette F, Paquin I, Bernstein N, Bouchain G, Vaisburg A, Jin Z, Gillespie J, Wang J, Fournel M, Yan PT, Trachy-Bourget MC, Kalita A, Lu A, Rahil J, MacLeod AR, Li Z, Besterman JM, Delorme D. 2008. Discovery of N-(2-aminophenyl)-4-[(4-pyridin-3-ylpyrimidin-2-ylamino) methyl]benzamide (MGCD0103), an orally active histone deacetylase inhibitor. *J Med Chem*. 51(14):4072-5.

[42]Garcia-Manero G, Assouline S, Cortes J, Estrov Z, Kantarjian H, Yang H, Newsome WM, Miller WH Jr, Rousseau C, Kalita A, Bonfils C, Dubay M, Patterson TA, Li Z, Besterman JM, Reid G, Laille E, Martell RE, and Minden M. 2011. Phase 1 study of the oral isotype specific histone deacetylase inhibitor MGCD0103 in leukemia. *Blood*. 112(4):981-9.

[43] Le Tourneau C and Siu LL. 2008. Promising antitumor activity with MGCD0103, a novel isotype-selective histone deacetylase inhibitor. *Expert Opin Investig Drugs*. 17(8):1247-54.

[44] Richards DA, Boehm KA, Waterhouse DM, Wagener DJ, Krishnamurthi SS, Rosemurgy A, Grove W, Macdonald K, Gulyas S, Clark M, Dasse KD. 2006. Gemcitabine plus CI-994 offers no advantage over gemcitabine alone in the treatment of patients with advanced pancreatic cancer: results of a phase II randomized, double-blind, placebo-controlled, multicenter study. *Ann Oncol*. 17(7):1096-102.

[45] LoRusso PM, Demchik L, Foster B, Knight J, Bissery MC, Polin LM, Leopold WR 3rd, Corbett TH. 1996. Preclinical antitumor activity of CI-994. *Invest New Drugs*. 14(4):349-56.

[46] Foster BJ, Jones L, Wiegand R, LoRusso PM, Corbett TH. 1997. Preclinical pharmacokinetic, antitumor and toxicity studies with CI-994 (correction of CL-994) (N-acetyldinaline). *Invest New Drugs*. 15(3):187-94.

[47] Riva L, Blaney SM, Dauser R, Nuchtern JG, Durfee J, McGuffey L, Berg SL. 2000. Pharmacokinetics and cerebrospinal fluid penetration of CI-994 (N-acetyldinaline) in the nonhuman primate. *Clin Cancer Res.* 6(3):994-7.

[48] Prakash S, Foster BJ, Meyer M, Wozniak A, Heilbrun LK, Flaherty L, Zalupski M, Radulovic L, Valdivieso M, LoRusso PM. 2001. Chronic oral administration of CI-994: a phase 1 study. *Invest New Drugs.* 19(1):1-11.

[49] Hooker JM, Kim SW, Alexoff D, Xu Y, Shea C, Reid A, Volkow N, Fowler JS.2010. Histone deacetylase inhibitor, MS-275, exhibits poor brain penetration: PK studies of [C]MS-275 using Positron Emission Tomography. *ACS Chem Neurosci.* 1(1):65-73.

[50] Acharya MR, Sparreboom A, Sausville EA, Conley BA, Doroshow JH, Venitz J, Figg WD. 2006. Interspecies differences in plasma protein binding of MS-275, a novel histone deacetylase inhibitor. *Cancer Chemother Pharmacol.* 57(3):275-81.

[51] Ryan QC, Headlee D, Acharya M, Sparreboom A, Trepel JB, Ye J, Figg WD, Hwang K, Chung EJ, Murgo A, Melillo G, Elsayed Y, Monga M, Kalnitskiy M, Zwiebel J, Sausville EA. 2005. Phase I and pharmacokinetic study of MS-275, a histone deacetylase inhibitor, in patients with advanced and refractory solid tumors or lymphoma. *J Clin Oncol.* 23(17):3912-22.

[52] Acharya MR, Karp JE, Sausville EA, Hwang K, Ryan Q, Gojo I, Venitz J, Figg WD, Sparreboom A. 2006. Factors affecting the pharmacokinetic profile of MS-275, a novel histone deacetylase inhibitor, in patients with cancer. *Invest New Drugs.* 24(5):367-75.

[53] Cai YY, Yap CW, Wang Z, Ho PC, Chan SY, Ng KY, Ge ZG, Lin HS. 2010. Solubilization of vorinostat by cyclodextrins. *J Clin Pharm Ther.* 35(5):521-6

[54] http://www.accessdata.fda.gov/scripts/cder/drugsatfda/index.cfm?fuseaction=Searc h.Drug Details

[55] Sandhu P, Andrews PA, Baker MP, Koeplinger KA, Soli ED, Miller T, and Baillie TA .2007. Disposition of vorinostat, a novel histone deacetylase inhibitor and anticancer agent, in preclinical species. *Drug Metab Lett* 1(2):153-61.

[56] Kelly WK, Richon VM, O'Connor O, Curley T, MacGregor-Curtelli B, Tong W, Klang M, Schwartz L, Richardson S, Rosa E, Drobnjak M, Cordon-Cordo C, Chiao JH, Rifkind R, Marks PA, Scher H. 2003. Phase I clinical trial of histone deacetylase inhibitor: suberoylanilide hydroxamic acid administered intravenously. *Clin Cancer Res.* 9:3578-88.

[57] Kelly WK, O'Connor OA, Krug LM, Chiao JH, Heaney M, Curley T, MacGregore-Cortelli B, Tong W, Secrist JP, Schwartz L, Richardson S, Chu E, Olgac S, Marks PA, Scher H, Richon VM. 2005. Phase I study of an oral histone deacetylase inhibitor, suberoylanilide hydroxamic acid, in patients with advanced cancer. *J Clin Oncol.* 23(17):3923-31.

[58] Rubin EH, Agrawal NG, Friedman EJ, Scott P, Mazina KE, Sun L, Du L, Ricker JL, Frankel SR, Gottesdiener KM, Wagner JA, Iwamoto M. 2006. A study to determine the effects of food and multiple dosing on the pharmacokinetics of vorinostat given orally to patients with advanced cancer. *Clin Cancer Res.* 12(23):7039-45.

[59] Balliet RM, Chen G, Gallagher CJ, Dellinger RW, Sun D, and Lazarus P.2009. Characterization of UGTs active against SAHA and association between SAHA glucuronidation activity phenotype with UGT genotype. *Cancer Res.* 69(7):2981-9.

[60] Konsoula Z, Cao H, Velena A, and Jung M. 2009. Pharmacokinetics-pharmacodynamics and antitumor activity of mercaptoacetamide-based histone deacetylase inhibitors. *Mol Cancer Ther.* 8(10):2844-51.

[61] Giles F, Fischer T, Cortes J, Garcia-Manero G, Beck J, Ravandi F, Masson E, Rae P, Laird G, Sharma S, Kantarjian H, Dugan M, Albitar M, and Bhalla K. 2006. A phase I study of intravenous LBH589, a novel cinnamic hydroxamic acid analogue histone deacetylase inhibitor, in patients with refractory hematologic malignancies. *Clin Cancer Res.* 12(15):4628-35

[62] Prince HM, Bishton MJ, Johnstone RW. 2009. Panobinostat (LBH589): a potent pan-deacetylase inhibitor with promising activity against hematologic and solid tumors. *Future Oncol.* 5(5):601-12.

[63] Clive S, Woo MM, Stewart M, Nydam T, Hirawat S, and Kagan M. 2009. Elucidation of the metabolic and elimination pathways of panabinostat (LBH589) using [14C]-panabinostat. *J Clin Oncol.* ASCO Annual Meeting Proceedings. 27(15S). Abstract number 2549.

[64] M. DeJonge, M. M. Woo, D. Van der Biessen, P. Hamberg, S. Sharma, L. C. Chen, N. Myke, L. Zhao, S. Hirawat, J. 2009. drug interaction study between ketoconazole and panobinostat (LBH589), an orally active histone deacetylase inhibitor, in patients with advanced cancer. *J Clin Oncol.* ASCO Annual Meeting Proceedings. 27(15S). Abstract number 2501.

[65] Furlan A, Monzani V, Reznikov LL, Leoni F, Fossati G, Modena D, Mascagni P, Dinarello CA. 2011. Pharmacokinetics, Safety and Inducible Cytokine Responses during a Phase 1 Trial of the Oral Histone Deacetylase Inhibitor ITF2357 (givinostat). *Mol Med..* doi: 10.2119/molmed.2011.00020

[66] Urbinati G, Marsaud V, Plassat V, Fattal E, Lesieur S, Renoir JM. 2010. Liposomes loaded with histone deacetylase inhibitors for breast cancer therapy. *Int J Pharm.* 397(1-2):184-93

[67] Plumb JA, Finn PW, Williams RJ, Bandara MJ, Romero MR, Watkins CJ, La Thangue NB, Brown R. 2003. Pharmacodynamic response and inhibition of growth of human tumor xenografts by the novel histone deacetylase inhibitor PXD101. *Mol Cancer Ther.* 2(8):721-8.

[68] Warren KE, McCully C, Dvinge H, Tjørnelund J, Sehested M, Lichenstein HS, Balis FM. 2008. Plasma and cerebrospinal fluid pharmacokinetics of the histone deacetylase inhibitor, belinostat (PXD101), in non-human primates. *Cancer Chemother Pharmacol.* 62(3):433-7.

[69] Steele NL, Plumb JA, Vidal L, Tjørnelund J, Knoblauch P, Buhl-Jensen P, Molife R, Brown R, de Bono JS, Evans TR. 2011. Pharmacokinetic and pharmacodynamic properties of an oral formulation of the histone deacetylase inhibitor Belinostat (PXD101). *Cancer Chemother Pharmacol.* 67(6):1273-9.

[70] Marquard L, Petersen KD, Persson M, Hoff KD, Jensen PB, Sehested M. 2008. Monitoring the effect of belinostat in solid tumors by H4 acetylation. *APMIS.* 116(5):382-92.

[71] Steele NL, Plumb JA, Vidal L, Tjørnelund J, Knoblauch P, Rasmussen A, Ooi CE, Buhl-Jensen P, Brown R, Evans TR, DeBono JS. 2008. A phase 1 pharmacokinetic and pharmacodynamic study of the histone deacetylase inhibitor belinostat in patients with advanced solid tumors. *Clin Cancer Res.* 14(3):804-10.

[72] Kelly WK, Yap T, Lee J, Lassen U, Crowley E, Clarke A, Hawthorne T, Buhl-Jensen P, and de Bono J. 2007. A phase I study of oral belinostat (PXD101) in patients with advanced solid tumors. *J Clin Oncol* 25(18S), ASCO Annual Meeting Proceedings. Abstract 14092

[73] Cashen A, Juckett M, Jumonville A, Litzow M, Flynn PJ, Eckardt J, Laplant B, Laumann K, Erlichman C, Dipersio J. 2011. Phase II study of the histone deacetylase inhibitor belinostat (PXD101) for the treatment of myelodysplastic syndrome (MDS). *Ann Hematol.* May 3. [Epub ahead of print]

[74] Wang L, Goh BC, Lwin TW, Lee H, S Chan SL, Lim RS, Chan AT, and Yeo W. 2010. Phase I pharmacokinetics and metabolic pathway of belinostat in patients with hepatocellular carcinoma. *J Clin Oncol* 28(15S), ASCO Annual Meeting Proceedings. Abstract 2585

[75] Cai X, Zhai HX, Wang J, Forrester J, Qu H, Yin L, Lai CJ, Bao R, Qian C. 2010. Discovery of 7-(4-(3-ethynylphenylamino)-7-methoxyquinazolin-6-yloxy)-N-hydroxyheptanamide (CUDC-101) as a potent multi-acting HDAC, EGFR, and HER2 inhibitor for the treatment of cancer. *J Med Chem.* 53(5):2000-9.

[76] Lai CJ, Bao R, Tao X, Wang J, Atoyan R, Qu H, Wang DG, Yin L, Samson M, Forrester J, Zifcak B, Xu GX, DellaRocca S, Zhai HX, Cai X, Munger WE, Keegan M, Pepicelli CV, Qian C. 2010. CUDC-101, a multitargeted inhibitor of histone deacetylase, epidermal growth factor receptor, and human epidermal growth factor receptor 2, exerts potent anticancer activity. *Cancer Res.* 70(9):3647-56

[77] Arts J, King P, Mariën A, Floren W, Beliën A, Janssen L, Pilatte I, Roux B, Decrane L, Gilissen R, Hickson I, Vreys V, Cox E, Bol K, Talloen W, Goris I, Andries L, Du Jardin M, Janicot M, Page M, van Emelen K, Angibaud P. 2009. JNJ-26481585, a novel "second-generation" oral histone deacetylase inhibitor, shows broad-spectrum preclinical antitumoral activity. *Clin Cancer Res.* 15(22):6841-51

[78] Postel-Vinay S, Kristeleit R, Fong P, Venugopal B, Crawford D, Van Beÿsterveldt L, Fourneau N, Hellemans P, Evans J, and De-Bono J. 2009. Preliminary results of an open-label phase I pharmacokinetic/pharmacodynamic study of JNJ26481585: Early evidence of antitumor activity. *J Clin Oncol* 27, 2009 (abstract e13504)

[79] Buggy JJ, Cao ZA, Bass KE, Verner E, Balasubramanian S, Liu L, Schultz BE, Young PR, Dalrymple SA. 2006. CRA-024781: a novel synthetic inhibitor of histone deacetylase enzymes with antitumor activity in vitro and in vivo. *Mol Cancer Ther.* 5(5):1309-17.

[80] Undevia SD, Janisch L, Schilsky RL, Loury D, Balasubramanian S, Mani C, Sirisawad M, Buggy JJ, Miller RA, and Ratain MJ. 2008. Phase I study of the safety, pharmacokinetics (PK) and pharmacodynamics (PD) of the histone deacetylase inhibitor (HDACi) PCI-24781. *J Clin Oncol* 26: (abstr 14514)

[81] Jayaraman R, Pilla Reddy V, Khalid Pasha M, Wang H, Sangthongpitag K, Yeo P, Hu C, Wu X, Xin L, Goh E, New L, and Ethirajulu K. 2011. Preclinical Metabolism and Disposition of SB939(Pracinostat), an Orally Active Histone Deacetylase (HDAC) Inhibitor, and Prediction of Human Pharmacokinetics. Drug Metab Dispos. doi: 10.1124/dmd.111.04155

[82] Yong WP, Goh BC, Soo RA, Toh HC, Ethirajulu K, Wood J, Novotny-Diermayr V, Lee SC, Yeo WL, Chan D, Lim D, Seah E, Lim R, and Zhu J .2011. Phase 1 and pharmacodynamic study of an orally administered novel inhibitor of histone deacetylases, SB939, in patients with refractory solid malignancies. *Ann Oncol* doi: 10.1093/annonc/mdq784 In press.

[83] Jayaraman R, Khalid Pasha M, Yeo P, Sangthongpitag K, Wang H, Hentze H, Novotny-Diermayr V, Wood J and Ethirajulu K. 2009. Pharmacokinetic/Pharmacodynamic (PK/PD) relationships of novel HDAC inhibitors in an HCT-116 mouse xenograft tumor model. *AACR*: 100th Annual Meeting, Abstract no 2924

Part 2

Anti-Infectives

microRNAs as Therapeutic Targets to Combat Diverse Human Diseases

Elizabeth Hong-Geller and Nan Li

Bioscience Division, Los Alamos National Laboratory, Los Alamos, NM
USA

1. Introduction

For decades, control of cellular behavior was thought to be the exclusive purview of protein-based regulators. However, the recent discovery of small RNAs (sRNAs) as a universal class of powerful RNA-based regulatory biomolecules has the potential to revolutionize our understanding of gene regulation in practically all biological functions, as sRNAs have been found in diverse organisms from bacteria to plants to man. A class of sRNAs in eukaryotes, termed microRNAs (miRNAs), has been found to modulate a wide variety of cellular functions, including cell growth, cell differentiation, and apoptosis. miRNAs function as regulators by base-pairing with trans-encoded mRNAs to prevent translation of mRNA into protein at the post-transcriptional level. By modulating the expression levels of target genes, miRNAs enable rapid adaptation of cellular physiology in response to specific environmental changes. It is estimated that at least ~30% of the human genome is regulated by miRNAs. (Lewis, et al., 2005) In this review, we will discuss recent discoveries that implicate miRNA function in host immunity, including specific miRNA expression in immune cells and their regulation of immune cell development, miRNA regulation of innate and acquired immune response, and viral-encoded miRNAs. These recent advances have strong potential to translate fundamental research in miRNA function into clinical applications. We will also describe the challenges in bringing another RNA interference (RNAi) methodology, small interfering RNA (siRNA), to clinical trials. This analysis will serve as a practical roadmap for development of novel miRNA-based therapies to combat infectious disease by reducing the host inflammatory response and the downstream effects of pathogen infection.

2. miRNA biogenesis and mechanism of action

Most miRNAs are transcribed by RNA polymerase II as either polycistronic or monocistronic transcription units called primary miRNAs (pri-miRNAs), in which one or more hairpin structures with ~33bp stem regions and terminal loops are embedded. (Fig. 1) (Lee, et al., 2004) These pri-miRNAs are capped and polyadenylated and can be as long as several kilobases. (Cai, et al., 2004) Hairpin structures embedded within pri-miRNA transcripts are recognized and excised by the microprocessor complex in the nucleus, which consists of the RNase III-like enzyme Drosha and double-stranded RNA (dsRNA) binding protein DGCR8 (DiGeorge syndrome critical region gene 8). (Landthaler, et al., 2004, Lee, et

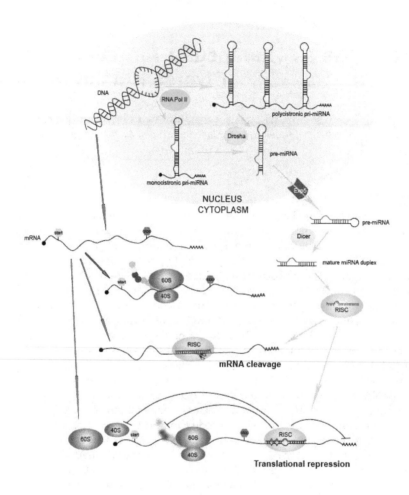

Fig. 1. miRNA biogenesis and mechanism of action. miRNAs are initially transcribed as either polycistronic or monocistronic long primary miRNA transcripts (pri-miRNAs), and then undergo a series of maturation steps including: (1) cleavage by the enzyme Drosha into the intermediate precursor miRNAs (pre-miRNAs), (2) transport from the nucleus to the cytoplasm via Exportin 5, and (3) final processing by the enzyme Dicer into the mature miRNA duplexes for loading into the RNA-induced silencing complex (RISC). Plant miRNAs pair extensively with their target mRNAs, resulting in direct cleavage of the mRNAs. Mammalian miRNAs exhibit partial complementarity with the 3′ untranslated region (UTR) of target mRNAs, causing translational repression, which may lead to mRNA degradation.

al., 2003) The released hairpin structure is typically ~65-70 nt and is referred to as a precursor miRNA (pre-miRNA). (Lee, et al., 2002) Pre-miRNAs are then exported into the cytoplasm by Exportin-5 (EXP5) in a Ran-GTP dependent manner. (Yi, et al., 2003) In the cytoplasm, the end opposite to Drosha cleavage in the mature miRNA is cleaved by another RNase III enzyme, Dicer, yielding a 22-25nt duplex. (Hutvagner, et al., 2001, Ketting, et al., 2001) Once the mature miRNA duplex is created, one strand of the duplex is loaded into a multi-protein complex, RNA-induced silencing complex (RISC), to direct subsequent miRNA:mRNA target interaction and gene silencing. (Bartel, 2004, Filipowicz, et al., 2008) This strand is called the guide strand (miRNA), while the other strand is termed the passenger strand (miRNA*), which usually undergoes degradation. There are cases where both strands can mediate subsequent gene silencing. The determination of guide/passenger strand is believed to depend on the thermodynamic stability of the base pairing at the ends of the duplex. The strand whose 5′ end displays less stability will become the guide strand. (Khvorova, et al., 2003) The catalytic component of RISC is the Argonaute (AGO) protein, which mediates binding and silencing of the target mRNAs. (Pillai, et al., 2004)

In general, miRNAs down-regulate translation by binding to the miRNA response elements (MREs) in the 3′UTR (3′ untranslated region) of their mRNA targets to cause inhibition of mRNA translation, and in some cases, mRNA destabilization. (Filipowicz, et al., 2008) Complementarity between miRNAs and MREs have been shown to be near perfect in plants, but only partial in animals. Multiple mechanisms of action have been proposed. AGO proteins in RISC may inhibit translation initiation by competing with eIF4E for mRNA m^7G cap-recognition. (Kiriakidou, et al., 2007, Mathonnet, et al., 2007) Alternatively, RISC may inhibit translation initiation by preventing the assembly of 80S ribosomes via recruitment of eIF6. (Chendrimada, et al., 2007) There is also evidence that RISC can repress translation post-initiation by causing ribosome drop-off or nascent polypeptide degradation during the elongation step. (Petersen, et al., 2006) Finally, miRNAs can accelerate mRNA destabilization. miRNA-associated targets were found to be enriched in P-bodies, compartmentalized cytoplasmic foci where mRNA decay occurs (Sheth and Parker, 2003), and to be associated with deadenylase, decapping enzymes and exonucleases. (Behm-Ansmant, et al., 2006, Liu, et al., 2005)

miRNA target identification in animals is relatively difficult because of imperfect miRNA:MRE complementarity. One important finding is the so-called "seed rule", in which extensive Watson-Crick base paring between the "seed" region (2-7 nt from the 5′ end) of the miRNA and its target, remarkably reduces the number of false positive predictions. (Lewis, et al., 2003, Lim, et al., 2005) The seed rule has been widely applied as the fundamental criteria by most current prediction algorithms to screen for potential miRNA target genes. Nevertheless, considerable evidence exists to argue that the seed pairing is either not required or not sufficient for predicting miRNA:mRNA interactions. (Didiano and Hobert, 2006) Other features within 3′UTRs, in addition to seed pairing, have been demonstrated to be important determinants, including overall thermodynamic stability of miRNA:mRNA duplex, total number of MREs within the 3′UTR, accessibility of the MRE, position of the MRE related to the stop codon, and local AU rich elements. (Hon and Zhang, 2007, Kertesz, et al., 2007, Li, et al., 2008) Thus, current computational target prediction is far from established, and predicted target candidates need to be experimental verified.

Both biogenesis and function of miRNAs are subject to tight regulation. Almost every aspect of miRNA biogenesis, from transcription and processing to subcellular localization and stability, can be regulated in a sequence-specific and cell-specific manner. Such regulation is believed to be important for many developmental and physiological processes. For example, the transcription factors Myogenin and MyoD1 induce expression of miR-1 and miR-133 specifically during myogenesis. (Rao, et al., 2006) During stem cell differentiation, the levels of pri-let-7 remain constant, while the levels of mature let-7 duplex increase. (Piskounova, et al., 2008) Interestingly, post-transcriptional suppression of let-7 in undifferentiated cells is mediated by its target Lin-28. Lin-28 not only blocks microprocessor cleavage in the nucleus by directly binding to the loop region of pri-let-7, (Piskounova, et al., 2008) but also prevents Dicer cleavage in the cytoplasm by promoting polyuridylation and degradation of pre-let-7. (Heo, et al., 2009) The nuclear export of miRNA is usually the rate-limiting step of miRNA biosynthesis. (Grimm, et al., 2006) Some pre-miRNAs such as human pre-miR-31, pre-miR-128, and pre-miR-105 are retained in the nucleus instead of being processed into mature miRNAs in certain cell types. (Lee, et al., 2008) Finally, although the degradation of miRNAs is not well-understood, the enrichment of guide strands but not passenger strands in the cells clearly indicates the existence of an as-yet unknown mechanism that quickly and selectively turns over these small RNAs. A family of exoribonucleases that degrades miRNAs have been identified in *A. thaliana*. (Ramachandran and Chen, 2008) Furthermore, under certain conditions, miRNA-mediated silencing can be reversed or blocked. (Kedde, et al., 2007, Schratt, et al., 2006) For example, mir-122-mediated repression of CAT1 (cationic amino acid transporter 1) can be alleviated in human cells lines as a response to starvation or other types of cell stress. (Bhattacharyya, et al., 2006)

3. miRNAs and the host immune system

Mammalian systems have developed a complex system of checks and balances to regulate gene expression in order to respond to pathogen infection. In the last several years, miRNAs are increasingly becoming implicated in the regulation of both immune cell development and function. Proper functioning of the immune system requires elaborate control of both innate and adaptive immune response in order to defend against various pathogens while maintaining self tolerance. miRNAs are required for normal immune system function by helping to maintain this balance. miR-146a is upregulated in human monocytes upon exposure to lipopolysaccharide (LPS), a cell wall component of Gram negative bacteria and established activator of innate immunity. Its upregulation is dependent on NF-κB, a key transcription factor that regulates practically all aspects of the innate immune response, such as synthesis of pro-inflammatory cytokines, including TNFα and IL-1β, and regulation of immune cell migration. Interestingly, TRAF6 (TNF receptor-associated factor 6) and IRAK1 (IL-1 receptor-associated kinase 1), two components of the Toll-like receptor 4 (TLR4) signaling pathway that act upstream of NF-κB, were found to be targets of miR-146a. These findings suggest that miRNAs function in the negative feedback regulation of TLR signaling in order to ensure appropriate strength and duration of the innate immune response. (Taganov, et al., 2006) Another inflammatory mediator, miR-155, is induced by LPS (Ceppi, et al., 2009, O'Connell, et al., 2007, Tili, et al., 2007) and nucleic acids, including poly(I:C) (polyriboinosinic:polyribocytidylic acid) and hypomethylated DNA (O'Connell, et al., 2007), implicating function in both bacterial and viral infection. miR-155 is proposed to fine tune inflammatory cytokine production through negative feedback loops by targeting TAB2 (Ceppi, et al., 2009), FADD (fas-associated death domain protein), IKKε (IκB kinase ε), and Ripk1 (receptor-interacting serine-threonine kinase 1). (Tili, et al., 2007)

In addition to innate immunity, the adaptive immune response is also subject to regulation by miRNAs, in particular miR-155. miR-155-deficient dendritic cells exhibited impaired ability in antigen presentation and T cell activation, suggesting its involvement in bridging innate and adaptive immunity. (Rodriguez, et al., 2007) miR-155 restricts Th2 but not Th1 lineage commitment after CD4+ T cell activation (Rodriguez, et al., 2007, Thai, et al., 2007), and is also required for the differentiation and proliferation of regulatory T helper cells, which function to self-limit the immune response. (Kohlhaas, et al., 2009, Lu, et al., 2009) Furthermore, miR-155 was induced in B lymphocytes upon activation and regulates the germinal center response and generation of immunoglobulin class-switched plasma cells. (Teng, et al., 2008, Thai, et al., 2007, Vigorito, et al., 2007) Naïve B lymphocytes express only immunoglobulin M (IgM) isotype antibodies on the cell surface as a result of V(D)J DNA recombination. Upon activation, B lymphocytes undergo somatic hypermutation (SHM), gene conversion (GCV), affinity maturation, and class-switched recombination (CSR) to produce a vast antibody repertoire with increased diversity, higher antigen-binding affinity, and different isotypes. miR-155 has been shown to regulate expression of activation-induced cytidine deaminase (AID), which catalyzes the SHM, GCV and CSR processes by deaminating cytosine to introduce U:G mismatches in Ig genes. (Teng, et al., 2008) Disruption of miR-155-AID interaction in vivo results in quantitative and temporal alteration of AID expression and defective antibody maturation. Another target of miR-155, the transcription factor PU.1, has been reported to be involved in the reduction of IgG1-switched plasma cells in a miR-155 deficient mouse model. (Vigorito, et al., 2007)

Several miRNAs have also been implicated in different immune development processes. miR-223 is activated by the myeloid transcription factors PU.1 and C/EBP (CCAAT/enhancer-binding protein) and has been shown to control granulocyte development. (Fazi, et al., 2005, Johnnidis, et al., 2008) miR-150 is an important regulator of B cell differentiation through targeting of the transcription factor c-Myb. (Xiao, et al., 2007, Zhou, et al., 2007) Finally, miR-181a modulates T cell receptor sensitivity and signaling strength during positive and negative selection, most likely through downregulation of phosphatases. (Li, et al., 2007)

4. miRNAs and viruses

Interestingly, miRNAs have been identified in various members of the herpesvirus family, such as Epstein-Barr virus (EBV), herpes simplex virus 1 (HSV-1), Kaposi's sarcoma-associated herpesvirus (KSHV), and human cytomegalovirus (HCMV), during both the latent and the productive stage of the viral life cycle. These viral miRNAs share the same biogenesis and execution pathways as their cellular counterparts, and downregulate either viral or host mRNAs in order to evade the host immune system or to control the transition from latent to the productive replication stage. (Cullen, 2009) For example, the degradation of EBV DNA polymerase mRNA by miR-BART2 (Barth, et al., 2008), the suppression of HSV-1 immediate early proteins ICP0 and ICP4 by miR-H2-3p and miR-H6 (Umbach, et al., 2008), and the downregulaton of HCMV viral immediate-early protein IE1 by miR-UL112-1 (Murphy, et al., 2008), help to establish and maintain viral latency. KSHV miRNA miR-K12-6-3p contributes to the formation of Kaposi's sarcoma tumors in vivo by downregulation of host gene THBS1 (thrombospondin 1). (Samols, et al., 2007) Downregulation of host MICB mRNA (major histocompatibility complex class I polypeptide-related sequence B), a ligand for natural killer cells, by HCMV miRNA miR-UL112-1 protects infected cells from natural killer cells. (Stern-Ginossar, et al., 2007) Another host antiviral gene CXCL11 (CXC-chemokine ligand 11), a target of EBV miRNA miR-BHRF1-3, is downregulated to protect infected B cells from being targeted by cytotoxic T cells. (Xia, et al., 2008)

5. Targeting miRNA expression to modulate gene expression

Medical countermeasures that exploit miRNA function have focused on therapies for cancer. Different approaches have been developed to manipulate expression levels of miRNAs and determine downstream effects on disease. (Fig. 2) A number of studies have demonstrated that specific miRNAs exhibit altered expression levels in tumors, and that "normalization" of miRNA expression in cancer cells may have a therapeutic effect. To up-regulate miRNA expression, either miRNA mimics or miRNA expression vectors can be overexpressed in target cells and tissues. Mirna Therapeutics has reported the systemic delivery of mimics for miR-34 and let-7 via a neutral lipid emulsion, as a strategy for miRNA replacement therapy to inhibit tumor growth and metastasis in a mouse model. (Trang, et al., 2011, Wiggins, et al., 2010) Both miR-34 and let-7 are natural tumor suppressors that exhibit reduced expression in different cancers. Introduction of the mimics in mice led to ~60% reduction in tumor area compared to control mice. These results offer a novel therapeutic strategy for cancer by restoring miR-34 and let-7 expression to wild-type levels to reduce tumor growth. Given that miR-34 and let-7 levels are reduced in a number of different cancers, it may be the case that synthetic miRNA mimics can have broad applicability as anti-cancer agents.

Inhibitory agents that down-regulate miRNA expression, termed antagomirs, have been developed to pair with mature miRNAs through sequence complementarity and block miRNA-mediated gene regulation. (Hutvagner, et al., 2004, Krutzfeldt, et al., 2005) Development of antagomirs that contain locked nucleic acids (LNAs), a backbone modification in which the ribose moiety has been locked by an oxymethylene bridge connecting the C(2') and C(4') atoms of the ribose, have yielded unusually stable oligonucleotides with high duplex melting temperatures for more robust therapeutic studies. Their relatively small size, high affinity, and potential for systemic delivery without complicated delivery vehicles has established LNA oligos as a favorite platform for design of RNA-based drug candidates. Antagomirs against miR-16, miR-122, miR-192, and miR-194, conjugated to cholesterol, have been intravenously administered in mice, and corresponding miRNA levels exhibited marked reduction in multiple organs and tissues. A systemically administered unconjugated LNA-anti-miR-122 oligonucleotide led to specific, dose-dependent silencing of miR-122 in non-human primates. (Elmen, et al., 2008) This particular anti-miR was composed of 15 nucleotides, which covered the seed sequence in the 3' UTR of miR-122 and adjacent nucleotides. In a recent study, 7-mer and 8-mer anti-miRs that only targeted the seed sequence exhibited potent inhibition of miR-21, which exhibits elevated levels in a variety of cancers. (Obad, et al., 2011) These short anti-miRs form strong hybrids with their target miRNAs and sterically block miRNA function. Injection of anti-miR-21 into mice yielded sequestration of the hybrid complex in the main organs and resultant upregulation of a miR-21 gene target. Their enhanced stability and relatively small size positions these seed-directed anti-miRs as potentially strong drug candidates to target specific miRNAs or miRNA families that function in disease onset.

Viral miRNAs are potential anti-viral candidates for therapeutic development and can serve as diagnostic markers for viral infection or specific stages of disease. The host miR-122, which has two recognition sites in the 5′ UTR of the hepatitis C virus (HCV) genome, is required for virus replication. (Jopling, et al., 2005) Use of specific antagonists that target miR-122 resulted in a reduction in HCV in the liver of a primate model, demonstrating the therapeutic utility of this strategy.(Lanford, et al., 2010) The anti-miR-122 treatment provided continued efficacy in the animals up to several months after the treatment period with no adverse effects or evidence of viral rebound. Based on these studies, Santaris Pharma A/S has initiated the first miRNA-targeted Phase 2a clinical trial, based on the miR-122-inhibitory drug, Miravirsen, to assess safety and tolerability in up to 55 treatment-naïve patients infected with HCV. Designed using LNA technology, Miravirsen sequesters miR-122 from HCV, thus inhibiting replication of the virus. Secondary validation studies, including drug pharmacokinetics and effect on viral load, will be assessed. miRNA technology has also been applied to vaccine development for influenza virus. A miRNA-responsive element (MRE) was introduced into the viral nucleoprotein gene to control the level of viral attenuation via miR-124, which targets the MRE sequence. The resulting viruses produced a species-specific vaccine that generated high levels of neutralizing antibodies in the host. (Perez, et al., 2009)

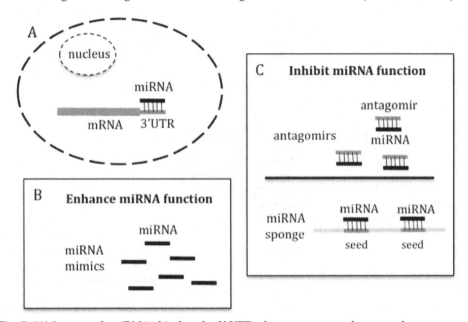

Fig. 2. (A) In general, miRNAs bind to the 3′ UTR of target genes to downregulate gene expression. (B) miRNA mimics provide increased numbers of miRNAs by overexpression or synthetic copies to enhance miRNA function. (C) Inhibition of miRNA function can be achieved by usage of (1) antagomirs, stable complementary oligonucleotides, that hybridize to target miRNAs, or with (2) miRNA sponges, which provide alternative binding platforms to levels sequester miRNAs.

Artificial miRNA decoys, termed miRNA "sponges", provide alternative binding platforms for the miRNAs and inhibit their ability to bind and suppress their endogenous targets. The miRNA sponges often contain a strong promoter to drive expression of binding sites for the miRNA either in a non-coding transcript or in the 3'UTR of a reporter gene, like GFP. (Brown and Naldini, 2009, Ebert, et al., 2007) Since the interaction between miRNAs and target genes is largely dependent on the seed region of the miRNA, design of the miRNA sponges that incorporate the seed sequence can interact with all members of a miRNA seed family. Both individual miRNAs and large seed families, such as miR-155 and the let-7 family, respectively, have been successfully targeted for continuous loss of miRNA function in multiple mammalian cell lines. (Bolisetty, et al., 2009, Kumar, et al., 2008) Compared to miRNA antisense oligonucleotides, a major advantage of miRNA sponges is the potential for stable integration for continual expression in the genome. Stable transfection of miRNA sponges in cultured cells led to partial derepression of miRNA target gene expression in a variety of cell systems, including mesenchymal stem cells (Huang, et al., 2010) and cancer cell models. (Bonci, et al., 2008, Valastyan, et al., 2009) A high expression level is often required for sufficient inhibition of endogenous miRNAs, given the much lower transgene copy number in stable lines compared to transient plasmid transfection. Forty integrated copies of a miRNA sponge targeting miR-223 driven by a weak promoter were needed to sufficiently suppress miR-223 expression. (Gentner, et al., 2009) Stable expression of sponges also enables miRNA loss-of-function studies that can span days to weeks. After 6 days, neurons that express anti-miR-92 sponges exhibited derepression of a potassium chloride cotransporter and electrophysiological changes in response to GABA treatment. (Barbato, et al., 2010) Both miR-144 and miR-451 were found to be required for erythropoiesis in bone marrow reconstitution experiments 3-4 weeks after transplantation of cells expressing miRNA sponges. (Papapetrou, et al., 2010)

6. RNAi therapeutics: Development of siRNAs for disease therapy

The potential development of new therapies for infectious disease using RNAi-based strategies has attracted the attention of biotechnology entrepreneurs. Multiple small companies have entered the field to transition RNAi from molecular biology tool to next-generation nucleotide-based drugs for treatment of disease. In the last ten years, there have been a growing number of clinical trials based on siRNAs, ~20 bp short interfering RNAs that silence target genes by directing their cognate mRNAs for degradation by the RISC complex. (Davidson and McCray, 2011, Vaishnaw, et al., 2010) Some programs involve local delivery of siRNAs to target tissues, including the eye, kidney, and liver, while others aim to achieve systemic delivery in the body. As with any novel strategy for drug development, there still remain technical challenges that need to be overcome before RNAi-based technology can successfully transition into robust therapies, including minimization of off-target effects (OTE) and systemic delivery of siRNAs in the body. A summary of these challenges and the methods that have been utilized to move the field of RNAi-based therapeutics forward is summarized in Table 1. Given that miRNA-based therapies will most likely face similar challenges that are currently being addressed by the more mature siRNA-anchored drug companies, we provide an overview of the strategies utilized in siRNA-based drug discovery.

6.1 Off-target effects

All RNAi-based therapeutics remain vulnerable to the potential of OTE, in which expression of non-targeted genes is unintentionally modulated. OTE can be categorized into sequence-dependent and sequence-independent effects. In the case of sequence-dependence, the siRNAs can bind to bystander mRNAs that exhibit partial sequence complementarity but is unrelated to the target gene. This type of OTE can be mitigated through use of bioinformatics screening algorithms to design siRNA sequences that exhibit rare or no direct complementarity to other genome sequences aside from the target gene. In sequence-independent OTE, the siRNAs may have inherent immunostimulatory properties or the endogenous miRNA pathway may be saturated, especially in the case of overexpression of heterologous siRNAs. For example, RNAs have been shown to stimulate the Toll-like receptor (TLR) (Kleinman, et al., 2008) and retinoic acid inducible gene (RIG)-I pathways. (Yoneyama, et al., 2004) Since there does not exist any a priori knowledge about which signaling pathways are activated by specific siRNAs, it may be necessary to evaluate a panel of pro-inflammatory markers to downselect siRNAs with comparatively reduced immunostimulatory properties in preclinical assays. RNAi-based therapies also need to be cautious about the level of exogenous siRNAs expressed in the host. In mouse studies, PolII promoter-driven expression of plasmid-based short hairpin RNA (shRNA) constructs in the liver induced host mortality, which has been attributed to saturation of the transport factor, Exportin 5, that ferries miRNAs from the nucleus to the cytoplasm. (Grimm, et al., 2006) Thus, it is necessary to determine the lowest possible concentration of siRNAs that can still be therapeutically effective for introduction into the host. OTEs and non-specific immunostimulatory responses can also be mitigated using different siRNA backbone modifications, including 2'-O-Me modifications (Jackson, et al., 2006) or DNA substitutions. (Ui-Tei, et al., 2008) Once candidate siRNAs have passed a threshold efficacy level in *in vitro* cell culture studies, leads are then assessed using good laboratory practice (GLP)-compliant preclinical toxicological studies with animal models such as rodents and non-human primates.

6.2 siRNAs enter clinical trials

Alnylam Pharmaceuticals currently has several advanced RNAi-based therapeutic programs that target multiple diseases. Alnylam has completed Phase II clinical trials on ALN-RSV01, a siRNA-based inhaled treatment for respiratory syncytial virus (RSV) that targets the nucleocapsid encoding gene in the virus. (Alvarez, et al., 2009) Lung transplant patients exhibited improved symptom scores and overall lung function. Alnylam has also developed ALN-VSP, a cocktail for two siRNAs that target vascular endothelial growth factor and kinesin spindle protein, as a systemically delivered liver cancer therapy. In Phase I trials, ALN-VSP was well tolerated and reduced tumor blood flow in patients. Finally, Alnylam has initiated a Phase I study of ALN-TTR01, a siRNA therapeutic that targets transthryretin (TTR), a carrier for thyroid hormones and retinol binding proteins, which is mutated in hereditary TTR-mediated amyloidosis. Pre-clinical trials have demonstrated that ALN-TTR01 can cause regression of amyloid deposits and silence the TTR gene.

Other companies have multiple RNAi-based drugs in the R&D pre-clinical and Phase I pipelines, targeting a wide range of disease conditions, including age-related macular degeneration (AMD) and various cancers. (Vaishnaw, et al., 2010) In addition to the Alnylam siRNA drug against RSV, there have been some inroads into development of RNAi-based therapies to treat infectious disease. For example, Tacere Therapeutics has developed a RNAi-based cocktail that targets three separate conserved regions of the Hepatitis C virus (HCV) and can be delivered to liver cells via intravenous administration using encapsidation in an adeno-associated protein coat. In animal studies, this therapeutic agent targeted and cleaved HCV at three different sites simultaneously without toxicity. In a pilot Phase I/II clinical trial, Benitec Ltd., in collaboration with City of Hope National Medical Center, demonstrated long-term expression of three RNA-based anti-HIV moieties (tat/rev short hairpin RNA, TAR decoy, and CCR5 ribozyme) in hematopoietic progenitor cells that support the development of an RNA-based cell therapy platform for HIV. (DiGiusto, et al., 2010) The gene-modified stem cells had been infused into HIV-positive patients via autologous bone marrow transplantation to treat AIDS-related lymphomas. In another study, intranasal delivery of siRNAs in a SARS coronavirus (SCV) rhesus macaque model was also effective in reducing SARS-like physiological symptoms, RNA expression of SCV genes, and lung histopathology associated with viral disease. (Li, et al., 2005)

Challenge	Methods to address challenge
RNA stability	Locked nucleic acids (LNA)
	Short (7-8-mer) seed-directed anti-miRs
Off-target effects	
Sequence-dependent	Bioinformatic screening algorithms
Sequence-independent	Evaluation of immunostimulatory properties
	Reduction of RNA expression levels
	Use of different RNA backbone modifications
	DNA sequence substitution
Systemic delivery	
Chemical modifications	Cholesterol
	Chitosan
	Lipophilic molecules (e.g. bile acids)
Packaging carriers	Lipid nanoparticles (LNPs, SNALPs)
	Multiple lipid bi-layer nanoparticles (Atuplex)
	Transferrin-decorated cyclodextrin particles
	Nanoparticles decorated with leukocyte receptor antibody
	Dynamic polyconjugates

Table 1. Transition of RNAi-based approaches to the therapeutic arena

It is also informative to describe siRNA-based clinical trials that were terminated prematurely due to conclusions that the study was unlikely to yield an effective drug. Bevasiranib (Opko Health Inc.) and AGN211745 (Allergan Inc.) were developed to target the vascular endothelial growth factor (VEGF) pathways to treat patients with AMD via the intravitreal route. The overgrowth of blood vessels behind the retina causes irreversible loss of vision. Despite initial positive reports of efficacy demonstrating reduced neovascularization upon direct ocular injection of VEGF siRNA (Shen, et al., 2006), both studies were terminated during Phase II/III of clinical trials, amid suggestions that the two siRNAs activated TLR3 to mediate its effects in preclinical models, rather than direct inhibition of target gene expression. (Kleinman, et al., 2008, Vaishnaw, et al., 2010)

6.3 Delivery of stable siRNAs into the body

A major technical challenge for RNAi-based therapy is drug stability in the body and efficient systemic delivery in sufficient quantity to have a therapeutic effect. Given their size and negative charge, siRNAs cannot easily cross the host cell membrane. Unmodified siRNAs injected into the body may be subject to RNase-mediated degradation and rapid renal excretion. Thus, therapeutic siRNAs are often chemically modified and/or packaged into carriers for delivery into the host. Various means of delivery have been tested in murine and non-human primate models, including in nanoparticles, complexed with polyconjugates, attached to cholesterol groups, or conjugated with cell surface receptors. (Table 1)

Tekmira Pharmaceuticals Corp. has developed stable nucleic acid lipid nanoparticles (LNPs, formerly referred to as SNALPs), composed of several non-covalently associated components, including an ionizable lipid, polyethylene glycol (PEG)-lipid, cholesterol, and a neutral lipid. LNPs containing siRNAs that target several Zaire Ebola (ZEBOV) viral proteins were delivered into a lethal non-human primate macaque model of ZEBOV-mediated hemorrhagic fever. (Geisbert, et al., 2010) All macaques given seven post-exposure treatments were protected against ZEBOV, demonstrating the efficacy of LNP-mediated siRNA therapy for emerging viral infections. Tekmira has also applied LNP-based delivery to a Phase I trial involving 23 patients with mild hypercholesterolemia. Alnylam Pharmaceuticals has also reported systemic delivery of siRNAs that target apolipoprotein B (ApoB), encapsulated in LNPs, by intravenous injection in cynomolgus monkeys. (Zimmermann, et al., 2006) A single injection was shown to last for more than 11 days, induced significant reductions in serum cholesterol and low-density lipoprotein levels, and resulted in greater than 90% target knockdown with no detectable toxicity. Silence Therapeutics has developed an independent nanoparticle approach, the AtuPlex technology, that embeds therapeutic siRNAs into multiple lipid bi-layer structures to provide systemic delivery to specific tissues. Pfizer and Quark Pharmaceuticals are currently testing delivery of therapeutic siRNAs using the Silence technology to treat AMD and diabetic macular edema in two separate Phase II trials. Pre-clinical data has indicated that therapy decreases onset of known endpoints in AMD.

Calando Pharmaceuticals has initiated a Phase I clinical trial that utilizes receptor-mediated delivery of siRNAs encapsulated in cyclodextrin particles decorated with transferrin. Cancer cells, which often overexpress the transferrin receptor, are thus more likely to take up the particles for targeted therapeutic delivery. The trial targeted a subunit of ribonucleotide reductase, an enzyme required for DNA synthesis, to inhibit cancer and tumor growth. Tumor biopsies from melanoma patients show the presence of intracellularly localized nanoparticles. Furthermore, mRNA and protein levels for ribonucleotide reductase in tumors were decreased compared to pre-dosing tissue. (Davis, et al., 2010) Another targeted receptor-based strategy is siRNA delivery to a specific class of leukocytes involved in gut inflammation. A cyclin D1 (Cyd-1)-targeted siRNA was loaded into stabilized nanoparticles, the surfaces of which incorporated an antibody specific for a receptor expressed by the leukocytes. The targeted siRNA-containing nanoparticles down-regulated the cyclin D1 target, suppressed leukocyte proliferation, and reversed experimentally-induced colitis in mice. (Peer, et al., 2008)

Cholesterol carriers enable improved siRNA uptake in the liver, with the cholesterol easily bound by low-density lipoprotein (LDL) in serum and robust LDL uptake in the liver.

(Soutschek, et al., 2004) An siRNA targeting apolipoprotein B (apoB) has been conjugated to cholesterol in order to load siRNAs into circulating LDLs for enhanced stability and to increase receptor-mediated uptake into target hepatocytes. (Soutschek, et al., 2004, Wolfrum, et al., 2007) ApoB siRNAs have also been complexed with dynamic polyconjugates, PEG, and the liver-targeting ligand N-acetyl galactosamine to achieve site-directed delivery and potent ApoB knock-down. (Rozema, et al., 2007) Lipophilic siRNAs can also bind high-density lipoprotein (HDL) and target to tissues with HDL receptors, such as gut and brain. (Chen, et al., 2010, Wolfrum, et al., 2007) Oral delivery of glucan-encapsulated siRNA particles has been reported to target Map4k4 in gut macrophages to protect mice from LPS-induced toxicity. (Aouadi, et al., 2009) Finally, the polymer chitosan has mucoadhesive properties and has been used for intranasal delivery of siRNAs specific to a BCR/ABL-1 junction sequence, into bronchiolar epithelial cells in mice, resulting in ~40% reduction of target gene expression. (Howard, et al., 2006)

7. Conclusions: Strategies and future of miRNA therapeutic applications

Recent advances in the understanding of miRNA structure and function has enabled development of novel miRNA-based strategies for combating human infectious disease. The technologies that have already been developed for stabilization and drug delivery of siRNA-based therapeutics will no doubt accelerate transition of miRNAs into the therapeutic arena. Given that miRNAs are thought to regulate tens to hundreds of genes in the cell, caution must be taken since there may be unintended downstream consequences on cell function by seemingly small alterations in miRNA expression. A recent development that may greatly advance anti-miR therapeutics is the silencing of miRNA families with short LNA antagomirs that specifically target the miRNA seed sequences. (Obad, et al., 2011) The relatively short 7-8 nucleotide lengths of these LNA sequences may bypass the need for carrier formulation for systemic administration in the host and reduce the manufacturing costs of RNAi therapeutics. Further research, including clinical trials, will determine the efficacy of these short antagomirs for treatment of human disease.

Several companies have been established to specifically develop high-impact medicines based on miRNAs, including Santaris Pharma A/S, Mirna Therapeutics, and Regulus Therapeutics. As aforementioned, Santaris has developed a LNA-based anti-miR-122 drug, Miravirsen, to inhibit HCV infection in Phase II clinical trials. Mirna Therapeutics has demonstrated intravenous administration of a neutral lipid emulsion to facilitate systemic delivery of tumor suppressor miRNA mimics modeled after the natural tumor suppressors let-7 and miR-34 to inhibit tumor growth. (Trang, et al., 2011) Regulus Therapeutics is focusing on both miR-21 as a potential target to reverse fibrosis and cancer onset and miR-122 to reduce cholesterol levels and inhibit HCV infection. Other studies in the laboratory have implicated miRNAs in key organ function. For example, the cardiac-specific miR-208 is required for cardiomyocyte hypertrophy, fibrosis and expression of bMHC in response to stress and hypothyroidism. (van Rooij, et al., 2007) This momentum in development of RNAi-based drug strategies represents an exciting time for translational research that links fundamental bioscience discovery in cancer and infectious disease to therapeutic treatment. The overall promise of miRNAs as a powerful new approach to induce sequence-specific inhibition of gene expression has generated enormous enthusiasm and hope in the biomedical community that miRNA-based therapeutic treatment of disease can become a reality in the near future.

8. Acknowledgements

The writing of this review was supported by a Los Alamos National Laboratory LDRD-DR grant to study small RNAs in host-pathogen interactions.

9. References

Alvarez, R., Elbashir, S., Borland, T., Toudjarska, I., Hadwiger, P., John, M., Roehl, I., Morskaya, S. S., Martinello, R., Kahn, J., Van Ranst, M., Tripp, R. A., DeVincenzo, J. P., Pandey, R., Maier, M., Nechev, L., Manoharan, M., Kotelianski, V.&Meyers, R. (2009) RNA interference-mediated silencing of the respiratory syncytial virus nucleocapsid defines a potent antiviral strategy. *Antimicrob Agents Chemother*, 53, 9, 3952-62.

Aouadi, M., Tesz, G. J., Nicoloro, S. M., Wang, M., Chouinard, M., Soto, E., Ostroff, G. R.&Czech, M. P. (2009) Orally delivered siRNA targeting macrophage Map4k4 suppresses systemic inflammation. *Nature*, 458, 7242, 1180-4.

Barbato, C., Ruberti, F., Pieri, M., Vilardo, E., Costanzo, M., Ciotti, M. T., Zona, C.&Cogoni, C. (2010) MicroRNA-92 modulates K(+) Cl(-) co-transporter KCC2 expression in cerebellar granule neurons. *J Neurochem*, 113, 3, 591-600.

Bartel, D. (2004) MicroRNAs: genomics, biogenesis, mechanism, and function. *Cell*, 116, 281-297.

Barth, S., Pfuhl, T., Mamiani, A., Ehses, C., Roemer, K., Kremmer, E., Jaker, C., Hock, J., Meister, G.&Grasser, F. A. (2008) Epstein-Barr virus-encoded microRNA miR-BART2 down-regulates the viral DNA polymerase BALF5. *Nucleic Acids Res*, 36, 2, 666-75.

Behm-Ansmant, I., Rehwinkel, J., Doerks, T., Stark, A., Bork, P.&Izaurralde, E. (2006) mRNA degradation by miRNAs and GW182 requires both CCR4:NOT deadenylase and DCP1:DCP2 decapping complexes. *Genes Dev*, 20, 14, 1885-98.

Bhattacharyya, S. N., Habermacher, R., Martine, U., Closs, E. I.&Filipowicz, W. (2006) Relief of microRNA-mediated translational repression in human cells subjected to stress. *Cell*, 125, 6, 1111-24.

Bolisetty, M. T., Dy, G., Tam, W.&Beemon, K. L. (2009) Reticuloendotheliosis virus strain T induces miR-155, which targets JARID2 and promotes cell survival. *J Virol*, 83, 23, 12009-17.

Bonci, D., Coppola, V., Musumeci, M., Addario, A., Giuffrida, R., Memeo, L., D'Urso, L., Pagliuca, A., Biffoni, M., Labbaye, C., Bartucci, M., Muto, G., Peschle, C.&De Maria, R. (2008) The miR-15a-miR-16-1 cluster controls prostate cancer by targeting multiple oncogenic activities. *Nat Med*, 14, 11, 1271-7.

Brown, B. D.&Naldini, L. (2009) Exploiting and antagonizing microRNA regulation for therapeutic and experimental applications. *Nat Rev Genet*, 10, 8, 578-85.

Cai, X., Hagedorn, C. H.&Cullen, B. R. (2004) Human microRNAs are processed from capped, polyadenylated transcripts that can also function as mRNAs. *Rna*, 10, 12, 1957-66.

Ceppi, M., Pereira, P. M., Dunand-Sauthier, I., Barras, E., Reith, W., Santos, M. A.&Pierre, P. (2009) MicroRNA-155 modulates the interleukin-1 signaling pathway in activated human monocyte-derived dendritic cells. *Proc Natl Acad Sci U S A*, 106, 8, 2735-40.

Chen, Q., Butler, D., Querbes, W., Pandey, R. K., Ge, P., Maier, M. A., Zhang, L., Rajeev, K. G., Nechev, L., Kotelianski, V., Manoharan, M.&Sah, D. W. (2010) Lipophilic siRNAs mediate efficient gene silencing in oligodendrocytes with direct CNS delivery. *J Control Release*, 144, 2, 227-32.

Chendrimada, T. P., Finn, K. J., Ji, X., Baillat, D., Gregory, R. I., Liebhaber, S. A., Pasquinelli, A. E.&Shiekhattar, R. (2007) MicroRNA silencing through RISC recruitment of eIF6. *Nature*, 447, 7146, 823-8.

Cullen, B. R. (2009) Viral and cellular messenger RNA targets of viral microRNAs. *Nature*, 457, 7228, 421-5.

Davidson, B. L.&McCray, P. B., Jr. (2011) Current prospects for RNA interference-based therapies. *Nat Rev Genet*, 12, 5, 329-40.

Davis, M. E., Zuckerman, J. E., Choi, C. H., Seligson, D., Tolcher, A., Alabi, C. A., Yen, Y., Heidel, J. D.&Ribas, A. (2010) Evidence of RNAi in humans from systemically administered siRNA via targeted nanoparticles. *Nature*, 464, 7291, 1067-70.

Didiano, D.&Hobert, O. (2006) Perfect seed pairing is not a generally reliable predictor for miRNA-target interactions. *Nat Struct Mol Biol*, 13, 9, 849-51.

DiGiusto, D. L., Krishnan, A., Li, L., Li, H., Li, S., Rao, A., Mi, S., Yam, P., Stinson, S., Kalos, M., Alvarnas, J., Lacey, S. F., Yee, J. K., Li, M., Couture, L., Hsu, D., Forman, S. J., Rossi, J. J.&Zaia, J. A. (2010) RNA-based gene therapy for HIV with lentiviral vector-modified CD34(+) cells in patients undergoing transplantation for AIDS-related lymphoma. *Sci Transl Med*, 2, 36, 36ra43.

Ebert, M. S., Neilson, J. R.&Sharp, P. A. (2007) MicroRNA sponges: competitive inhibitors of small RNAs in mammalian cells. *Nat Methods*, 4, 9, 721-6.

Elmen, J., Lindow, M., Schutz, S., Lawrence, M., Petri, A., Obad, S., Lindholm, M., Hedtjarn, M., Hansen, H. F., Berger, U., Gullans, S., Kearney, P., Sarnow, P., Straarup, E. M.&Kauppinen, S. (2008) LNA-mediated microRNA silencing in non-human primates. *Nature*, 452, 7189, 896-9.

Fazi, F., Rosa, A., Fatica, A., Gelmetti, V., De Marchis, M. L., Nervi, C.&Bozzoni, I. (2005) A minicircuitry comprised of microRNA-223 and transcription factors NFI-A and C/EBPalpha regulates human granulopoiesis. *Cell*, 123, 5, 819-31.

Filipowicz, W., Bhattacharyya, S. N.&Sonenberg, N. (2008) Mechanisms of post-transcriptional regulation by microRNAs: are the answers in sight? *Nat Rev Genet*, 9, 2, 102-14.

Geisbert, T. W., Lee, A. C., Robbins, M., Geisbert, J. B., Honko, A. N., Sood, V., Johnson, J. C., de Jong, S., Tavakoli, I., Judge, A., Hensley, L. E.&Maclachlan, I. (2010) Postexposure protection of non-human primates against a lethal Ebola virus challenge with RNA interference: a proof-of-concept study. *Lancet*, 375, 9729, 1896-905.

Gentner, B., Schira, G., Giustacchini, A., Amendola, M., Brown, B. D., Ponzoni, M.&Naldini, L. (2009) Stable knockdown of microRNA in vivo by lentiviral vectors. *Nat Methods*, 6, 1, 63-6.

Grimm, D., Streetz, K. L., Jopling, C. L., Storm, T. A., Pandey, K., Davis, C. R., Marion, P., Salazar, F.&Kay, M. A. (2006) Fatality in mice due to oversaturation of cellular microRNA/short hairpin RNA pathways. *Nature*, 441, 7092, 537-41.

Grimm, D., Streetz, K. L., Jopling, C. L., Storm, T. A., Pandey, K., Davis, C. R., Marion, P., Salazar, F.&Kay, M. A. (2006) Fatality in mice due to oversaturation of cellular microRNA/short hairpin RNA pathways. *Nature*, 441, 7092, 537.

Heo, I., Joo, C., Kim, Y. K., Ha, M., Yoon, M. J., Cho, J., Yeom, K. H., Han, J.&Kim, V. N. (2009) TUT4 in concert with Lin28 suppresses microRNA biogenesis through pre-microRNA uridylation. *Cell*, 138, 4, 696-708.

Hon, L. S.&Zhang, Z. (2007) The roles of binding site arrangement and combinatorial targeting in microRNA repression of gene expression. *Genome Biol*, 8, 8, R166.

Howard, K. A., Rahbek, U. L., Liu, X., Damgaard, C. K., Glud, S. Z., Andersen, M. O., Hovgaard, M. B., Schmitz, A., Nyengaard, J. R., Besenbacher, F.&Kjems, J. (2006) RNA interference in vitro and in vivo using a novel chitosan/siRNA nanoparticle system. *Mol Ther*, 14, 4, 476-84.

Huang, J., Zhao, L., Xing, L.&Chen, D. (2010) MicroRNA-204 regulates Runx2 protein expression and mesenchymal progenitor cell differentiation. *Stem Cells*, 28, 2, 357-64.

Hutvagner, G., McLachlan, J., Pasquinelli, A. E., Balint, E., Tuschl, T.&Zamore, P. D. (2001) A cellular function for the RNA-interference enzyme Dicer in the maturation of the let-7 small temporal RNA. *Science*, 293, 5531, 834-8.

Hutvagner, G., Simard, M. J., Mello, C. C.&Zamore, P. D. (2004) Sequence-specific inhibition of small RNA function. *PLoS Biol*, 2, 4, E98.

Jackson, A. L., Burchard, J., Leake, D., Reynolds, A., Schelter, J., Guo, J., Johnson, J. M., Lim, L., Karpilow, J., Nichols, K., Marshall, W., Khvorova, A.&Linsley, P. S. (2006) Position-specific chemical modification of siRNAs reduces "off-target" transcript silencing. *RNA*, 12, 7, 1197-205.

Johnnidis, J. B., Harris, M. H., Wheeler, R. T., Stehling-Sun, S., Lam, M. H., Kirak, O., Brummelkamp, T. R., Fleming, M. D.&Camargo, F. D. (2008) Regulation of progenitor cell proliferation and granulocyte function by microRNA-223. *Nature*, 451, 7182, 1125-9.

Jopling, C. L., Yi, M., Lancaster, A. M., Lemon, S. M.&Sarnow, P. (2005) Modulation of hepatitis C virus RNA abundance by a liver-specific MicroRNA. *Science*, 309, 5740, 1577-81.

Kedde, M., Strasser, M. J., Boldajipour, B., Oude Vrielink, J. A., Slanchev, K., le Sage, C., Nagel, R., Voorhoeve, P. M., van Duijse, J., Orom, U. A., Lund, A. H., Perrakis, A., Raz, E.&Agami, R. (2007) RNA-binding protein Dnd1 inhibits microRNA access to target mRNA. *Cell*, 131, 7, 1273-86.

Kertesz, M., Iovino, N., Unnerstall, U., Gaul, U.&Segal, E. (2007) The role of site accessibility in microRNA target recognition. *Nat Genet*, 39, 10, 1278-84.

Ketting, R. F., Fischer, S. E., Bernstein, E., Sijen, T., Hannon, G. J.&Plasterk, R. H. (2001) Dicer functions in RNA interference and in synthesis of small RNA involved in developmental timing in C. elegans. *Genes Dev*, 15, 20, 2654-9.

Khvorova, A., Reynolds, A.&Jayasena, S. D. (2003) Functional siRNAs and miRNAs exhibit strand bias. *Cell*, 115, 2, 209-16.

Kiriakidou, M., Tan, G. S., Lamprinaki, S., De Planell-Saguer, M., Nelson, P. T.&Mourelatos, Z. (2007) An mRNA m7G cap binding-like motif within human Ago2 represses translation. *Cell*, 129, 6, 1141-51.

Kleinman, M. E., Yamada, K., Takeda, A., Chandrasekaran, V., Nozaki, M., Baffi, J. Z., Albuquerque, R. J., Yamasaki, S., Itaya, M., Pan, Y., Appukuttan, B., Gibbs, D., Yang, Z., Kariko, K., Ambati, B. K., Wilgus, T. A., DiPietro, L. A., Sakurai, E., Zhang, K., Smith, J. R., Taylor, E. W.&Ambati, J. (2008) Sequence- and target-independent angiogenesis suppression by siRNA via TLR3. *Nature*, 452, 7187, 591-7.

Kohlhaas, S., Garden, O. A., Scudamore, C., Turner, M., Okkenhaug, K.&Vigorito, E. (2009) Cutting edge: the Foxp3 target miR-155 contributes to the development of regulatory T cells. *J Immunol*, 182, 5, 2578-82.

Krutzfeldt, J., Rajewsky, N., Braich, R., Rajeev, K. G., Tuschl, T., Manoharan, M.&Stoffel, M. (2005) Silencing of microRNAs in vivo with 'antagomirs'. *Nature*, 438, 7068, 685-9.

Kumar, M. S., Erkeland, S. J., Pester, R. E., Chen, C. Y., Ebert, M. S., Sharp, P. A.&Jacks, T. (2008) Suppression of non-small cell lung tumor development by the let-7 microRNA family. *Proc Natl Acad Sci U S A*, 105, 10, 3903-8.

Landthaler, M., Yalcin, A.&Tuschl, T. (2004) The human DiGeorge syndrome critical region gene 8 and Its D. melanogaster homolog are required for miRNA biogenesis. *Curr Biol*, 14, 23, 2162-7.

Lanford, R. E., Hildebrandt-Eriksen, E. S., Petri, A., Persson, R., Lindow, M., Munk, M. E., Kauppinen, S.&Orum, H. (2010) Therapeutic silencing of microRNA-122 in primates with chronic hepatitis C virus infection. *Science*, 327, 5962, 198-201.

Lee, E. J., Baek, M., Gusev, Y., Brackett, D. J., Nuovo, G. J.&Schmittgen, T. D. (2008) Systematic evaluation of microRNA processing patterns in tissues, cell lines, and tumors. *Rna*, 14, 1, 35-42.

Lee, Y., Ahn, C., Han, J., Choi, H., Kim, J., Yim, J., Lee, J., Provost, P., Radmark, O., Kim, S.&Kim, V. N. (2003) The nuclear RNase III Drosha initiates microRNA processing. *Nature*, 425, 6956, 415-9.

Lee, Y., Jeon, K., Lee, J. T., Kim, S.&Kim, V. N. (2002) MicroRNA maturation: stepwise processing and subcellular localization. *Embo J*, 21, 17, 4663-70.

Lee, Y., Kim, M., Han, J., Yeom, K. H., Lee, S., Baek, S. H.&Kim, V. N. (2004) MicroRNA genes are transcribed by RNA polymerase II. *Embo J*, 23, 20, 4051-60.

Lewis, B. P., Burge, C. B.&Bartel, D. P. (2005) Conserved seed pairing, often flanked by adenosines, indicates that thousands of human genes are microRNA targets. *Cell*, 120, 1, 15-20.

Lewis, B. P., Shih, I. H., Jones-Rhoades, M. W., Bartel, D. P.&Burge, C. B. (2003) Prediction of mammalian microRNA targets. *Cell*, 115, 7, 787-98.

Li, B. J., Tang, Q., Cheng, D., Qin, C., Xie, F. Y., Wei, Q., Xu, J., Liu, Y., Zheng, B. J., Woodle, M. C., Zhong, N.&Lu, P. Y. (2005) Using siRNA in prophylactic and therapeutic regimens against SARS coronavirus in Rhesus macaque. *Nat Med*, 11, 9, 944-51.

Li, N., Flynt, A. S., Kim, H. R., Solnica-Krezel, L.&Patton, J. G. (2008) Dispatched Homolog 2 is targeted by miR-214 through a combination of three weak microRNA recognition sites. *Nucleic Acids Res*, 36, 13, 4277-85.

Li, Q. J., Chau, J., Ebert, P. J., Sylvester, G., Min, H., Liu, G., Braich, R., Manoharan, M., Soutschek, J., Skare, P., Klein, L. O., Davis, M. M.&Chen, C. Z. (2007) miR-181a is an intrinsic modulator of T cell sensitivity and selection. *Cell*, 129, 1, 147-61.

Lim, L. P., Lau, N. C., Garrett-Engele, P., Grimson, A., Schelter, J. M., Castle, J., Bartel, D. P., Linsley, P. S.&Johnson, J. M. (2005) Microarray analysis shows that some microRNAs downregulate large numbers of target mRNAs. *Nature*, 433, 7027, 769-73.

Liu, J., Valencia-Sanchez, M. A., Hannon, G. J.&Parker, R. (2005) MicroRNA-dependent localization of targeted mRNAs to mammalian P-bodies. *Nat Cell Biol*, 7, 7, 719.

Lu, L. F., Thai, T. H., Calado, D. P., Chaudhry, A., Kubo, M., Tanaka, K., Loeb, G. B., Lee, H., Yoshimura, A., Rajewsky, K.&Rudensky, A. Y. (2009) Foxp3-dependent microRNA155 confers competitive fitness to regulatory T cells by targeting SOCS1 protein. *Immunity*, 30, 1, 80-91.

Mathonnet, G., Fabian, M. R., Svitkin, Y. V., Parsyan, A., Huck, L., Murata, T., Biffo, S., Merrick, W. C., Darzynkiewicz, E., Pillai, R. S., Filipowicz, W., Duchaine, T. F.&Sonenberg, N. (2007) MicroRNA inhibition of translation initiation in vitro by targeting the cap-binding complex eIF4F. *Science*, 317, 5845, 1764-7.

Murphy, E., Vanicek, J., Robins, H., Shenk, T.&Levine, A. J. (2008) Suppression of immediate-early viral gene expression by herpesvirus-coded microRNAs: implications for latency. *Proc Natl Acad Sci U S A*, 105, 14, 5453-8.

O'Connell, R. M., Taganov, K. D., Boldin, M. P., Cheng, G.&Baltimore, D. (2007) MicroRNA-155 is induced during the macrophage inflammatory response. *Proc Natl Acad Sci U S A*, 104, 5, 1604-9.

Obad, S., Dos Santos, C. O., Petri, A., Heidenblad, M., Broom, O., Ruse, C., Fu, C., Lindow, M., Stenvang, J., Straarup, E. M., Hansen, H. F., Koch, T., Pappin, D., Hannon, G. J.&Kauppinen, S. (2011) Silencing of microRNA families by seed-targeting tiny LNAs. *Nat Genet*, 43, 4, 371-8.

Papapetrou, E. P., Korkola, J. E.&Sadelain, M. (2010) A genetic strategy for single and combinatorial analysis of miRNA function in mammalian hematopoietic stem cells. *Stem Cells*, 28, 2, 287-96.

Peer, D., Park, E. J., Morishita, Y., Carman, C. V.&Shimaoka, M. (2008) Systemic leukocyte-directed siRNA delivery revealing cyclin D1 as an anti-inflammatory target. *Science*, 319, 5863, 627-30.

Perez, J. T., Pham, A. M., Lorini, M. H., Chua, M. A., Steel, J.&tenOever, B. R. (2009) MicroRNA-mediated species-specific attenuation of influenza A virus. *Nat Biotechnol*, 27, 6, 572-6.

Petersen, C. P., Bordeleau, M. E., Pelletier, J.&Sharp, P. A. (2006) Short RNAs repress translation after initiation in mammalian cells. *Mol Cell*, 21, 4, 533-42.

Pillai, R. S., Artus, C. G.&Filipowicz, W. (2004) Tethering of human Ago proteins to mRNA mimics the miRNA-mediated repression of protein synthesis. *Rna*, 10, 10, 1518-25.

Piskounova, E., Viswanathan, S. R., Janas, M., LaPierre, R. J., Daley, G. Q., Sliz, P.&Gregory, R. I. (2008) Determinants of microRNA processing inhibition by the developmentally regulated RNA-binding protein Lin28. *J Biol Chem*, 283, 31, 21310-4.

Ramachandran, V.&Chen, X. (2008) Degradation of microRNAs by a family of exoribonucleases in Arabidopsis. *Science*, 321, 5895, 1490-2.

Rao, P. K., Kumar, R. M., Farkhondeh, M., Baskerville, S.&Lodish, H. F. (2006) Myogenic factors that regulate expression of muscle-specific microRNAs. *Proc Natl Acad Sci U S A*, 103, 23, 8721-6.

Rodriguez, A., Vigorito, E., Clare, S., Warren, M. V., Couttet, P., Soond, D. R., van Dongen, S., Grocock, R. J., Das, P. P., Miska, E. A., Vetrie, D., Okkenhaug, K., Enright, A. J.,

Dougan, G., Turner, M.&Bradley, A. (2007) Requirement of bic/microRNA-155 for normal immune function. *Science*, 316, 5824, 608-11.

Rozema, D. B., Lewis, D. L., Wakefield, D. H., Wong, S. C., Klein, J. J., Roesch, P. L., Bertin, S. L., Reppen, T. W., Chu, Q., Blokhin, A. V., Hagstrom, J. E.&Wolff, J. A. (2007) Dynamic PolyConjugates for targeted in vivo delivery of siRNA to hepatocytes. *Proc Natl Acad Sci U S A*, 104, 32, 12982-7.

Samols, M. A., Skalsky, R. L., Maldonado, A. M., Riva, A., Lopez, M. C., Baker, H. V.&Renne, R. (2007) Identification of cellular genes targeted by KSHV-encoded microRNAs. *PLoS Pathog*, 3, 5, e65.

Schratt, G. M., Tuebing, F., Nigh, E. A., Kane, C. G., Sabatini, M. E., Kiebler, M.&Greenberg, M. E. (2006) A brain-specific microRNA regulates dendritic spine development. *Nature*, 439, 7074, 283-9.

Shen, J., Samul, R., Silva, R. L., Akiyama, H., Liu, H., Saishin, Y., Hackett, S. F., Zinnen, S., Kossen, K., Fosnaugh, K., Vargeese, C., Gomez, A., Bouhana, K., Aitchison, R., Pavco, P.&Campochiaro, P. A. (2006) Suppression of ocular neovascularization with siRNA targeting VEGF receptor 1. *Gene Ther*, 13, 3, 225-34.

Sheth, U.&Parker, R. (2003) Decapping and decay of messenger RNA occur in cytoplasmic processing bodies. *Science*, 300, 5620, 805-8.

Soutschek, J., Akinc, A., Bramlage, B., Charisse, K., Constien, R., Donoghue, M., Elbashir, S., Geick, A., Hadwiger, P., Harborth, J., John, M., Kesavan, V., Lavine, G., Pandey, R. K., Racie, T., Rajeev, K. G., Rohl, I., Toudjarska, I., Wang, G., Wuschko, S., Bumcrot, D., Koteliansky, V., Limmer, S., Manoharan, M.&Vornlocher, H. P. (2004) Therapeutic silencing of an endogenous gene by systemic administration of modified siRNAs. *Nature*, 432, 7014, 173-8.

Stern-Ginossar, N., Elefant, N., Zimmermann, A., Wolf, D. G., Saleh, N., Biton, M., Horwitz, E., Prokocimer, Z., Prichard, M., Hahn, G., Goldman-Wohl, D., Greenfield, C., Yagel, S., Hengel, H., Altuvia, Y., Margalit, H.&Mandelboim, O. (2007) Host immune system gene targeting by a viral miRNA. *Science*, 317, 5836, 376-81.

Taganov, K. D., Boldin, M. P., Chang, K. J.&Baltimore, D. (2006) NF-kappaB-dependent induction of microRNA miR-146, an inhibitor targeted to signaling proteins of innate immune responses. *Proc Natl Acad Sci U S A*, 103, 33, 12481-6.

Teng, G., Hakimpour, P., Landgraf, P., Rice, A., Tuschl, T., Casellas, R.&Papavasiliou, F. N. (2008) MicroRNA-155 is a negative regulator of activation-induced cytidine deaminase. *Immunity*, 28, 5, 621-9.

Thai, T. H., Calado, D. P., Casola, S., Ansel, K. M., Xiao, C., Xue, Y., Murphy, A., Frendewey, D., Valenzuela, D., Kutok, J. L., Schmidt-Supprian, M., Rajewsky, N., Yancopoulos, G., Rao, A.&Rajewsky, K. (2007) Regulation of the germinal center response by microRNA-155. *Science*, 316, 5824, 604-8.

Tili, E., Michaille, J. J., Cimino, A., Costinean, S., Dumitru, C. D., Adair, B., Fabbri, M., Alder, H., Liu, C. G., Calin, G. A.&Croce, C. M. (2007) Modulation of miR-155 and miR-125b levels following lipopolysaccharide/TNF-alpha stimulation and their possible roles in regulating the response to endotoxin shock. *J Immunol*, 179, 8, 5082-9.

Trang, P., Wiggins, J. F., Daige, C. L., Cho, C., Omotola, M., Brown, D., Weidhaas, J. B., Bader, A. G.&Slack, F. J. (2011) Systemic Delivery of Tumor Suppressor microRNA Mimics Using a Neutral Lipid Emulsion Inhibits Lung Tumors in Mice. *Mol Ther*, 19, 1116-22.

Trang, P., Wiggins, J. F., Daige, C. L., Cho, C., Omotola, M., Brown, D., Weidhaas, J. B., Bader, A. G.&Slack, F. J. (2011) Systemic Delivery of Tumor Suppressor microRNA Mimics Using a Neutral Lipid Emulsion Inhibits Lung Tumors in Mice. *Mol Ther*,

Ui-Tei, K., Naito, Y., Zenno, S., Nishi, K., Yamato, K., Takahashi, F., Juni, A.&Saigo, K. (2008) Functional dissection of siRNA sequence by systematic DNA substitution: modified siRNA with a DNA seed arm is a powerful tool for mammalian gene silencing with significantly reduced off-target effect. *Nucleic Acids Res*, 36, 7, 2136-51.

Umbach, J. L., Kramer, M. F., Jurak, I., Karnowski, H. W., Coen, D. M.&Cullen, B. R. (2008) MicroRNAs expressed by herpes simplex virus 1 during latent infection regulate viral mRNAs. *Nature*, 454, 7205, 780-3.

Vaishnaw, A. K., Gollob, J., Gamba-Vitalo, C., Hutabarat, R., Sah, D., Meyers, R., de Fougerolles, T.&Maraganore, J. (2010) A status report on RNAi therapeutics. *Silence*, 1, 1, 14.

Valastyan, S., Reinhardt, F., Benaich, N., Calogrias, D., Szasz, A. M., Wang, Z. C., Brock, J. E., Richardson, A. L.&Weinberg, R. A. (2009) A pleiotropically acting microRNA, miR-31, inhibits breast cancer metastasis. *Cell*, 137, 6, 1032-46.

van Rooij, E., Sutherland, L. B., Qi, X., Richardson, J. A., Hill, J.&Olson, E. N. (2007) Control of stress-dependent cardiac growth and gene expression by a microRNA. *Science*, 316, 5824, 575-9.

Vigorito, E., Perks, K. L., Abreu-Goodger, C., Bunting, S., Xiang, Z., Kohlhaas, S., Das, P. P., Miska, E. A., Rodriguez, A., Bradley, A., Smith, K. G., Rada, C., Enright, A. J., Toellner, K. M., Maclennan, I. C.&Turner, M. (2007) microRNA-155 regulates the generation of immunoglobulin class-switched plasma cells. *Immunity*, 27, 6, 847-59.

Wiggins, J. F., Ruffino, L., Kelnar, K., Omotola, M., Patrawala, L., Brown, D.&Bader, A. G. (2010) Development of a lung cancer therapeutic based on the tumor suppressor microRNA-34. *Cancer Res*, 70, 14, 5923-30.

Wolfrum, C., Shi, S., Jayaprakash, K. N., Jayaraman, M., Wang, G., Pandey, R. K., Rajeev, K. G., Nakayama, T., Charrise, K., Ndungo, E. M., Zimmermann, T., Koteliansky, V., Manoharan, M.&Stoffel, M. (2007) Mechanisms and optimization of in vivo delivery of lipophilic siRNAs. *Nat Biotechnol*, 25, 10, 1149-57.

Xia, T., O'Hara, A., Araujo, I., Barreto, J., Carvalho, E., Sapucaia, J. B., Ramos, J. C., Luz, E., Pedroso, C., Manrique, M., Toomey, N. L., Brites, C., Dittmer, D. P.&Harrington, W. J., Jr. (2008) EBV microRNAs in primary lymphomas and targeting of CXCL-11 by ebv-mir-BHRF1-3. *Cancer Res*, 68, 5, 1436-42.

Xiao, C., Calado, D. P., Galler, G., Thai, T. H., Patterson, H. C., Wang, J., Rajewsky, N., Bender, T. P.&Rajewsky, K. (2007) MiR-150 controls B cell differentiation by targeting the transcription factor c-Myb. *Cell*, 131, 1, 146-59.

Yi, R., Qin, Y., Macara, I. G.&Cullen, B. R. (2003) Exportin-5 mediates the nuclear export of pre-microRNAs and short hairpin RNAs. *Genes Dev*, 17, 24, 3011-6.

Yoneyama, M., Kikuchi, M., Natsukawa, T., Shinobu, N., Imaizumi, T., Miyagishi, M., Taira, K., Akira, S.&Fujita, T. (2004) The RNA helicase RIG-I has an essential function in double-stranded RNA-induced innate antiviral responses. *Nat Immunol*, 5, 7, 730-7.

Zhou, B., Wang, S., Mayr, C., Bartel, D. P.&Lodish, H. F. (2007) miR-150, a microRNA expressed in mature B and T cells, blocks early B cell development when expressed prematurely. *Proc Natl Acad Sci U S A*, 104, 17, 7080-5.

Zimmermann, T. S., Lee, A. C., Akinc, A., Bramlage, B., Bumcrot, D., Fedoruk, M. N., Harborth, J., Heyes, J. A., Jeffs, L. B., John, M., Judge, A. D., Lam, K., McClintock, K., Nechev, L. V., Palmer, L. R., Racie, T., Rohl, I., Seiffert, S., Shanmugam, S., Sood, V., Soutschek, J., Toudjarska, I., Wheat, A. J., Yaworski, E., Zedalis, W., Koteliansky, V., Manoharan, M., Vornlocher, H. P.&MacLachlan, I. (2006) RNAi-mediated gene silencing in non-human primates. *Nature*, 441, 7089, 111-4.

7

Antitubercular Drugs Development: Recent Advances in Selected Therapeutic Targets and Rational Drug Design

Virgilio Bocanegra-García[4], Abraham García[2], Jose Prisco Palma-Nicolás[3],
Isidro Palos[1] and Gildardo Rivera[4]
[1]*Universidad Autónoma de Tamaulipas, Reynosa,*
[2]*Facultad de Ciencias Químicas, Universidad Autónoma de Nuevo León, Monterrey,*
[3]*Instituto de Fisiología Celular, Universidad Nacional Autónoma de México DF,*
[4]*Centro de Biotecnología Genomica, Instituto Politécnico Nacional, Reynosa,*
México

1. Introduction

Mycobacterium tuberculosis, the causative agent of tuberculosis (TB), is a remarkably successful pathogen that has latently infected a third of the world population (Zhang et al., 2006). Infection occurs via aerosol, and inhalation of a few droplets containing *M. tuberculosis* bacilli is enough for lung infection (Hassan et al., 2006). After infection, *M. tuberculosis* pathogenesis occurs in two stages. The first is an asymptomatic state that can persist for many years in the host, called latent TB. The second stage requires only a weakened immune response to become activated (Zhang, 2004), then the bacteria begins replicating and causing characteristic symptoms such as cough, chest pain, fatigue and unexplained weight loss. If left untreated, the disease eventually culminates in death. The emergence of Human Immunodeficiency Virus (HIV) and the resultant Acquired Immune Deficiency Syndrome (AIDS) pandemic underlined the importance of reactivation of the disease and its potentially catastrophic outcome since over 50% of deaths among HIV-infected patients results from co-infection with *M. tuberculosis* with the two pathogens inducing each other's replication, thus accelerating the collapse of the immune system (Cole & Alzari, 2007).

While it is impossible to determine the exact number of cases, the latest World Health Organization (WHO) survey estimates that close to 2 million deaths occur every year, that there are approximately 8 million new cases annually, and that every third individual on the planet has been exposed to or infected by *M. tuberculosis* (Dye, 2006; Cole & Alzari, 2007).

Although TB can be treated and even cured with chemotherapy, treatment is exceedingly lengthy and takes 6-9 months (Blumberg, et al., 2003). In addition to significant toxicity, lengthy therapy also causes poor patient compliance, which is a frequent cause for selection of drug resistant and often deadly multidrug resistant TB (MDR-TB) bacteria (Zang et al., 2006).

Currently, TB chemotherapy is made up of a cocktail of first-line drugs, isoniazid (INH), Rifampicin (RIF), pyrazinamide (PZA) and ethambutol (EMB), which are given for six months (Blumberg et al., 2006). If this treatment fails as a result of bacterial drug resistance or intolerance to one or more drugs, second-line drugs are used, such as *para*-aminosalicilate (PAS), kanamycin, fluoroquinolones, capreomycin, ethionamide and cycloserine. These are generally less effective or more toxic with serious side effects (Blumberg et al., 2006). This second-line treatment can also result ineffective since MDR-strains that exhibit resistance to these second-line drugs are currently on the rise (Zhang & Amzel, 2002)

Treatment is also made quite difficult by the presence of metabolically silent, persistent or dormant bacteria within host lesions. These are not susceptible to the anti-mycobacterial drugs that usually kill growing but not persistent bacteria (Zhang, 2004). While there are many reasons for drug resistance, including prescription of inadequate regimens, an uncertain drug supply, and ineffective drugs, duration of lengthy treatments is one of the major contributors because some TB patients prematurely stop their therapy after an initial, rapid heath improvement, thereby favoring the emergence of drug-resistant strains (Cole & Alzari, 2007)

2. Anti-TB drug targets

Despite the relative efficacy of current treatment, the various antibiotics that constitute first- and second-line drugs for TB therapy target only a small number of core metabolic processes such as Deoxyribonucleic acid (DNA) and Ribonucleic acid (RNA) synthesis, cell wall synthesis, and energy metabolism pathways (Zhang, 2005). New classes of drugs with additional drug targets that are difficult to overcome by mutation are urgently needed (Hansan et al., 2006). Desirable new targets should be involved in vital aspects of bacterial growth, metabolism and viability whose inactivation would lead to bacterial death or an inability to persist, thus therapy could be shortened and drug resistant strains could be eliminated or drastically reduced (Mdluli & Spigelman, 2006; Duncan, 2004). Moreover, targets involved in the pathogenesis of the disease process should also be considered for drug development (Zhang et al., 2006; Palomino et al., 2009).

The discovery of the complete genome sequence of TB bacteria helped to identify several important drug targets (Cole et al., 1998). Various groups have used this genomic information to identify and validate targets as the basis for development of new Anti-TB agents. Besides, mycobacterial genetic tools, such as transposon mutagenesis, gene knockout, and gene transfer, greatly facilitate target identification.

2.1 Cell wall biosynthesis related targets

Cell wall biosynthesis is a particularly good source of molecular targets because the biosynthetic enzymes do not have homologues in the mammalian system (Mdluli & Spigelman, 2006). The cell wall of *M. tuberculosis* is very important for its survival within constrained conditions such as those inside of human macrophages. The biosynthesis of the cell wall components involves many important stages and different enzymes that are absent in mammals and could be attractive drug targets (Khasnobis et al., 2002; Brennan & Crick, 2007; Sarkar & Suresh, 2011). Recently, the 2C-methyl-D-erytrol 4-fosphate (MEP) pathway was found (Eoh et al., 2009) as a potential drug target since the end product of the pathway leads to the formation of isoprenoids, which are responsible for the synthesis of several cell wall components (Mahapatra et al., 2005; Anderson et al., 1972).

Peptidoglycan biosynthesis is another source of potential drug targets. For instance, alanine racemase and D-Ala-D-Ala-ligase catalyze the first and second committed steps in bacterial peptidoglycan biosynthesis, and since these steps are essential for important polymers, they are good drug targets. Both alanine racemase and D-Ala-D-Ala ligase are inhibited by D-cycloserine, a second line anti-TB drug (Strych et al., 2001; Feng & Barletta, 2003). Another good drug target is the pyridoxal 5'-phosphate containing enzyme Alr that catalyzes the racemization of L-Alanine into D-Alanine, a major component in the biosynthesis of peptidoglycan (LeMagueres et al., 2005). Arabinogalactan biosynthesis, a novel arabionofuranosyl transferase that catalyzes the addition of the first key arabinofuranosyl redisude of the galactan core, is not sensitive to EMB, but is essential for viability (Sassetti et al., 2003). The ribosyltransferase that catalyzes the first committed step in the synthesis of decaprenyl-phosphoryl-D-arabinose, the lipid donor of mycobacterial d-arabinofuranosyl residues, has also recently been characterized and shown essential for growth (Huang et al., 2005)

2.2 Mycolic acid biosynthesis related targets
Within the mycobacteria lipid metabolism, mycolic acids are essential structural components of the mycobacterial cell wall (Brennan, 2003). The early stage of fatty acid biosynthesis, which generates the precursors of mycolic acids, is a rich source of antibacterial targets (Heath et al., 2001). It is also the site of action of INH and ethionamide (Quemard et al., 1995; Larsen et al., 2002). *M. tuberculosis* has both types of fatty acids synthase (FAS) systems found in nature, FAS-I and FAS-II. FAS I is the system responsible for de novo synthesis of C16-C26 fatty acids and the FAS II system extends these fatty acids up to C56 chains to make precursors of mycolic acids, which are essential for growth.
Since enoil-ACP reductase (InhA) is the target of INH, it is reasonable to assume that all steps in the FAS-II pathway will be essential for the viability of *M. tuberculosis*. Many of the individual enzymes of the FAS-II system have been expressed, purified and characterized (Kremer et al., 2001; Choi et al., 2000; Scardale et al 2001; Benerjee et al 1998; Marrakchi et al.,2002; Marrakchi et al., 2000; Slayden & Barry, 2002).

2.3 Energy production related targets
Isocitrate lyase (ICL) is an important enzyme in this category and also an important drug target. ICL is involved in energy production via the metabolism of acetyl-CoA and propionial CoA of the glyoxilate pathway. Inactivation of the *icl* gene leads to attenuation of both persistent and virulent strains of *M. tuberculosis*. However, *M. tuberculosis* has a salvage pathway, so a suitable anti-TB drug for this target must address both the main and salvage pathways (McKinney et al., 2000; Savi et al., 2008)

2.4 Amino acid biosynthesis related drug targets
Amino acid biosynthesis is another important target for developing anti-TB drugs. The shikimate pathway is very important and is involved in the synthesis of aromatic amino acids in algae, fungi, bacteria, and higher plants; however, it is absent in the mammalian system (Sarkar & Suresh, 2011). The final product of the shikimate pathway, chorismate, is a key biosynthetic intermediate involved in generating aromatic amino acids and other metabolites. The entire pathway is essential in *M. tuberculosis* (Parish & Stoker 2002). This feature makes the pathway an attractive target for developing anti-TB drugs with minimum cross reactivity (Ducati et al., 2007). Other enzymes of this pathway are also likely to be essential, and shikimate dehydrogenase (Magalhaes et al., 2002), and 5-enolpyruvylshikimate 3-phosphate synthase (Oliverira et al., 2001) have been characterized

in detail. The biosynthesis of non-aromatic amino acids is also emerging as a potential drug target. The impact of amino acids such as lysine (Pavelka & Jacobs, 1999), proline, tryptophan and leucine (Smith et al., 2001) is evident from the fact that knocked out *M. tuberculosis* strains of the genes required for amino acid biosynthesis showed less virulence (Pavelka et al., 2003; Smith et al., 2001). Another attractive target of the lysine biosynthesis pathway is the enzyme dihydrodipicolinate reductase, for which potent inhibitors have been identified (Paiva et al., 2001).

2.5 Cofactor-related drug targets

Several cofactor biosynthetic pathways and pathways requiring some cofactors are good candidates for identification of new drug targets. Folate derivatives are cofactors utilized in the biosynthesis of essential molecules including purines, pyrimidines, and amino acids. While bacteria synthesize folate de novo, mammals must assimilate preformed folate derivatives through an active transport system (Mdluli & Spigelman, 2006). Dihydrofolate reductase, which catalyses the reduction of dihydrofolate to tetrahydrofolate, a key enzyme in folate utilization whose inhibition may affect the growth of *M. tuberculosis* (Gerum et al., 2002), and dehydropteroate synthase are validated targets of the widely used antibacterial sulfonamide, trimethoprim (Huovinen et al., 1995).

Two enzymes involved in the de novo biosynthesis of NAD that affects the NADH/NAD+ ratio upon which *M. tuberculosis* is dependent, have been studied as possible drug targets (Bellinzoni et al., 2002). Genomic analysis studies have suggested that the riboflavin biosynthesis pathway is essential in *M. tuberculosis* (Morgunova et al., 2005) and the lumazine synthase pathway has been validated as a target for anti-TB drug discovery.

2.6 DNA metabolism

Differences in mammalian and mycobacterial thymidin monophosphate kinase have been studied and exploited in an attempt to find selective inhibitors for this drug target (Haouz et al., 2003; Vanheusden et al., 2002). Other targets are ribonucleotide reductases that catalyze the first committed step in DNA synthesis and have differences with corresponding mammalian enzymes (Yang et al., 1994; Yang et al., 1997); DNA ligases, that play an important role in the replication and repair of DNA, are classified as NAD+ or ATP dependent. NAD+ dependent ligases are only found in some viruses and eubacteria (Mdluli & Spigelman, 2006). LigA is essential for growth of *M. tuberculosis* (Gong et al., 2004) and inhibitors that distinguish between the two types of ligases and have anti-TB activity have been identified (Srivastava et al., 2005). DNA gyrase has also been validated as a target for *M. tuberculosis*, since this is the only type II topoisomerase that it possesses (Cole et al., 1998). Its inhibition by fluoroquinolones results in highly mycobactericidal activity.

2.7 Menaquinone biosynthesis

It appears that menaquinone is the only quinone in *M. tuberculosis*, so its biosynthesis is essential for growth. The menaquinone pathway is not present in humans, and bacterial homologues of MenA-E and MenH have been described in *M. tuberculosis*, so this pathway is another promising drug target (Meganathan, 2001).

2.8 Other potential drug targets in *M. tuberculosis*

The tubercle bacillus produces no less than 20 cythochrome p450 enzymes, some of which appear to play essential roles (Cole & Alzari, 2007). Antifungal azole drugs target these enzymes and the cytochrome p450 homologues in the bacteria. Drugs like miconazole and clotrimazole are active against *M. tuberculosis* (McLean et al., 2007; Ahmad et al., 2006; Sun et al., 1999 TD). Subsequent crystallization studies of the *M. tuberculosis* cytochrome p450 enzyme system evoked studies to evaluate new drugs (Leys et al., 2003).

Peptide deformylase inhibitors may be effective against *M. tuberculosis* since peptide deformylase catalyzes the hydrolytic removal of the B-terminal formyl group from nascent proteins. It is a metalloprotease essential for maturation of nascent polypeptides in bacteria but not essential for humans, making it an attractive target for antibacterial drug development (Teo et al., 2006); however, it has little effect on slow growing TB bacteria (Khasnobis et al., 2002).

Another important set of emerging drug targets are the components of the siderophore biosynthesis of *M. tuberculosis* (Monfeli et al., 2007). Upon infection, as a part of the defense mechanism, the host has several mechanisms to withdraw or control the free extracellular, as well as intracellular, iron concentration (Weinberga & Miklossy, 2008; Ferreras et al., 2005). Mycobacteria have an unusual reliance on serine/threonine protein kinases as the main component of signal transduction pathways (Av-Gay & Everett, 2000), and there is considerable activity around this transduction system since some of these enzymes are essential for growth (Fernandez et al., 2006). *M. tuberculosis* synthesizes mycothiol in a multistep process involving four enzymatic reactions for protection against the damaging effects of reactive oxygen species. This pathway is absent in humans, and it has been shown to be essential to *M. tuberculosis* (Sareen et al., 2003).

3. Rational drug design

One of the design strategies for new anti-TB compounds is based on the development of analogs of first-line and/or second line drugs. In this section we review the strategies employed and analyze structure-activity relationships (SAR), which have led to the development of new anti-TB agents. In addition, we review new pharmacophore groups. One problem that must be considered in the design of anti-TB compounds is that there is a subpopulation of bacteria in a persistent non-replicating state. This is considered a major contributing factor to long drug treatments for TB. For this reason, it is important to determine if compounds have potential activity against these bacteria at the onset of design. We should also consider the physicochemical properties that directly affect the pharmacokinetics and pharmacodynamics of drugs. An example of this is the influence of stereoisomers on biological activity, because individual enantiomers have significant differences in activity, although sometimes the activity of some enantiomers cannot be explained.

3.1 Isoniazid derivatives

One of the strategies frequently used in medicinal chemistry to develop new drugs is "hybridization", a method that has been proposed particularly for new anti-TB drugs. An example is the design of molecules based on INH or PZA, incorporating NR1R2 groups derived from a second anti-TB molecule or possibly other nucleophilic groups to provide anti-TB activity. With special interest compounds 1 and 2 (figure 1) were obtained. These could be considered prodrugs because they contain two conventional drugs that are bound by a CH fragment. Although the results of activity are very similar to those presented by INH and PZA, the hydrolysis of new compounds ensures prolonged release of the active drugs (Imramovsky et al., 2007).

A variety of compounds derived from INH that include mostly a hydrazine fragment have been determined. Following this strategy and considering the inclusion of an oxadiazole moiety, Navarrete et al, developed new agents with high anti-TB activity (3, figure 1). Due to the substitution in 5-position on the oxadiazole ring, the compounds obtained showed high lipophilicity, hypothesizing that this lipophilicity could facilitate passage of these compounds through the *M. tuberculosis* bacterial membrane (Navarrete-Vazquez et al., 2007). Also, structural modification of the hydrazide moiety on INH (4, figure 1) provided lipophilic adaptations of the drug that blocked the N-acetylation process, obtained high levels of *in vitro* activity against *M. tuberculosis* and macrophages infected, as well as low toxicity (Hearn et al., 2009).

Another strategy in drug design is the formation of molecules that mimic the natural substrate of an enzyme. Delaine et al designed a new series of bi-substrate-type inhibitors based on a covalent association between molecules mimicking the INH substrate and the NAD cofactor that could provide compounds with a high affinity and selectivity for the INH catalytic site (5 and 6, figure 1). In these compounds, the authors determined that incorporating a lipophilic component into the nicotinamide hemiamidal framework provides more active derivatives (Delaine et al., 2010).

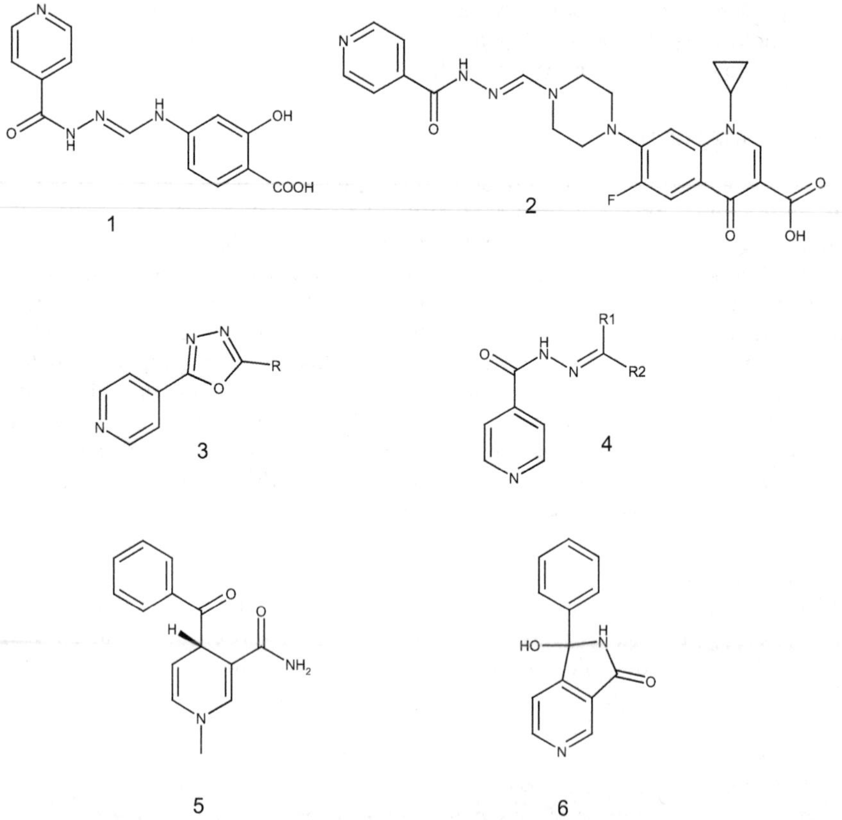

Fig. 1. Structure of compounds derivatives of anti-TB first line drugs.

3.2 Ethambutol derivatives

Amino alcohols that include EMB, which is used for pharmacological TB treatment, are an important class of compounds with various applications. This compound has been widely studied determining that the 1,2-ethylenediamine moiety is the EMB pharmacophore, possibility due to chelate bond formation with divalent metal ions such as copper. Based on EMB, a second-generation agent has been developed, a compound called SQ109 (7, figure 2), which is being tested in clinical trials. It is a drug that exhibits potent activity against *M. tuberculosis* strains, including multidrug resistant strains *in vitro* and *in vivo*. Unfortunately, SQ109 has poor bioavailability of only 12% and 3.8% in rats and dogs, respectively. Studies indicate that this compound undergoes oxidation, epoxidation and *N*-dealkylation, which cause its low bioavailability; therefore strategies have been designed to improve its bioavailability minimizing this first-pass effect. Prodrugs based on carbamate groups are a good option for reducing this effect. Considering this Meng and colleagues developed a new series of analogues based on carbamate prodrugs of SQ109 (8, figure 2) that provide good chemical stability as substrates of plasma esterase. The results of bioavailability of these compounds show a five-fold increase of the SQ109 reference compound (Meng et al., 2009). Alternatively, Zhang has carried out the synthesis of new analogues of S2824 (9, figure 2), a second-generation compound derived from EMB. The results show that new analogues with a homopiperazine ring (10, figure 2) have high *in vitro* activity against both sensitive and drug-resistant *M. tuberculosis* strains (Zhang et al., 2009).

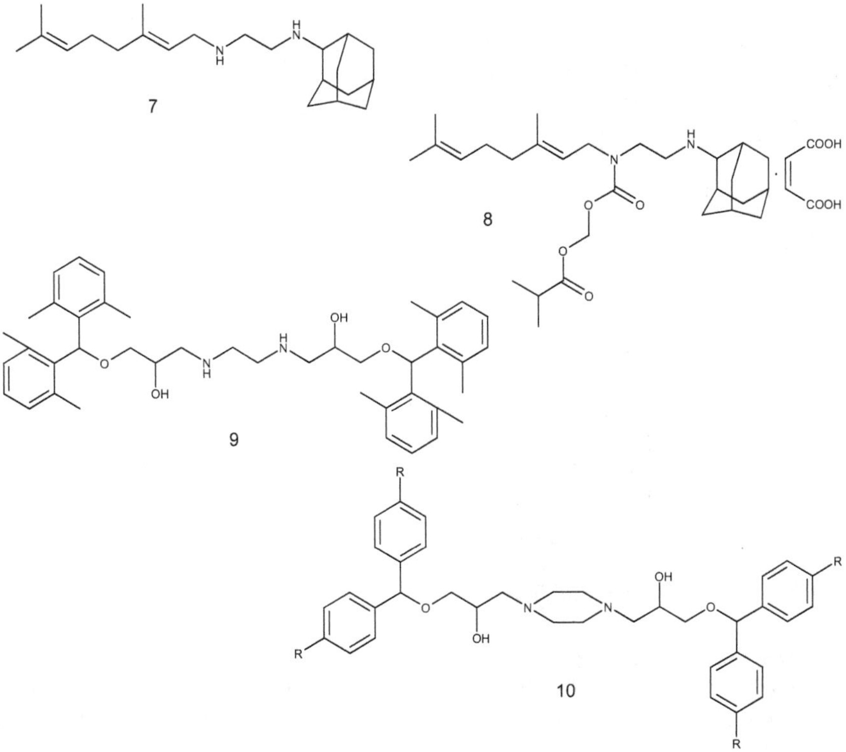

Fig. 2. Structure of SQ109 and analogs.

In the design of new 1,2-diamine derivatives (11, figure 3) compounds with 35 times more activity than EMB have been synthesized. Interestingly, studies show that they do not have the same target as EMB. An SAR analysis has determined that the presence of an β-hydroxy group on the amine increases anti-TB activity; however, the distance between oxygen and nitrogen atoms in EMB are the same as between both atoms in the hydroxyethylamine suggesting a good relationship between both structures (12, figure 3). In a new series of EMB analogs obtained by Cunico et al, it was determined that the sulfonamide moiety reduces activity against *M. tuberculosis*, and that the amino alcohol moiety on hidroxyethylsulfonamide is crucial for anti-TB activity, where the presence of a carbamate moiety leads to a loss of activity. Consistent with this, it has been reported that if compounds lose the basicity of the amino group (12, figure 3), this results in a loss of activity (Cunico et al., 2011). Finally, EMB has served as a proposal for tripartite hybridization (chloroquine, isoxyl and ethambutol) for the development of new anti-TB agents (13, figure 3), which exhibit high activity against *M. tuberculosis* (Nava-Zuazo et al., 2010).

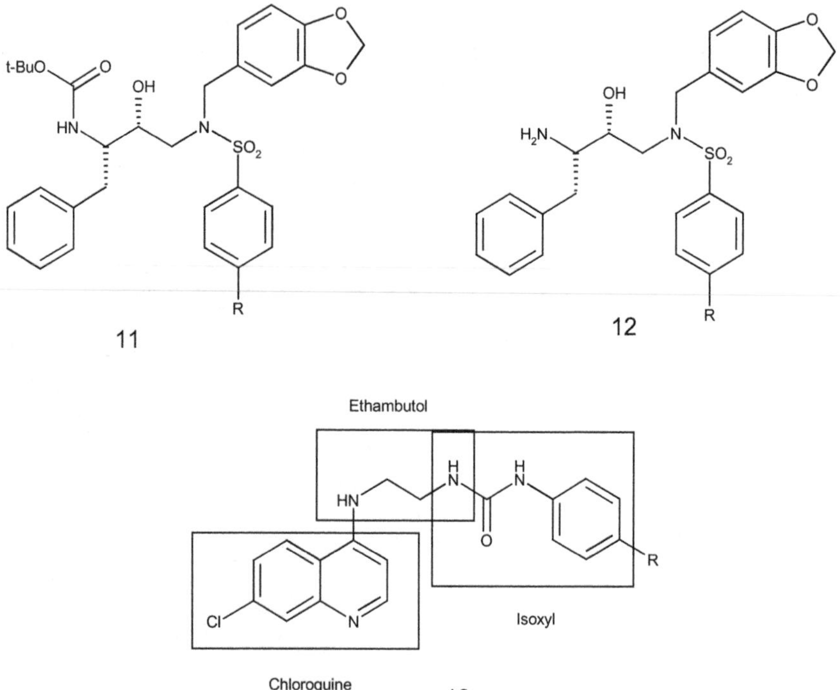

Fig. 3. Ethambutol analogs as anti-TB agents.

3.3 Salicylanilides derivatives

salicylanilides (SAL) derivatives have been of great interest in medicinal chemistry, although their mechanism of action still unknown. It is postulated that they serve as epidermal growth factor receptor protein kinase (EGFR PTK) inhibitors. Such compounds have generally been designed to compete with adenosine triphosphate (ATP) in binding with the catalytic domain of tyrosine kinase. Recent studies specify that selective inhibitors of interleukin-12p40 production also have a specific role in the initiation, expansion, and control of the cellular response to TB. Following the development of SAL derivatives, Imramovský´s group obtained a series of compounds (14, figure 4) with activity similar to INH. Through a SAR study, they established that positions R1 and R2 showed Cl and Br atoms that are necessary for high activity against TB and that the benzyl and isopropyl substituent at R3 increases activity (Imramovský et al., 2009).

In addition, in various SAL derivatives that have been developed it has been shown that electron withdrawing groups on the salicyloyl ring and hydrophobic groups on the anilide ring, as well as the 2-hydroxy group, are essential for optimal antimicrobial effect. Halogen-substituted SAL in both parties maintains the requirements and forms of more active derivatives that show anti-TB activity. However, its unsuitable physical properties led to the generation of prodrugs of SAL derivatives with better bioavailability, and due to a high degree of lipophilicity, more efficient transport through M. tuberculosis cell membranes. Considering this, Imramovský and colleagues obtained compounds (15, figure 4) with interesting activity against M. tuberculosis. They showed a level of inhibition of 89%-99% and an MIC of 3.13 µg/mL. Although, they demonstrated that lipophilicity is a secondary parameter in anti-TB activity, they also demonstrated that in these compounds the stereoisomer effect is important for anti-TB activity; however, in this case the difference is not determined for individual R/S isomers (Imramovský et al., 2009).

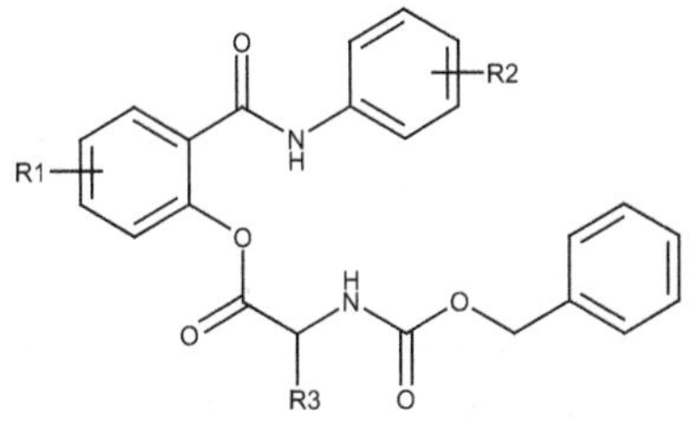

14

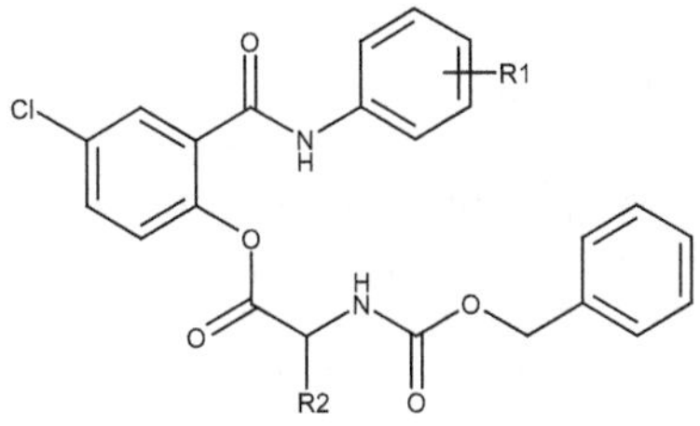

15

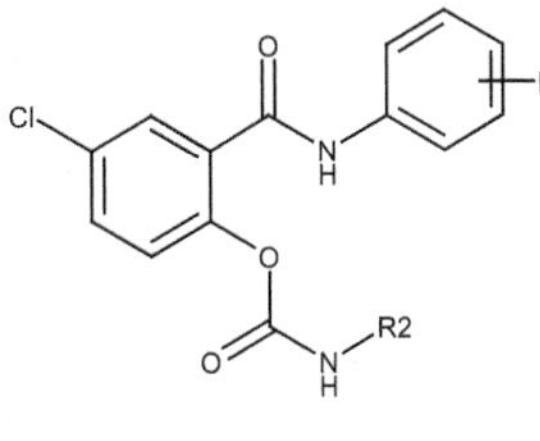

16

Fig. 4. General structure of salicylanilides derivatives with anti-TB activity.

Using the hybridization strategy, Ferriz et al obtained a new series of derivatives with SAL and carbamate groups, which have been used as antibacterial and antiviral agents. Thus the hybridization of two moieties could produce a new series with changes in their pharmacokinetic and pharmacodynamic properties. Ferriz et al postulated that carbamate could be protecting these molecules against first-pass metabolism, increasing their activity profile. The series obtained show that Cl atoms at 3 and 4-position on the aniline ring increase *M. tuberculosis* biological activity. Interestingly, the presence of an alkyl chain also increases the biological activity of these compounds, which suggests the importance of carbamate group (16, figure 4). Although these kinds of compounds are consistent with the Lipinski rules, it is speculated that due to their high lipophilicity, these molecules have high permeability, making their release more effective (Ferriz et al., 2009).

Another strategy using SAL derivatives has been the formation of cyclic derivatives, which could serve as antibacterial agents with a dual inhibition system. Thus, following this design strategy a new series of benzoxazinediones derivatives was obtained, where a thioxo group replaced one or two oxo groups. The substitution of an oxo group by the thioxo group (17, figure 5) strongly increased anti-TB activity, although a second substitution with the thioxo group had only a small effect on activity (18, figure 5) (Petrlikova et al., 2010).

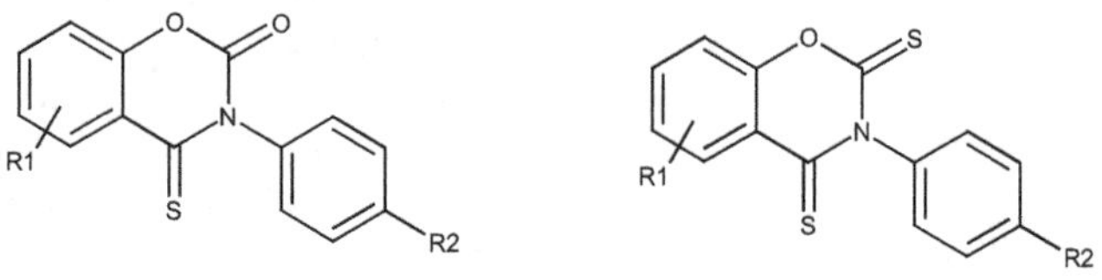

17   18

Fig. 5. General structure of 1,3-benzoxazine derivatives.

3.4 Quinoline derivatives

A quinoline ring is one of the moieties frequently used in new drug design. It has been considered a pharmacophore for the design of anti-TB agents. Diarilquinoline, denominated TMC207 (19, figure 6), is an adenosine ATP synthase inhibitor that is one of the most important quinoline derivatives with anti-TB activity. TMC207 is currently in Phase II clinical trials. Also, butanamide has been established as an important pharmacophore with good antibacterial activity and the carbohydrazone moiety is also known as a pharmacophore group. Based on the above, the design of new quinoline derivatives with active carbohydrazine and butanamide moieties in 3 and 4-position, respectively, has been carried out. The SAR study of these compounds shows that the presence of a trifluoromethyl group at 8-position increases activity; however, the introduction of a fluoro group in 6-position partially decreases activity (20, figure 6) considering these type of compounds non-toxic (Eswaran et al., 2009). Following the development of mefloquine analogs (21, figure 6) in a series of compounds (22, figure 6), good anti-TB activity has been attributed to the presence of pharmacologically active heterocyclic groups such as pyrazole, imidazole, and indole rings on the quinoline ring. Surprisingly, compounds with a hetoaromatic pyrazole ring have activity against resistant strains, which can be attributed to the presence of substituents (electron donating groups) that stabilize the pyrazole ring, making the quinoline ring a more active entity (Eswaran et al., 2010).

The conformational restriction-like strategy in flexible drugs is extensively used in medicinal chemistry. This helped determine steric requirements of receptor-drug interaction and identification of new structures with high efficiency and selectivity. Based on this, Goncalves et al studied the conformational restriction of the piperidinyl ring of mefloquine through the construction of an oxazolidine ring and different substituents on the phenyl ring (23, figure 6).

Conformational restriction showed that the introduction of an oxazolidine core in the mefloquine structure enhances anti-TB activity. Although, the activity of these compounds is affected by substituents on the aromatic ring bound to C-17 of the oxazolidenyl nucleus. Compounds that show hydroxyl or methoxyl groups, which are both electron donators and capable of forming strong hydrogen bonds, in general are active. In contrast, with one exception, compounds with nitro or halogenated groups (electron withdrawing groups and capable of forming only weak hydrogen bonds), are inactive (Goncalves et al., 2010). Thus, mefloquine has been used to design anti-TB agents. Modifications in previous reports included introduction of a hydrazone linker into mefloquine at 4-position, substitution of a piperidine with a piperazine ring and extension of the basic terminus of the piperazine ring at 4-position. Additionally, isoxazole is emerging as one of the most powerful hits in high-throughput screening (HTS) against *M. tuberculosis*. Both types of compounds show an aromatic ring, a two-atom linker and a five or six member ring. Hybridization strategies have been the basis for the design of new chemical entities by Mao et al (24, figure 6). One problem that has been detected in this type of compounds is poor penetration of acid derivatives through the *M. tuberculosis* cell wall. It is suggested that these compounds may act as prodrugs when ester derivatives generate acid derivatives (24, figure 6). SAR studies of these compounds show that when a methyl group replaces a trifluoromethyl group, it is 10 times less active, suggesting that electronic effects may play an important role in anti-TB activity. Additionally, steric effects can affect anti-TB activity. Subsequently, making use of drug design strategies, the authors included ester bioisosteres, such as amides and oxadiazole, although none of these bioisosteres showed better activity than ester derivatives. It was determined that 2 and 8-trifluoromethyl groups on quinoline ring (24, figure 6) are essential for anti-TB activity against replicative bacteria (Mao et al., 2009).

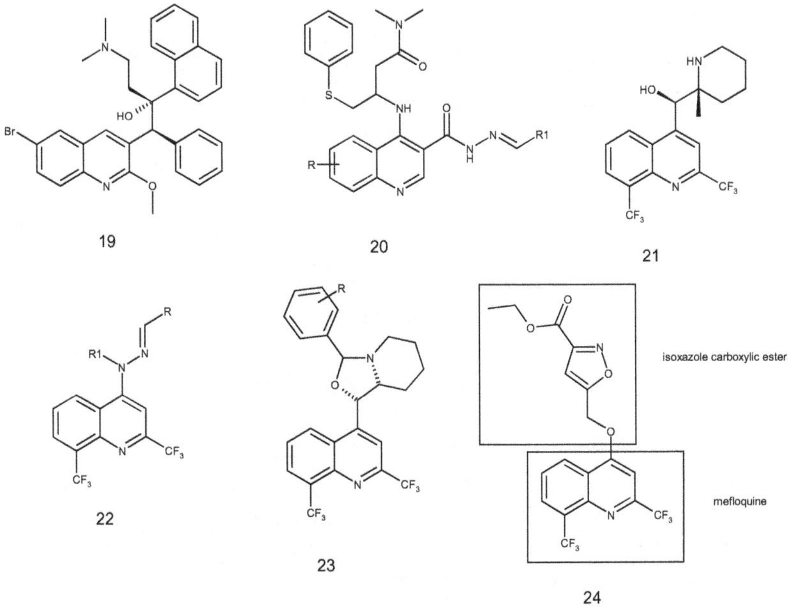

Fig. 6. Quinoline as scaffold for designing new anti-TB agents.

Isoxazole derivatives have also been reported as anti-TB agents, in particular compound 25 (figure 7) with an activity of 2.9 µM, which is comparable to INH and (RIF) (Kini et al., 2009). Thus, quinoline and oxazole ring hybridization has been used to develop a series of new anti-TB agents (26, figure 7) which have good activity due to the presence of aryl substituents at 2-position on quinoline ring. SAR studies show that the introduction of a 1,3-oxazole ring significantly increases activity, obtaining compounds that are more potent than INH (Eswaran et al., 2009). In search of a new moiety that confers anti-TB activity with low cytotoxicity, Yang and colleagues reported methoxybenzofuro[2,3-b]quinoline derivatives (27, figure 7), compounds that have a potent *M. tuberculosis* growth inhibition of 99% at low concentrations (0.20 µg/mL) and very low cytotoxicity against VERO cells with an Inhibitor concentration 50 (IC50) value of > 30.00 µg/mL (Yang et al., 2009).

Several studies have analyzed modifications in the quinolone ring, mainly at 3, 6 and 7-position. Wube et al proposed a new strategy for anti-TB agent development. They made a modification in the 2-position, including an aliphatic side chain with various degrees of unsaturation, lengths chains, and double bond positions (28, figure 7). Their results showed that increasing the chain length enhances anti-TB activity, showing optimal activity with 14 C atoms. If there is an increase of more carbon atoms in the chain, activity decreases dramatically. This behavior has also been described for ciprofloxacin derivatives where lipophilicity could play an important role in anti-TB activity. Other research has determined that the saturated aliphatic chain has less activity than unsaturated analogues. This means that unsaturation of an aliphatic chain is an essential structure for *in vitro* anti-TB activity (Wube et al., 2010).

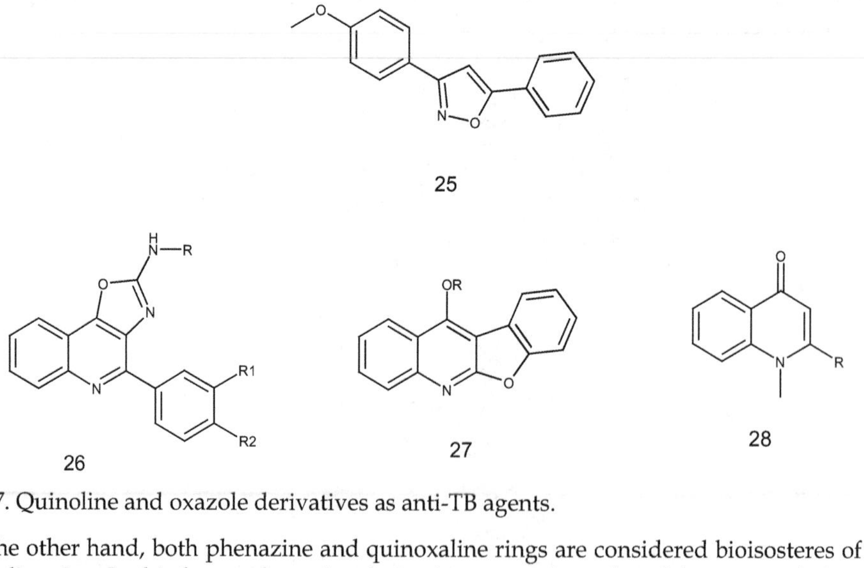

25

26   27   28

Fig. 7. Quinoline and oxazole derivatives as anti-TB agents.

On the other hand, both phenazine and quinoxaline rings are considered bioisosteres of the quinoline ring. In this focus, phenazine derivatives are a class of useful compounds for new anti-TB agent development, particularly Tubermicyn B and Clofazimine (phenazine derivatives). Likewise, De Logu et al developed new agents that show activity (29, figure 8) in a concentration range of 0.19 to 3.12 mg/L against *M. tuberculosis*-resistant clinical isolates. Interestingly, they found that this series of compounds were ineffective in inhibiting the growth of INH resistant strains. Compounds that had exocyclic groups, which confer different lipophilic and electronic properties, but with a size similar to INH, such as the phenylamide methyl lipophilic group in 4-position, were the most active. In contrast, the same group in 3-position reduced activity 100-fold. Also, phenazine derivatives with electron withdrawing groups in 2 and 3-position have values with similar biological activity. These results show the importance of the arylic moiety as a pharmacophore for phenazinecarboxamide anti-TB agents. While phenazine´s mechanism of action is still unknown, it is hypothesized that it could act as a cellular superoxide bismutase inhibitor. We know that the compound Lomofungin (1-carbomethoxy-5-formyl-4,6,8-trihydroxyphenazine) is capable of inhibiting DNA-dependent RNA polymerase, with both options being possible mechanisms of action of phenazine derivatives (De Logu et al., 2009). Quinoxalines are compounds with a broad spectrum of biological activities. Quinoxaline-N-oxide derivatives are known as *M. tuberculosis* bioreductor agents. In this type of compounds missing N-oxide groups have led to the loss of anti-TB activity. In this sense, Monge´s group developed over 500 derivatives of quinoxaline (30, figure 8), demonstrating the importance of this group for generating a new class of anti-TB drugs. Interestingly, this research group determined that the quinoxaline compounds obtained have activity on non-replicating bacteria, which could lead to shorter anti-TB therapies (Vicente et al., 2008).

Finally, a compound denominated ER-2 is a new analogue of quinoline derivatives (31, figure 8) that is a gyrase supercoiling inhibitor that has potency similar to Ciprofloxacin with a minimum inhibitory concentration 90 (MIC90) of 0.5 µg/mL (Sainath et al, 2009).

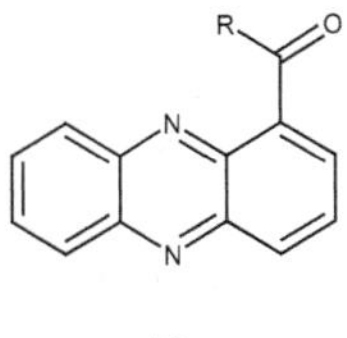

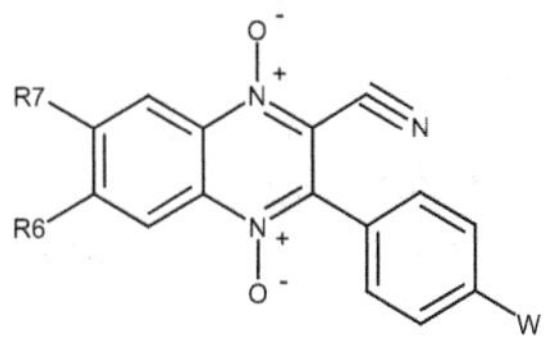

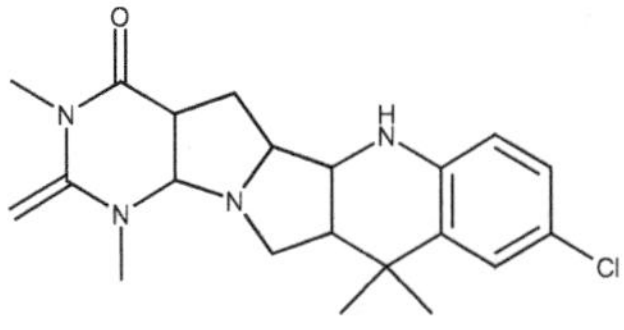

Fig. 8. General structure of phenazine-1-carboxamides, quinoline and quinoxaline derivatives.

3.5 Azoles derivatives

One of the most important strategies for effective anti-TB agent design has been the development of cell wall biosynthesis inhibitors. Azole derivatives have shown interesting anti-TB antimicrobial activity, inhibiting the bacteria by blocking lipid biosynthesis and/or additional mechanisms. Thus, by hybridization of 1,2,4-triazoles and a thiazole moiety, new anti-TB agents were discovered (32, figure 9). These molecules with a highly electronegative part at the sulfhydryl groups have emerged as new anti-TB compounds. Particularly, Schiff bases derivatives probably due to its ability to increase penetration into the bacterial cell (Shiradkar et al, 2006).

Benzimidazole is an important pharmacophore in drug discovery. Gill et al propose 1,2,3-triazole and benzimidazole ring hybridization as design strategies of new anti-TB agents. They have also considered the use of electron withdrawing groups in the benzimidazole ring, which are present in molecules with anti-TB activity. They obtained compound 33 (figure 9) that could be considered a lead series. Their optimization led to determine that substitutions with electron withdrawing groups produce a loss of anti-TB activity (Gill et al., 2008). A new strategy of hybridization between benzimidazole and a 1,2,4-triazole ring has obtained a series of compounds (34, figure 9). Using a SAR study, it was determined that these compounds enhance biological activity by increasing electronegativity of the molecule, but surprisingly when a trifluoromethyl group (high electronegativity) was introduced, it produced a substantial loss of activity, which could be due to a delay in intracellular transport (Jadhav et al., 2009). Following with the use of a benzimidazole ring as a drug design, Klimešova and cols replaced a nitrogen atom with a corresponding oxygen atom (isosteric) (35, figure 9) to obtain a series of benzylsulfanyl benzoxazole derivatives. They consider alkylsulfanyl derivatives of pyridine, benzimidazole and tetrazole as new anti-TB agents, which present anti-TB activity due to the presence of the alkylsulfanyl group bound to an electron deficient carbon atom in the heterocycle ring. Thus, a SAR study of these compounds indicates that anti-TB activity is attributed to the presence of a benzyl moiety at 2-position on the benzoxazole ring, denoting that anti-TB activity is not affected by electron withdrawing or electron donating susbstituents on the benzyl moiety. It is important to note that the presence of two nitro groups on benzyl led to the most active compound (MIC 2 μmol/L), which may be related to compounds such as PA-824 and OPC-67683, that also show nitro groups. Research postulated as a mechanism of action the generation of active species that act on biochemical targets. Additionally, regression coefficient values for log P show that anti-TB activity increases when lipophilicity decreases (Klimesova et al., 2008).

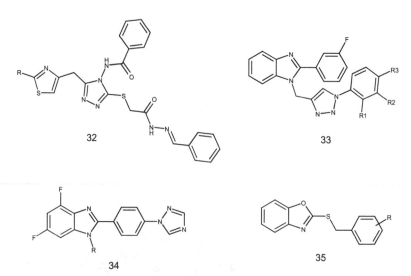

Fig. 9. Triazole and benzimidazole scaffold for designing new anti-TB agents.

Another strategy using 1,2,4-triazole and 1,3,4-thiadiazole rings, led to the development of new anti-TB agents (36, figure 10). Guzeldemerci et al obtained compounds that inhibit 90% *M. tuberculosis* with a concentration greater than 6.25 µg/mL. In addition, the benzothiazole moiety has been recognized for anti-TB design. Both benzothiazole and 1,2,4-triazole moiety were considered to obtain new structures based on hybridization (37, figure 10). Benzothiazole derivatives with 4-methoxy groups showed the best anti-TB activity; however, compounds obtained by hybridization with the 1,2,4-triazole-benzothiazole moiety with the best activity were those with an electron withdrawing substituent (Cl) on the benzothiazole ring (Patel et al., 2010).

Another moiety considered in anti-TB agent design has been isopropylthiazole. Based on this a series of isopropylthiazole derived triazolothiadiazoles, triazolothidiazines derivatives, and mannich bases were developed. The SAR study of the thiadiazoles series (38, figure 10) shows that these compounds have excellent activity against *M. tuberculosis* when they have fluorinated (highly electronegative) substituents that increase molecule lipophilicity, producing hydrophobic molecule interactions with specific binding sites on either receptors or enzymes (Suresh Kumar et al., 2010).

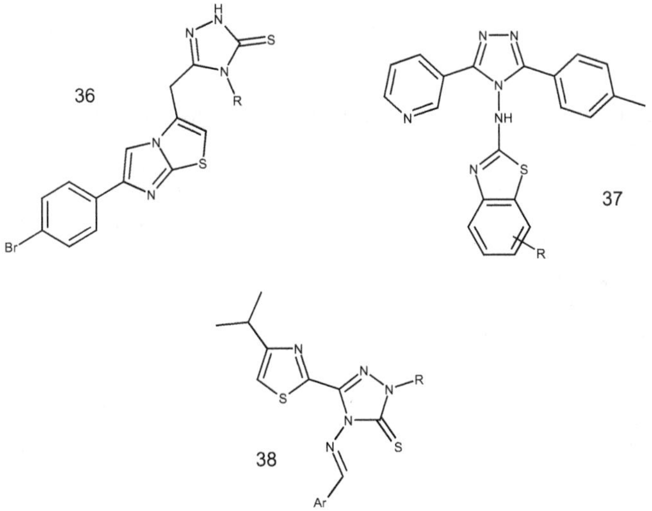

Fig. 10. Triazole derivatives as anti-TB agents.

One of the strategies employed in the development of new drugs is *in silico* screening based on drug structure, structural data of protein and a virtual library of compounds. With this strategy Izumizono et al identified 5 classes of compounds that have an affinity for the active site of enoyl-acyl carrier protein reductase. They determined that these compounds have a structural skeleton of dibenzofuran, acetoamide, triazole, furyl and methoxy phenyl groups (figure 11) that completely inhibit *M vanbaalenii* growth with no toxic effect on mammalian cells. Binding mode prediction determined that compounds 39, 40 and 41 form common hydrogen bonds with amino acid Lys 165 of the active site of the reductase protein. Lys 165 is an amino acid residue that is known to form hydrogen bonds with INH. This shows that hydrogen bond formation with Lys 165 tends to be effective in the design of new drugs. In drug-interaction, the triazole group of compound 39 forms hydrogen binds with the active side, and the methoxy and sulfonyl groups in compound 40 and the sulfonyl group in compound 41, respectively, form hydrogen bonds with Lys 165 (Izumizono et al., 2011).

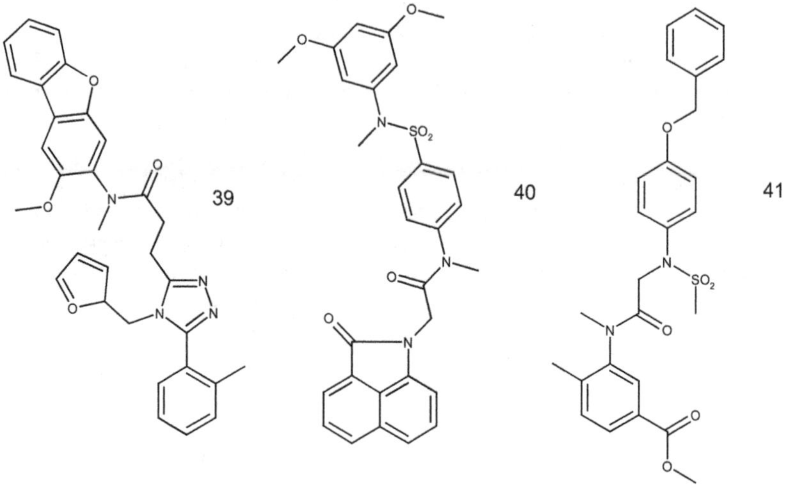

Fig. 11. Dibenzofurane, triazole, methylphenyl and acetamide moiety in compounds with anti-TB activity.

Other derivatives of azoles are pyrazoles. Their activity has been tested against M. tuberculosis. SAR studies show that the presence of a para-chlorobenzoyl moiety in C4-position on the pyrazole ring is essential for anti-TB activity. Results of a series of pyrazole derivatives, generally show that cyclohexylthio substituted pyrazole derivatives are more active than arylthio substituted systems. An excellent activity is presented when a para-nitrophenilthio ring is incorporated on a pyrazole ring (42, figure 12) (Manikannan et al, 2010).

Thiazoles are compounds that contains sulfur and nitrogen atom in its structure, and have been the basis of clinically used compounds. Therefore Samadhiya and colleagues consider it a basis of anti-TB agent design. In one study, which synthesized a series of new thiazoles (43, figure 12), it was demonstrated through SAR analysis that compounds with nitro groups show greater biological activity on M. tuberculosis than compounds with Cl and Br atoms, although these derivatives (Cl and Br) have better activity than other compounds. Finally, they found that the activity of the compound depends on the nature of the substituent groups (electron withdrawing) with the following sequence NO_2 > Cl > Br > OCH_3 < OH > CH_3 (Samdhiya et al., 2010).

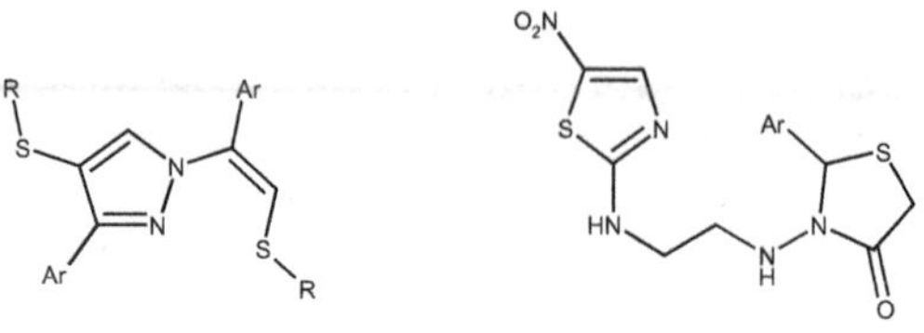

Fig. 12. General structure of pyrazoles and thiazoles derivatives as anti-TB agents.

On the other hand, hybridization of Spiro compound and pyrrolo[2,1-b]thiazole, an unusual ring with different biological properties, particularly permitted the obtention of pyrrolothiazoles derivatives (44, figure 13) that present a MIC of 0.007 µM against *M. tuberculosis*, being more potent than INH and Ciprofloxacin (Karthikeyan et al., 2010) .

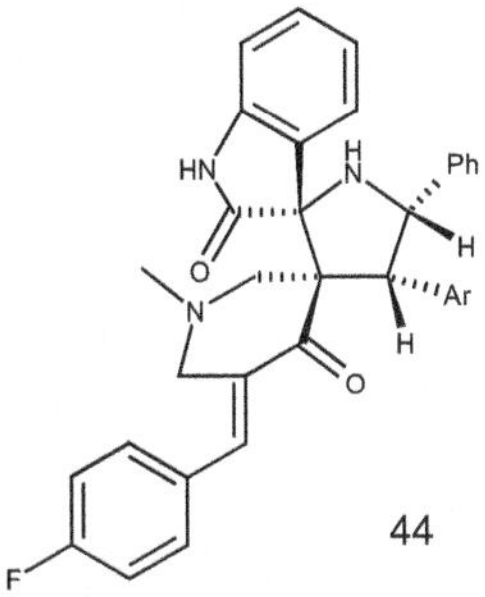

Fig. 13. Spiro-pyrrolothiazoles derivative with anti-TB activity.

3.6 Hydrazides/hydrazones derivatives

Hydrazide/hydrazone is a class of compounds that have been considered for new anti-TB drug design. An example is diflunisal, a hydrazide/hydrazone derivative, which has dual effect acting with antimicrobial/anti-inflammatory properties. Furthermore, in thiazolylhydrazone derivatives, SAR studies have found that substitutions on the phenyl ring affect anti-TB activity (45, figure 14) (Turan-Zitouni et al., 2008). Another example of a thiazolylhydrazine is compound 46 (figure 14), which has high anti-TB activity with a IC50 of 6.22 µg/mL and low toxicity (CC50> 40 µg/mL). Here, a pyridyl moiety plays a direct role related to anti-TB activity (Turan-Zitouni et al, 2010). Pyridine is a moiety known in the design of anti-TB agents. Considering this, and using hybridization technique, Sankar et al developed a series of compounds with potential anti-TB activity (47, figure 14), although in many cases as this, the use of this technique did not produce any agent with excellent activity against *M. tuberculosis* (Sankar et al, 2010).

New designs have been made by molecular hybridization of E-cinamic acid and guanylhydrazones. Based on an empirical analysis of SAR, Bairwa and colleagues determined that electronic and steric parameters have an important role in the activity of these compounds on *M. tuberculosis* (48, figure 14).They remain the basis of new anti-TB agents (Bairwa et al, 2010).

3.7 Nitrogen heterocyclic derivatives

Purines are an important group in the design of anti-TB agents. In these compounds (49, figure 15), activity depends on the substituents present in C2, C6 and N9 of the purine ring (Correia et al., 2009). In 6,9-disubtituted purine derivatives, activity increases substantially when a Cl atom is introduced in the 2-position. Interestingly, purine derivatives with thienyl substituents exhibit better activity in non-replicating bacteria, although in these compounds a Cl atom in 2-position is not beneficial for activity. Additionally, it has been determined that purine N-9 is important for activity, in the case of purine C-8, an atom can be exchanged without losing activity and a change in purine N-7 results in a loss of activity, although there are 7-deazapurines derivatives (50, figure 15) that could be compared with RIF (Khoje et al., 2010).

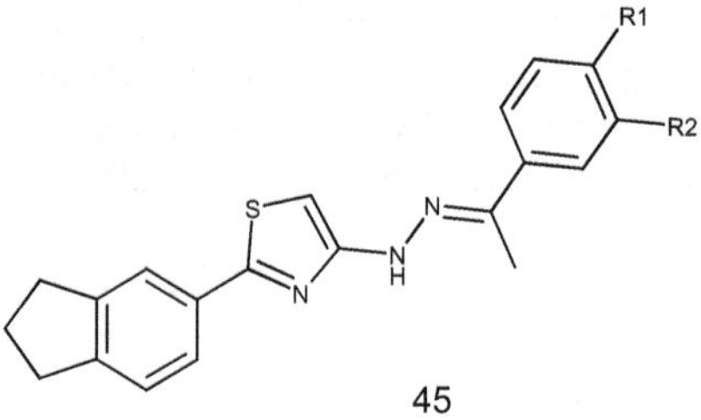

Fig. 14. Hydrazone derivatives as anti-TB agents.

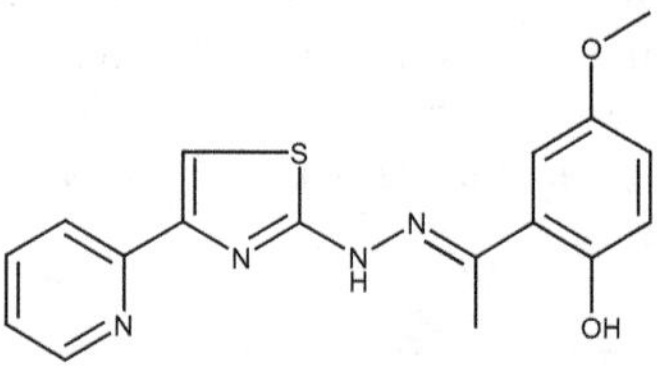

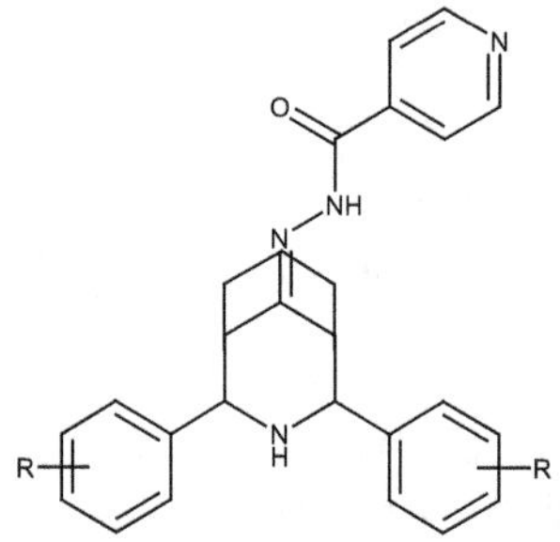

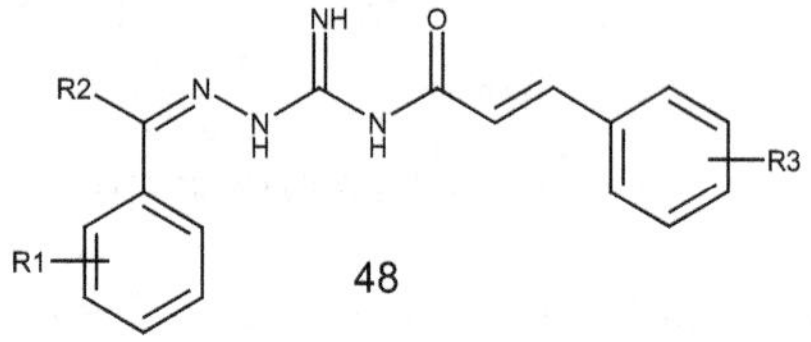

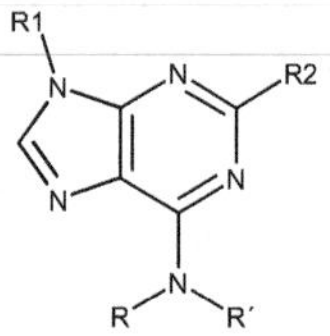

Fig. 15. Purine derivatives as anti-TB agents.

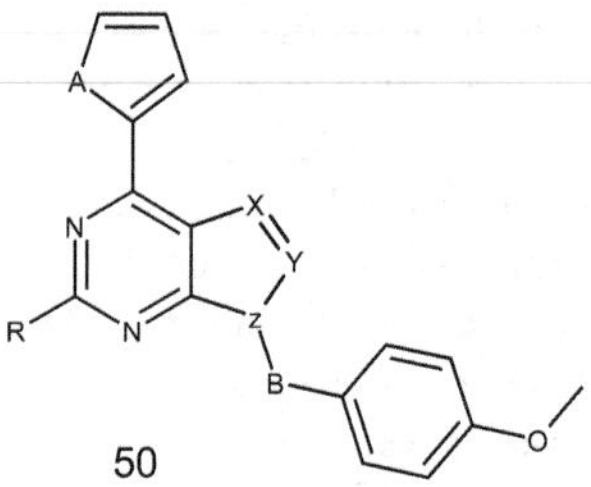

Heterocycles with one nitrogen atom, especially pyrimidines have potential therapeutic applications as anti-TB agents, but there are few reports. For this reason, the design of new pyrimidine derivatives is a viable option (51, figure 16). However, neither compound has an activity comparable to reference drugs, although it has been described that the substituent nature in 2-position can modulate cytotoxic activity (Singh et al, 2011).

On the other hand, thymidine monophosphate kinase of *M. tuberculosis* (TMPKmt) is a prominent target for the development of anti-TB drugs. TMPK is the last specific enzyme for dTTP synthesis and is a key enzyme in *M. tuberculosis* metabolism. This enzyme is different from human enzyme analogs (22% homology). TMPK inhibitors have been developed with single or multiple chemical modifications of the pyrimidine moiety and thymidylate sugar. In particular benzyl-thymine derivatives have been remarkable TMPK inhibitors, which has led to the proposal of new modifications such as: chain length in *para*-position on the benzyl ring, saturation of the alkyl chain, functionalization of the chain group and substitution at 5-

position of the core base. This has led to more selective compounds on TMKP that correspond to benzyl-pyrimidines substituted by a chain length of 4 carbons and a terminal carboxylic acid function. Docking of molecule 52 (figure 16) on TMPKmt showed that the hydrogen of the thymine and acid group can interact with Arg95 (Gasse et al., 2008).

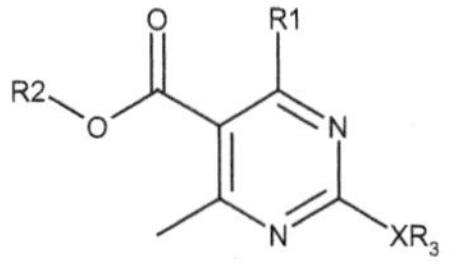

Fig. 16. General structure of pyrimidine derivatives as anti-TB agents.

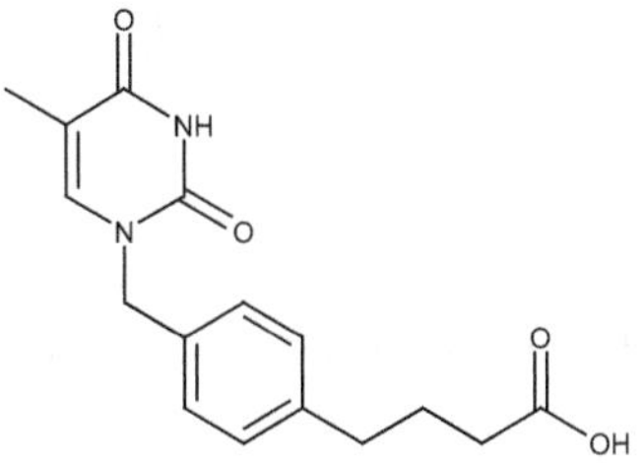

Pyridine derivatives have also been described as anti-TB agents, an example is compound 53 (figure 17), which presents inhibitory activity with an IC50 value of 0.38 µM, suggesting that its possible mechanism of action is through glutamine synthetase inhibition. This would be the first inhibitor compound not derived from amino acids (Odell et al, 2009). Another series of pyridine derivatives were developed by Fassihi et al who synthesized compound 54 (figure 17), a potent anti-TB agent with activity similar to RIF. The results of these compounds showed that an imidazole group as a substituent is equivalent to a nitro phenyl group, which has been reported in anti-TB agents derived from 1,4-dihydropyridinecarboxamides (Fassihi et al., 2009).

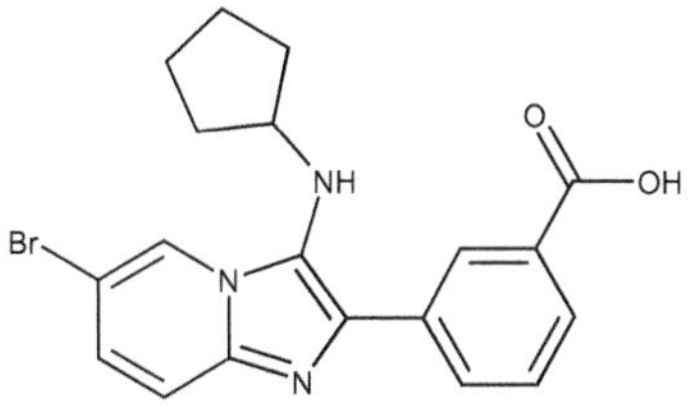

Fig. 17. Pyridine derivatives with potential activityanti-TB.

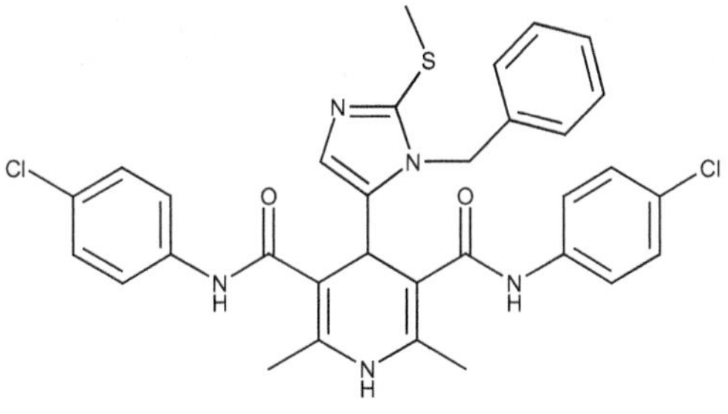

Another important heterocyclic for the design of anti-TB agents is the pyridazine moiety. In these compounds a relationship between Br, Cl and CH_3 substituents, respectively, with Br and vinyl has been found with a favorable anti-TB activity. In these compounds there is an influence of the substituents X in *para*-position on the aromatic ring, where the activity is increased in the following order: $CH_3 < Cl < Br$ with the activity being affected by the R1 substituents, where the most active compounds have a CH_3 group (55, figure 18) (Mantu et al., 2010).

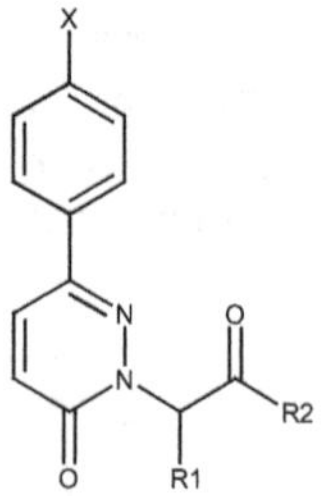

55

Fig. 18. N-substituted-pyridazinones derivatives.

3.8 Other derivatives

Several studies indicate that thiosemicarbazone derivatives can be used in TB therapy and prophylaxis. Previous studies of 1H-2-thiosemicarbazoneindolinone derivatives indicate that halogenation of R1, elongation of the alkyl chain in R2, substitutions of the alkyl chain in R2 with cyclohexyl or phenyl, and the presence of a substituent in R3, are more efficient for increasing anti-TB activity, while R1 substitutions with a nitro group produce the most active compounds. The presence of a morpholine ring in Schiff bases substituted in R1 with a nitro group also has a significant impact on anti-TB activity. The results of biological activity of this new series indicate that the elongation of the alkyl chain increases activity. This enhanced activity is related to lipophilicity properties and confirmed by values of Log P compounds. Also, replacement of the alkyl chain in R2 and phenyl unsubstituted ciclohexyl has led to more active compounds (56, figure 19). The absence of substitutions at N1 on the indole ring and increased lipophilicity appear to be responsible for high activity against *M. tuberculosis* (Guzel et al., 2008). An example of thiosemicarbazone-derived compounds that have exhibited important anti-TB activity with an IC50 value of 2.59 uM/mL, is compound 57 (figure 19) (Karali et al., 2007).

56   57

Fig. 19. General structure of 1H-indole-2,3-dione 3-thiosemicarbazone with anti-TB activity.

Other moieties used in the design of anti-TB agents are phenazine and benzothidiazine. In particular, benzothidiazine 1,1-dioxide constituents are an important class of anti-TB agents (58, figure 20). A SAR study of this series of compounds indicates that the furan/thiophene group linked to benzothidiazine through a methylen bridge exhibits good activity against TB. It is important to point out that a conjugated thiophene derivative shows moderate activity and is enhanced when it presents a nitrofuran group. However, elimination of the methylene group with a carbonyl group leads to a dramatic loss of activity. Finally, Kamal et al postulated piperazine-benzothidiazine with methylene linkage (59, figure 20) as an attractive moiety for the design of anti-TB agents (Kamal et al., 2010).

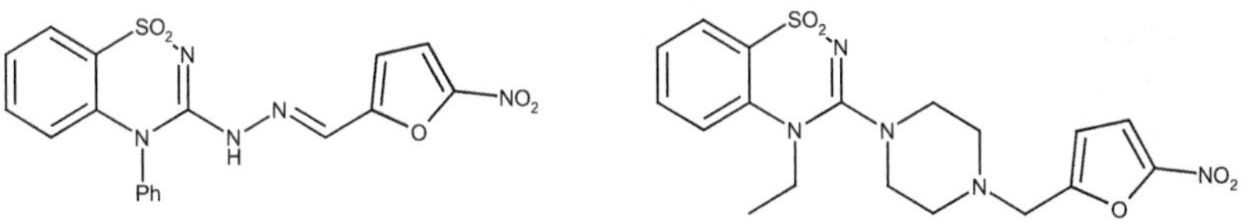

58   59

Fig. 20. Benzothiadiazine derivatives as anti-TB agents.

The creation of a hybrid compound has been a frequent strategy for the design of anti-TB agents. One example is compound 60 (figure 21), formed from dibenzofuran and 2,2-dimethylpyran subunits. SAR studies and modifications of benzofurobenzopyran have demonstrated less active compounds such as compound 61, where the furan B ring is replaced by an ether linker, a single carbon-carbon bond, a carbonyl group, a hydroxymethylene or a methylene group. Even modifications such as acylation and bromination in 5-position on the C ring have produced inactive compounds, thus, it has been suggested as a basis for the pharmacophore structure of compound 60. In this sense, Termenzi et al has carried out the synthesis of more derivatives of compound 60, finding that substitutions with a hydroxy, methoxy, or halogen group on benzofurobenzopyran increases anti-TB activity. Although, hydroxy compounds with good activity showed, unfortunately, cytotoxic activity on VERO cells. Halogenated compounds with a Cl or Br atom in 8, 9 and 11-position, exhibit increased potency compared with compound 60. SAR analysis shows that electronic effects of substituents on the A ring play a dramatic role in anti-TB activity. In addition, potency was significantly decreased when the A ring was substituted by an electron withdrawing group. In contrast, electron donating group substitutions such as hydroxy or methoxy show a significant increase in activity (62, figure 21). While all compounds showed a possible mechanism of action of interaction with lipid biosynthesis of the M. tuberculosis cell wall, a specific compound was an epoxy-mycolate synthesis inhibitor (Termentzi et al., 2010).

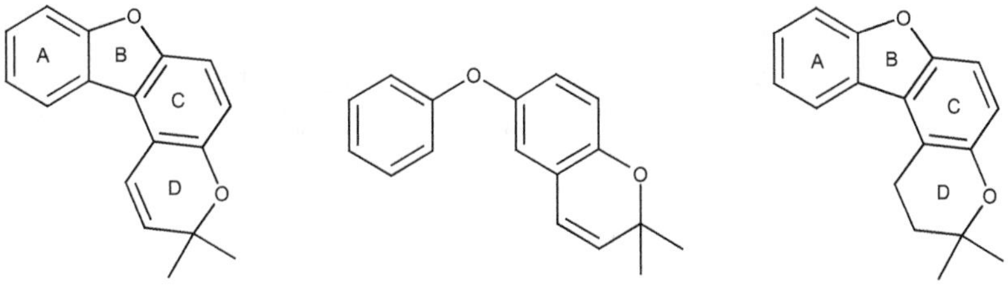

60   61   62

Fig. 21. Structure of benzofurobenzopyrane as anti-TB agents.

Other compounds containing a phthalimide moiety have been described as biophoro to design new prototypes of drug candidates with different biological activities. It has been shown that hybridization of both phthalimide (Thalidomide) and sulfonamide (Dapsone) moiety leads to compounds with activity against *M. leprae*. In this sense, the design of new products such as anti-TB agents is interesting. SAR study of a series of derivatives showed that if the pyrimidine ring is substituted in any position or changed by an isosteric, this decreases activity on *M. tuberculosis*. Amino group substitutions by another phthalimide ring also lead to a decrease in anti-TB activity (63, figure 22). Modifications in the pyridine ring decrease anti-TB activity. Introduction of a phthalimide group by molecular hybridization did not produce compounds with an activity similar to INH; however, it allows for compounds with MIC values similar to PZA (Santos et al., 2009).

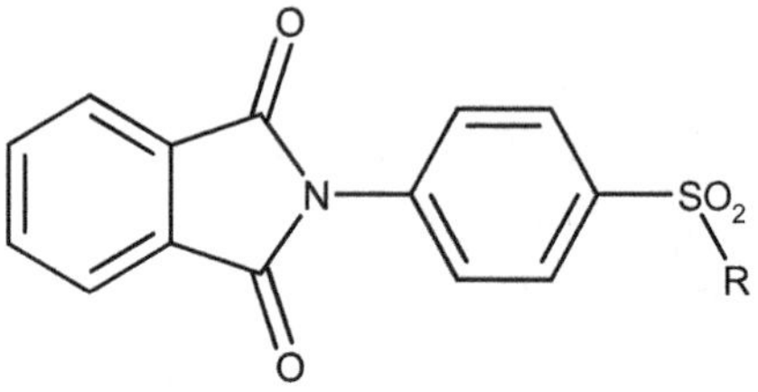

63

Fig. 22. Phthalimide derivatives as anti-TB agent.

Among families of compounds that act as inhibitors of the FAS-II system we can mention diphenyl ether systems that interact with enzyme-cofactor binary complex, but, recently new compounds such as indols, benzofuran and cinnamic acid derivatives have been reported. Development of new cinnamic acid derivatives would focus on more specific FAS-II inhibitors. From a series of compounds developed (figure 23) it was determined that addition of an alkyl chain increases anti-TB activity. The best results are associated with an acceptable lipophilicity parameter that appears when a geranyl chain is incorporated. This led to compound 64, the most active substance with an MIC of 0.1 μg/mL (Yoya et al., 2009).

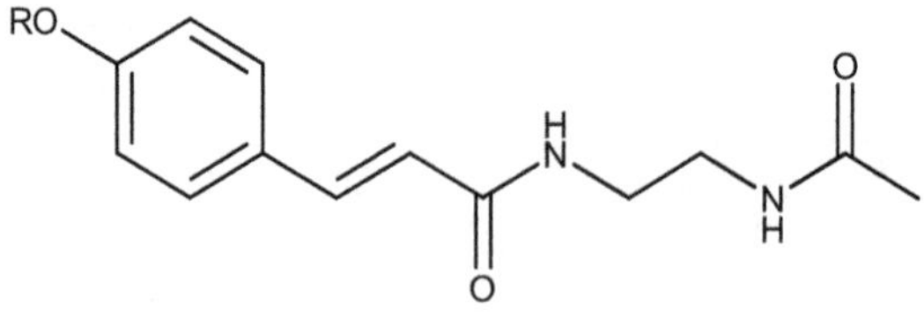

64

Fig. 23. Cinnamic derivatives.

It has also been shown that amide derivatives of fatty acids have anti-TB activity. Due to their nature these compounds are designed to penetrate bacterial cells, which can be useful for studying the mechanism of INH resistance as this can also be due to factors such as mutations in unknown genes, decreased permeability, or increased efflux (D'Oca et al., 2010).

4. Drugs in clinical trials

In drug design, bicyclic nitroimidazofurane derivatives that have anti-TB activity, such as CGI-17341 (65, figure 24) have been developed; however, this compound is mutagenic. This has led to the development of PA-824 (66, figure 24), which is currently in phase II clinical studies and has a long half-life. Its mechanism of action is to inhibit *M. tuberculosis* cell wall lipids and protein synthesis; however, it also inhibits non-replicating bacteria. Additionally, it was reported that PA-824 is a prodrug that is metabolized by *M. tuberculosis* before exercising its effect and may involve bioreduction of aromatic nitro groups to generate a radical intermediate nitro.

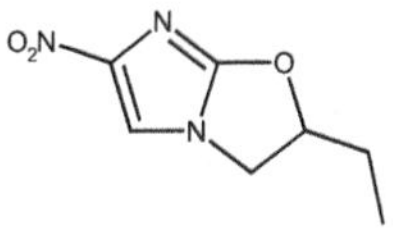

CGI-17341 (65)

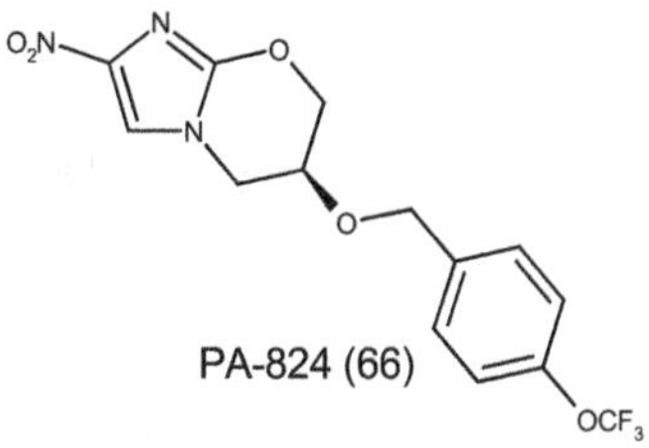

PA-824 (66)

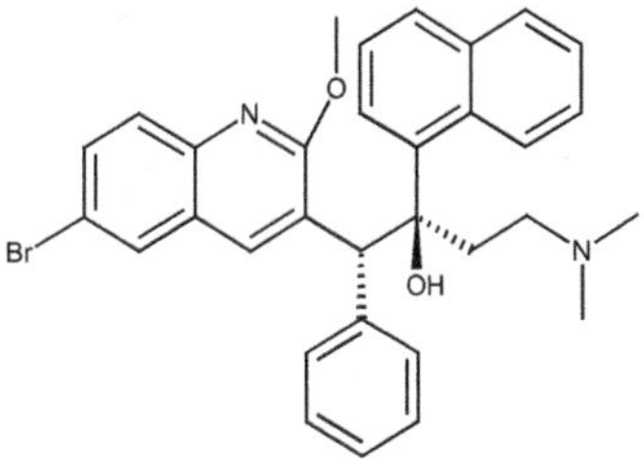

TMC-207 (68)

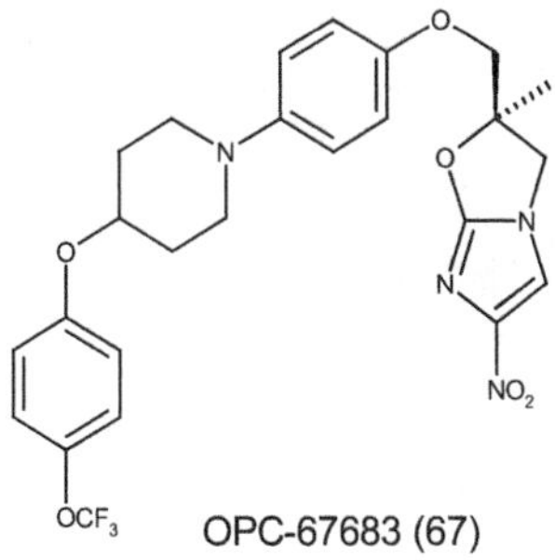

OPC-67683 (67)

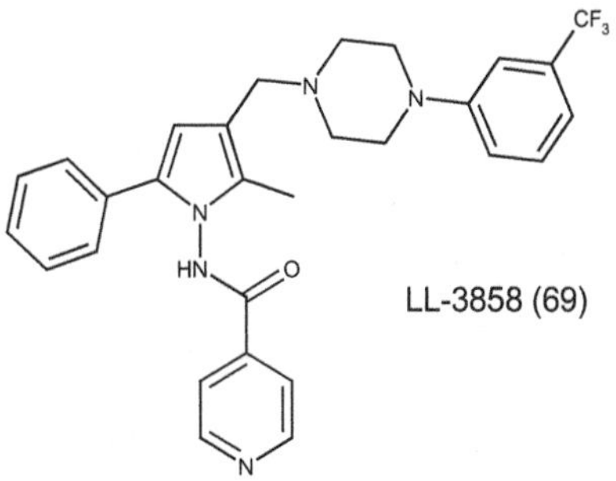

LL-3858 (69)

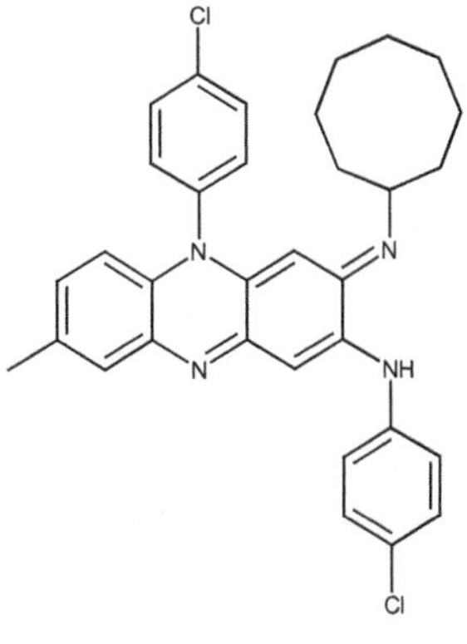

OPC-37306 (70)

Fig. 24. Anti-TB compounds in clinical trials.

The interest in derived oxazoles as anti-TB compounds led to the development of OPC-67683 (67, figure 24), which has excellent activity *in vitro* in sensitive and resistant *M. tuberculosis* strains. It has a long half-life and its mechanism of action involves inhibition of the synthesis of keto-mycolic, and methoxy-mycolic acid, although is possible another possible mechanism of action or interaction with another drug target in *M. tuberculosis*. OPC-67683 also acts as a prodrug, since *M. tuberculosis* metabolizes it and produces as a product desnitro-imidazooxazole metabolite.

TMC207 (68, figure 25) is a quinoline derivative with potent anti-TB activity in susceptible, DR and XDR strains. It is well absorbed in humans with a long half-life and is currently in phase II clinical studies. Its mechanism of action involves inhibition of ATP synthase that binds the *M. tuberculosis* membrane and there is a synergistic effect between TMC207 and PZA. Other compounds with very promising anti-TB activity are LL-3858 and OPC-37306 (69 and 70, figure 25) (Rivers et al., 2008). Some other examples of anti-TB compounds in clinical trials are showed in table 1 (Janin, 2007; Palomino et al., 2009; Shi & Sugawara, 2010)

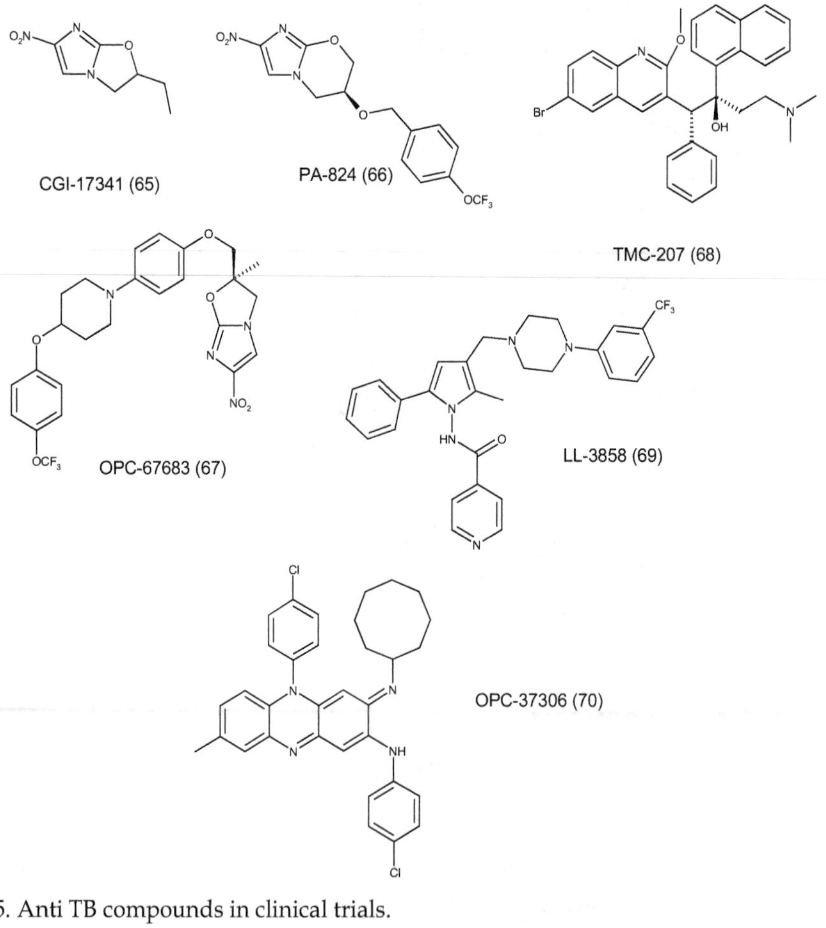

Fig. 25. Anti TB compounds in clinical trials.

Compound	Funding	Target	Mechanism of action	Resistance mechanisms	Clinical trial phase
a) Nitroimidazoxacines					
PA-824	GATB	F420 dependent nitroreductase	Inhibition of proteins and cell wall biosynthesis	Rv0407, Rv3547, Rv3261 and Rv3262 mutations	II
OPC-67683	Otsuka	Nitroreductase	Inhibition of mycolic acid and cell wall biosynthesis	Rv3547 mutations	II
b) Fluoroquinolones					
Moxifloxacin	Bayer, CDC, NIH, FDA	DNA girase	Inhibition of DNA biosynthesis	*gyrA* mutations	III
Gatifloxacine	NIH	DNA girase	Inhibition of DNA biosynthesis	*gyrA* mutations	III
c) Diarilquinolines					
TMC207	Tibotec	F1F0 ATP sintetase	Inhibition of ATP synthesis and disruption of membrane potential	*atp*E mutations	II
d) Oxazolidinones					
Linezolid	NIH, Pfizer	Ribosome	Inhibition of protein biosynthesis	rRNA 23S mutations	Pre-trial
e) Dietilamins					
SQ109	Sequella	Un known	Inhibition of cell wall biosynthesis	Unknown	I/II
f) Pirrols					
LL3858	Lupin	Unknown	Unknown	Unknown	I

Table 1. Some compounds under clinical trials

5. Conclusion

Tuberculosis remains the leading infectious disease worldwide, despite the availability of TB chemotherapy and the BCG vaccine. This is further demonstrated by the fact that half a year of treatment with multiple drugs is needed. Recent genetic and genomic tools as well as high-throughput screening, and structure-based drug design strategies have allowed the discovery of new anti-TB drugs. These are increasingly receiving more attention, and a large number of new compounds or derivatives from existing drugs are under investigation. With this and a better understanding of the unique biology of TB, more targets will be validated, and hopefully a pattern will emerge that will help us reach the goals of more potent compounds that allow multiple stages and drug targets to be addressed.

6. References

Ahmad, Z., Sharma, S., Khuller, GK., Singh, P., Faujdar, J., Katoch, VM. (2006). Antimycobacterial activity of econazole against multidrug-resistant strains of *Mycobacterium tuberculosis*. *International Journal of Antimicrobial Agents*, Vol. 28, No.6, (Dec 2006), pp. 543-544. ISSN: 0924-8579.

Anderson, RG., Hussey, H., Baddiley, J. (1972). The mechanism of wall synthesis in bacteria. The organization of enzymes and isoprenoid phosphates in the membrane. *The Biochemical Journal*. Vol. 127, No. 1 (Mar 1972), pp. 11-25. ISSN: 0264-6021.

Av-Gay, Y., Everett, M. (2000). The eukaryotic-like Ser/Thr protein kinases of *Mycobacterium tuberculosis*. *Trends in Microbiology*, Vol. 8, No.5, (May 2000), pp. 238-244. ISSN: 0966-842X.

Bairwa, R., Kakwani, M., Tawari, NR., Lalchandani, J., Ray, MK., Rajan, MG., Degani, MS. (2010). Novel molecular hybrids of cinnamic acids ad guanylhydrazones as potential antitubercular agents. *Bioorganic & Medicinal Chemistry Letters*, Vol.20, No.5 (Jan, 2010), pp. 1623-1625, ISSN 0960-894X.

Banerjee, A., Sugantino, M., Sacchettini, JC., Jacobs, WR. Jr. (1998). The mabA gene from the inhA operon of *Mycobacterium tuberculosis* encodes a 3-ketoacyl reductase that fails to confer isoniazid resistance. *Microbiology*, Vol. 144, No.10,(Oct 1998), pp. 2697-2704. ISSN: 1350-0872.

Bellinzoni, M., De Rossi, E., Branzoni, M., Milano, A., Peverali, FA., Rizzi, M., Riccardi, G. (2002). Heterologous expression, purification, and enzymatic activity of *Mycobacterium tuberculosis* NAD(+) synthetase. *Protein Expression and Purification*. Vol. 25, No.3, (Aug 2002), pp. 547-557. ISSN: 1046-5928.

Betts, JC., McLaren, A., Lennon, MG., Kelly, FM., Lukey, PT., Blakemore, SJ., Duncan, K. (2003). Signature gene expression profiles discriminate between isoniazid-, thiolactomycin-, and triclosan-treated *Mycobacterium tuberculosis*. *Antimicrobial Agents and Chemotherapy*. Vol. 47, No.9, (Sep 2003), pp. 2903-2913. ISSN: 1073-449X.

Blumberg, HM., Burman, WJ., Chaisson, RE., Daley, CL., Etkind, SC., Friedman, LN., Fujiwara, P., Grzemska, M., Hopewell, PC., Iseman, MD., Jasmer, RM., Koppaka, V., Menzies, RI., O'Brien, RJ., Reves, RR., Reichman, LB., Simone, PM., Starke, JR., Vernon, AA. (2003). American Thoracic Society, Centers for Disease Control and Prevention and the Infectious Diseases Society. American Thoracic Society/Centers for Disease Control and Prevention/Infectious Diseases Society of America: treatment of tuberculosis. *American Journal of Respiratory and Critical Care Medicine*. Vol. 167, No.4, (Feb 2003), pp. 603-662. ISSN: 1073-449X.

Brennan, PJ., Crick, DC. (2007). The cell-wall core of Mycobacterium tuberculosis in the context of drug discovery. *Current Topics in Medicinal Chemistry*, Vol. 7, No.5, (Feb 2007), pp. 475-88. ISSN: 1568-0266.

Choi, KH., Kremer, L., Besra, GS., Rock, CO. (2000). Identification and substrate specificity of beta -ketoacyl (acyl carrier protein) synthase III (mtFabH) from *Mycobacterium tuberculosis*. *The Journal Biological Chemistry*, Vol. 275, No.36, (Sep 2000), pp. 28201-28207. ISSN: 0021-9258.

Cole, ST., and Alzari PM. (2007) Towards new tuberculosis drugs. *Biochemical Society Transactions*, Vol. 35, Part 5 (Sep 2007), pp. 1321-1324. ISSN: 0300-5127.

Cole, ST., Brosch, R., Parkhill, J., Garnier, T., Churcher, C., Harris, D., Gordon, SV., Eiglmeier, K., Gas, S., Barry, CE. 3rd, Tekaia, F., Badcock, K., Basham, D., Brown,

D., Chillingworth, T., Connor, R., Davies, R., Devlin, K., Feltwell, T., Gentles, S., Hamlin, N., Holroyd, S., Hornsby, T., Jagels, K., Krogh, A., McLean, J., Moule, S., Murphy, L., Oliver, K.,Osborne, J., Quail, MA., Rajandream,MA., Rogers, J., Rutter, S., Seeger, K., Skelton, J., Squares, R., Squares, S., Sulston, JE., Taylor, K., Whitehead, S., Barrell, BG. (1998). Deciphering the biology of *Mycobacterium tuberculosis* from the complete genome sequence. *Nature*, Vol. 393, No.6685, (Jun 1998), pp 537-544. ISSN: 0028-0836.

Correia C., Carvalho MA., Proenca MF. (2009). Synthesis and in vitro activity of 6-amino-2,9-diarylpurines for *Mycobacterium tuberculosis*. *Tetrahedron*, Vol.65, No.34, (Aug, 2009), pp. 6903-6911, ISSN 0040-4020.

Cunico, W., Gomes CR., Ferreira, ML., Ferreira, TG., Cardinot, D., de Souza, MV., Lorenco, MC. (2011). Synthesis and anti-mycobacterial activity of novel amino alcohol derivatives. *European Journal of Medicinal Chemistry*. Vol.46, No.3, (Mar, 2011), pp. 974-978, ISSN 0223-5234.

D'Oca, Cda R., Coelho, T., Marinho, TG., Hack, CR., Duarte, Rda C., da Silva, PA., D'Oca, MG. (2010). Synthesis and antituberculosis activity of new fatty acid amides. *Bioorganic & Medicinal Chemistry Letters*, Vol.20, No.17, (Jul, 2010), pp. 5255-5257, ISSN 0960-894X.

De Logu, A., Palchykovska, LH., Kostina, VH., Sanna, A., Meleddu, R., Chisu, L., Alexeeva, IV., Shved, AD. (2009). Novel N-aryl- and N-hetryl phenazine-1-carboxamide as potential targets for the treatment of infections sustained by drug-resistant and multidrug-resistant *Mycobacterium tuberculosis*. *International Journal Of Antimicrobial Agents*. Vol.33, No.3 (Dec, 2008), pp. 223-229, ISSN 0924-8579.

Delaine, T., Bernades-Genisson, V., Quemard, A., Constant, P., Meunier, B., Bernadou, J. (2010). Development of isoniazid-NAD truncated adduct embedding a lipophilic fragment as potential bi-substrate InhA inhibitorsd and antimycobacterail agents. *European Journal of Medicinal Chemistry*, Vol.45, No. 10, (Oct, 2010), pp. 4554-4561, ISSN 0223-5234.

Ducati, RG., Basso, LA., Santos, DS. (2007). Mycobacterial shikimate pathway enzymes as targets for drug design. *Current Drug Targets*, Vol. 8, No. 3 (Mar 2007), pp. 423-35. ISSN: 1389-4501.

Duncan, K. (2004). Identification and validation of novel drug targets in tuberculosis. *Current Pharmaceutical Design*, Vol. 10, No.26, (Sep 2004) pp. 3185-94. ISSN: 1381-6128

Dye C. (2006). Global epidemiology of tuberculosis. *Lancet*, Vol. 367, No.9514, (Mar 2006), pp.938-40. ISSN: 0140-6736.

Eoh, H., Brennan, PJ., Crick, DC. (2009). The *Mycobacterium tuberculosis* MEP (2C-methyl-d-erythritol 4-phosphate) pathway as a new drug target. *Tuberculosis* (Edinburg, Scotland). Vol. 89, No. 1 (Jan 2009), pp. 1-11. ISSN:1472-9792.

Eswaran, S., Adhikari, AV., Chowdhury, IH., Pal, NK., Thomas, K. (2010). New quinoline derivatives: synthesis and investigation of antibacterial and antituberculosis properties. *European Journal Of Medicinal Chemistry*, Vol.45, No.8, (Apr, 2010), pp. 3374-3383, ISSN 0223-5234.

Eswaran, S., Adhikari, AV., Kumar, R. (2010). New 1,3-oxazolo[4,5-c]quinoline derivatives: Synthesis and evaluation of antibacterial and antituberculosis properties. *European*

Journal of Medicinal Chemistry, Vol.45, No.3, (Nov, 2009), pp. 957-966, ISSN 0223-5234.

Eswaran, S., Adhikari, AV., Pal, NK., Chowdhury, IH. (2010). Design and synthesis of some new quinoline-3-carbohydrazone derivatives as potential antimycobacterial agents. *Bioorganic & Medicinal Chemistry Letters*, Vol.20, No.3, (Dec, 2009), pp. 1040-1044, ISSN 0960-894X.

Fassihi A., Azadpour Z., Delbari N., Saghaie L., Memarian HR., Sabet R., Alborzi A., Miri R., Pourabbas B., Mardaneh J., Mousavi P., Moeinifard B., Sadeghi-aliabdi, H. (2009). Synthesis and antitubercular activity of novel 4-susbtituted imidazolyl-2.6-dimethyl-N3,N5-bisaryl-1,4-dihydropyridine-3,5-dicaroxamides. *European Journal of Medicinal Chemistry*, Vol.44, No.8, (Mar, 2009), pp. 3253-3258. ISSN 0223-5234.

Feng, Z., Barletta, RG. (2003). Roles of *Mycobacterium smegmatis* D-alanine:D-alanine ligase and D-alanine racemase in the mechanisms of action of and resistance to the peptidoglycan inhibitor D-cycloserine. *Antimicrobial Agents and Chemotherapy*, Vol. 47, No. 1 (Jan 2003), pp. 283-291 ISSN: 0066-4804.

Fernandez, P., Saint-Joanis, B., Barilone, N., Jackson, M., Gicquel, B., Cole, ST., Alzari, PM. (2006). The Ser/Thr protein kinase PknB is essential for sustaining mycobacterial growth. *Journal of Bacteriology*, Vol. 188, No.22, (Nov 2006), pp. 7778-7784. ISSN: 0021-9193.

Ferreras, JA., Ryu, JS., Di Lello, F., Tan, DS., Quadri, LE. (2005). Small-molecule inhibition of siderophore biosynthesis in *Mycobacterium tuberculosis* and *Yersinia pestis*. *Nature Chemical Biology*, Vol. 1, No.1, (Jun 2005), pp. 29-32. ISSN: 1552-4450.

Ferriz, JM., Vavrova, K., Kunc, F., Imramovsky, A., Stolarikova, J., Vavrikova, E., Vinsova, J. (2010). Salicylanilide carbamates: Antitubercular agents active against multidrug-resistant *Mycobacterium tuberculosis* strains. *Bioorganic & Medicinal Chemistry*, Vol.18, No.3, (Dec, 2009), pp. 1054-1061, ISSN 0968-0896.

Gasse, C., Douguet, D., Huteau, V., Marchal, G., Munier-Lehmann, H., Pochet, S. (2008). Substituted benzyl-pyrimidines targeting thymidine monophosphate kinase of *Mycobacterium tuberculosis*: Synthesis and in vitro anti-mycobacterial activity. *Bioorganic & Medicinal Chemistry*, Vol. 16, No.11, (Apr, 2008), pp. 6075-6085, ISSN 0968-0896.

Gerum, AB., Ulmer, JE., Jacobus, DP., Jensen, NP., Sherman, DR., Sibley, CH. (2002). Novel Saccharomyces cerevisiae screen identifies WR99210 analogues that inhibit *Mycobacterium tuberculosis* dihydrofolate reductase. *Antimicrobial Agents and Chemotherapy*, Vol. 46, No.11, (Nov 2002), pp. 3362-3369. ISSN: 0066-4804.

Gill, C., Jadhav, G., Shaikh, M., Kale, R., Ghawalkar, A., Nagargoje, D., Shiradkar, M. (2008). Clubbed [1,2,3] triazoles by fluorine benzimidazole: A novel approach to H37Rv inhibitors as a potential treatment for tuberculosis. *Bioorganic & Medicinal Chemistry Letters*, Vol.18, No.23, (Oct, 2008), pp. 6244-6247, ISSN 0968-0896.

Goncalves, RS., Kaiser, CR., Lourenco, MC., de Souza, MV., Wardell, JL., Wardell, SM., da Silva, AD. (2010). Synthesis and antitubercular activity of new mefloquine-oxazolidine derivatives. *European Journal of Medicinal Chemistry*. Vol.45, No.12, (Sep, 2010), pp. 6095-6100, ISSN 0223-5234.

Gong, C., Martins, A., Bongiorno, P., Glickman, M., Shuman, S. (2004). Biochemical and genetic analysis of the four DNA ligases of mycobacteria. *The Journal of Biological Chemistry*, Vol. 279, No.20, (May 2004), pp. 20594-20606. ISSN: 0021-9258.

Güzel, O., Karali, N., Salman, A. (2008). Synthesis and antituberculosis activity of 5-methyl/trifluoromethoxy-1H-indole-2,3-dione 3-thiosemicarbazone derivatives. *Bioorganic & Medicinal Chemistry*, Vol.16, No.19, (Aug, 2008), pp. 8976-8987, ISSN 0968-0896.

Haouz, A., Vanheusden, V., Munier-Lehmann, H., Froeyen, M., Herdewijn, P., Van Calenbergh, S., Delarue, M. (2003). Enzymatic and structural analysis of inhibitors designed against *Mycobacterium tuberculosis* thymidylate kinase. New insights into the phosphoryl transfer mechanism. *The Journal of Biological Chemistry*, Vol. 278, No. 7, (Feb 2003), pp. 4963-4971. ISSN: 0021-9258.

Hasan, S., Daugelat, S., Rao, PS., Schreiber, M. (2006). Prioritizing genomic drug targets in pathogens: application to *Mycobacterium tuberculosis*. *PLoS Computational Biology*, Vol. 2, No.6, (Jun 2006) Epub 2006: ISSN: 1553-734X.

Hearn MJ., Cynamon MH., Chen MF., Coppins R., Davis J., Joo-On Kang, H., Noble A., Tu-Sekine B., Terrot MS., Trombino D., Thai M., Webster ER., Wilson, R. (2009). Preparation and antitubercular activities in vitro and in vivo of novel Schiff bases of isoniazid. *European Journal of Medicinal Chemistry*, Vol.44, No.10, (Oct, 2009), pp. 4169-4178, ISSN 0223-5234.

Heath, RJ., White, SW., Rock, CO. (2001). Lipid biosynthesis as a target for antibacterial agents. *Progress in Lipid Research*. Vol. 40, No.6, (Nov 2001), pp. 467-497. ISSN: 0163-7827.

Huang, H., Scherman, MS., D'Haeze, W., Vereecke, D., Holsters, M., Crick, DC., McNeil, MR. (2005) Identification and active expression of the *Mycobacterium tuberculosis* gene encoding 5-phospho-{alpha}-d-ribose-1-diphosphate: decaprenyl phosphate 5-phosphoribosyltransferase, the first enzyme committed to decaprenylphosphoryl-d-arabinose synthesis. *The Journal Biological Chemistry*, Vol. 280, No. 26 (Jul 2005), pp. 24539-24543. ISSN: 0021-9258.

Huovinen, P., Sundström, L., Swedberg, G., Sköld, O. (1995). Trimethoprim and sulfonamide resistance. *Antimicrobial Agents and Chemotherapy*, Vol. 39, No.2, (Feb 1995), pp. 279-289. ISSN: 0066-4804.

Imramovsky, A., Polanc, S., Vinsova, J., kocevar, M., Jampilek, J., Reckova, Z., Kaustova, J. (2007). A new modification of anti-tubercular active molecules. *Bioorganic & Medicinal Chemistry*, Vol.15, No.7, (Apr, 2007), pp. 2551-2559, ISSN 0968-0896.

Imramovsky, A., Vinsova J., Ferriz, JM., Buchta, V., Jampilek, J. (2009). Salicylanilide esters of N-protected amino acids as novel antimicrobial agents. *Bioorganic & Medicinal Chemistry Letters*, Vol.19, No.2, (Nov, 2008), pp. 348-351, ISSN 0968-0896.

Imramovsky, A., Vinsova, J., Ferriz, JM., Dolezal, R., Jampilek, J., Kaustova, J., Kunc, F. (2009). New antituberculotics originated from salicylanilides with promising in vitro activity against atypical mycobacterial strains. *Bioorganic & Medicinal Chemistry*, Vol.17, No.10, (May, 2010), pp. 3572-3579, ISSN 0968-0896.

Izumizono, Y., Arevalo, S., Koseki, Y., Kuroki, M., Aoki, S. (2011). Identification of novel potential antibiotics for tuberculosis by in silico structure-based drug screening. *European Journal of Medicinal Chemistry*, Vol.46, No.5, (Feb, 2011), pp. 1849-1856, ISSN 0223-5234.

Jadhav GR., Shaikh MU., Kale RP., Shiradkar MR., Gill, CH. (2009). SAR study of clubbed [1,2,4]-triazolyl with fluorobenzimidazoles as antimicrobial and antitubeculosis agents. *European Journal of Medicinal Chemistry*, Vol.44, No.7, (Dec, 2008), pp. 2930-2935, ISSN 0223-5234.

Janin YL. (2007). Antituberculosis drugs: ten years of research. *Bioorganic and Medicinal Chemistry*, Vol. 15, No.7, (Apr 2007), pp. 2479-2513. ISSN: 0968-0896.

Kamal, A., Shett, RVCRNC., Azeeza, S., Ahmed, SK., Swapna, P., Reddy, AM., Khan, IA., Sharma, S., Abdullah, ST. (2010). Anti-tubercular agents. Part 5: Synthesis and biological evaluation of benzothiadiazine 1,1,-dioxide based congeners. *European Journal of Medicinal Chemistry*, Vol.45, No.10, (Jul, 2010), pp. 4545-4553, ISSN0223-5234.

Karali, N., Gürsoy, A., Kandemirli, F., Shvets, N., Kaynak, FB., Özbey., Kovalishyn, V., Dimoglo, A. (2007). Synthesis and structure-antituberculosis activity relationship of 1H-indole-2,3-dione derivatives. *Bioorganic & Medicinal Chemistry*, Vol.15, No.17, (Jun, 2007), pp. 5888-5904, ISSN 0968-0896.

Karthikeyan, SV., Bala, BD., Raja, VP., Perumal, S., Yogeeswari, P., Sriram, D. (2010). A highly atom economic, chemo-, regio and stereoselective synthesis and evaluation of spiro-pyrrolothiazoles as antitubercular agents. *Bioorganic & Medicinal Chemistry Letters*, Vol. 20, No.1, (Oct, 2009), pp. 350-353, ISSN 0960-894X.

Khasnobis, S., Escuyer, VE., Chatterjee, D. (2002). Emerging therapeutic targets in tuberculosis: post-genomic era. *Expert Opinion on Therapeutic Targets*, Vol. 6, No.1, (Feb 2002), pp. 21-40. ISSN: 1472-8222.

Khoje, AD., Kulendrn, A., Charnock, C., Wan, B., Franzblau, S., Gundersen, LL. (2010). Synthesis of non-purine analogs of 6-aryl-9-benzylpurines, and their antimycobacterial activities. Compounds modified in the imidazole ring. *Bioorganic & Medicinal Chemistry*, Vol.18, No.20, (Aug, 2010), pp. 7274-7282, ISSN 0968-0896.

Kini SG., bhat AR., Bryant B., Williamson J., Dayan FE. (2009). Synthesis, antitubercular activity and docking study of novel cyclic azole substituted diphenyl ether derivatives. *European Journal of Medicinal Chemistry*, Vol.44, No.2, (May, 2008), pp. 492-500, ISSN 0223-5234.

Klimesova, V., Koci, J., Waisser, K., Kaustova, J., Mollmann, U. (2009). Preparation and in vitro evaluation of benzylsulfanyl benzoxazole derivatives as potential antituberculosis agents. *European Journal of Medicinal Chemistry*, Vol.44, No.5, (Jul, 2008), pp. 2286-2293, ISSN 0223-5234.

Kremer, L., Nampoothiri, KM., Lesjean, S., Dover, LG., Graham, S., Betts, J., Brennan, PJ., Minnikin, DE., Locht, C., Besra, GS. (2001). Biochemical characterization of acyl carrier protein (AcpM) and malonyl-CoA:AcpM transacylase (mtFabD), two major components of *Mycobacterium tuberculosis* fatty acid synthase II. *The Journal Biological Chemistry*, Vol. 276, No.30, (Jul 2001), pp. 27967-27974. ISSN: 0021-9258.

Larsen, MH., Vilchèze, C., Kremer, L., Besra, GS., Parsons, L., Salfinger, M., Heifets, L., Hazbon, MH., Alland, D., Sacchettini, JC., Jacobs, WR Jr. (2002). Overexpression of inhA, but not kasA, confers resistance to isoniazid and ethionamide in *Mycobacterium smegmatis*, *M. bovis* BCG and *M. tuberculosis*. *Molecular Microbiology*, Vol. 46, No.2, (Oct 2002), pp. 453-466. ISSN: 0950-382X.

LeMagueres, P., Im, H., Ebalunode, J., Strych, U., Benedik, MJ., Briggs, JM., Kohn, H., Krause, KL. (2005). The 1.9 A crystal structure of alanine racemase from *Mycobacterium tuberculosis* contains a conserved entryway into the active site. *Biochemistry*, Vol. 44, No.5, (Feb 2005), pp. 1471-1481. ISSN: 0006-2960.

Leys, D., Mowat, CG., McLean, KJ., Richmond, A., Chapman, SK., Walkinshaw, MD., Munro, AW. (2003). Atomic structure of *Mycobacterium tuberculosis* CYP121 to 1.06 A reveals novel features of cytochrome P450. *The Journal Biological Chemistry*, Vol. 278, No.7, (Feb 2003), pp. 5141-5147. ISSN: 0021-9258.

Magalhães, ML., Pereira, CP., Basso, LA., Santos, DS. (2002). Cloning and expression of functional shikimate dehydrogenase (EC 1.1.1.25) from *Mycobacterium tuberculosis* H37Rv. *Protein Expression and Purification*, Vol. 26, No.1, (Oct 2002), pp. 59-64. ISSN: 1046-5928.

Mahapatra, S., Yagi, T., Belisle, JT., Espinosa, BJ., Hill, PJ., McNeil, MR., Brennan, PJ., Crick, DC. (2005). Mycobacterial lipid II is composed of a complex mixture of modified muramyl and peptide moieties linked to decaprenyl phosphate. *Journal Bacteriology*, Vol. 187, No.8, (Apr 2005), pp.2747-2757. ISSN: 0021-9193.

Manikannan, R., Venkatesan, R., Muthusubramanian., Yogeeswari, P., Sriram, D. (2010). Pyrazole derivatives from azines of substituted phenacyl aryl/cyclohexyl sulfides and their antimycobacterial activity. *Bioorganic & Medicinal Chemistry Letters*, Vol.20, No.23, (Oct, 2010), pp. 6920-6924, ISSN 0960-894X.

Mantu, D., Luca, MC., Moldoveanu, C., Zbancioc, G., Mangalagiu, II. (2010). Synthesis and antituberculosis activity of some new pyridazine derivatives. Part II. *European Journal of Medicinal Chemistry*. Vol.45, No.11, (Aug, 2010), pp. 5164-5168, ISSN 0223-5234.

Mao, J., Yuan, H., Wang, Y., Wan, B., Pak, D., He, R., Franzblau, SG. (2010). Synthesis and antituberculosis activity of novel mefloquine-isoxazole carboxylic esters as prodrugs. *Bioorganic & Medicinal Chemistry Letters*, Vol.20, No.3, (Nov, 2009), pp. 1263-1268, ISSN 0960-894X.

Marrakchi, H., Ducasse, S., Labesse, G., Montrozier, H., Margeat, E., Emorine, L., Charpentier, X., Daffé, M., Quémard, A. (2002). MabA (FabG1), a *Mycobacterium tuberculosis* protein involved in the long-chain fatty acid elongation system FAS-II. *Microbiology*, Vol. 148, No.4, (Apr 2002), pp. 951-960. ISSN: 1350-0872.

Marrakchi, H., Lanéelle, G., Quémard, A. (2000). InhA, a target of the antituberculous drug isoniazid, is involved in a mycobacterial fatty acid elongation system, FAS-II. *Microbiology*, Vol. 146, No.2, (Feb 2000), pp. 289-296. ISSN: 1350-0872.

McKinney, JD., Hönerzu Bentrup, K., Muñoz-Elías, EJ., Miczak, A., Chen, B., Chan, WT., Swenson, D., Sacchettini, JC., Jacobs, WR Jr., Russell, DG. (2000). Persistence of *Mycobacterium tuberculosis* in macrophages and mice requires the glyoxylate shunt enzyme isocitrate lyase. *Nature*, Vol. 406, No.6797, (Aug 2000), pp. 735-738. ISSN: 0028-0836 EISSN: 1476-4687.

McLean, KJ., Dunford, AJ., Neeli, R., Driscoll, MD., Munro, AW. (2007). Structure, function and drug targeting in *Mycobacterium tuberculosis* cytochrome P450 systems. *Archives of Biochemistry and Biophysics*, Vol. 464, No.2, (Aug 2007), pp. 228-240. ISSN: 0003-9861.

Mdluli, K., Spigelman, M. (2006). Novel targets for tuberculosis drug discovery. *Current Opinion Pharmacology*, Vol. 6, No.5, (Oct 2006), pp. 459-467. ISSN: 1471-4892.

Meganathan, R. (2001). Biosynthesis of menaquinone (vitamin K2) and ubiquinone (coenzyme Q): a perspective on enzymatic mechanisms. *Vitamins & Hormones*, Vol. 61, No.173, (Aug 2001), pp. 173-218. ISSN: 0083-6729.

Meng, Q., Luo, H., Lu, Y., Li, W., Zhang, W., Yao, Q. (2009). Synthesis and evaluation of carbamate prodrugs of SQ109 as antituberculosis agents. *Bioorganic & Medicinal Chemistry Letters*, Vol.19, No.10, (May, 2009), pp. 2808-2810, ISSN 0960-894X.

Monfeli, RR., Beeson, C. (2007). Targeting iron acquisition by *Mycobacterium tuberculosis*. *Infectious Disorders- Drug Targets*, Vol. 7, No.3, (Sep 2007), pp. 213-220. ISSN: 1871-5265.

Morgunova, E., Meining, W., Illarionov, B., Haase, I., Jin, G., Bacher, A., Cushman, M., Fischer, M., Ladenstein, R. (2005). Crystal structure of lumazine synthase from *Mycobacterium tuberculosis* as a target for rational drug design: binding mode of a new class of purinetrione inhibitors. *Biochemistry*, Vol. 44, No.8, (Mar 2005), pp. 2746-2758. ISSN: 0006-2960,

Navarrete-Vázquez, G., Molina-Salinas, GM., Duarte-Fajardo, ZV., Vargas-Villarreal, J., Estrada-Soto, S., Gonzalez-Salazar, F., Hernandez-Nuñez, E., Said-Fernández, S. (2007). Synthesis and antimycobacterial activity of 4-(5-substituted-1,3,4-oxadiazol-2-yl)pyridines. *Bioorganic & Medicinal Chemistry*, Vol.15, No.16, (Aug, 2007), pp. 5502-5508, ISSN 0968-0896

Nava-Zuazo, C., Estrada-Soto, S., Guerrero-Alvarez, J., Leon-Rivera, I., Molina-Salinas, GM., Said-Fernández, S., Chan-Bacab, MJ., Cedillo-Rivera, R., Moo-Puc, R., Mirón-Lopez, G., Navarrete-Vázquez, G. (2010). Design, synthesis and in vitro anti protozoal, antimycobaterial activities of N-{2-[(7-chloroquinolin-4-yl)amino]ethyl} ureas. *Bioorganic & Medicinal Chemistry*, Vol.18, No.17, (Sep, 2010), pp. 6398-6403, ISSN 0968-0896.

Odell LR., Nilsson MT., Gising J., Lagerlund O., Muthas D., Nordqvist A., Karlen A., Larhed M. (2009). Functionalized 3-amino-imidazol[1,2-a]pyridines: A novel class of drug-like *Mycobacterium tuberculosis* glutamine synthase inhibitors. *Bioorganic & Medicinal Chemistry Letters*, Vol.19, No.16, (Jun, 2009), pp. 4790-4793, ISSN 0960-894X.

Oliveira, JS., Pinto. CA., Basso. LA., Santos. DS. (2001). Cloning and overexpression in soluble form of functional shikimate kinase and 5-enolpyruvylshikimate 3-phosphate synthase enzymes from *Mycobacterium tuberculosis*. *Protein Expression and Purification*, Vol. 22, No.3, (Aug 2001), pp. 430-435. ISSN: 1046-5928.

Paiva, AM., Vanderwall, DE., Blanchard, JS., Kozarich, JW., Williamson, JM., Kelly TM. (2001). Inhibitors of dihydrodipicolinate reductase, a key enzyme of the diaminopimelate pathway of *Mycobacterium tuberculosis*. *Biochimica et Biophysica Acta*, Vol. 1545, No. (Feb 2001), pp. 67-77. ISSN: 0006-3002.

Palomino, JC., Ramos, DF., da Silva PA. (2009). New anti-tuberculosis drugs: strategies, sources and new molecules. *Current Medicinal Chemistry*, Vol. 16, No.15, (Jan 2009), pp. 1898-1904. ISSN: 0929-8673.

Parish, T., Stoker, NG. (2002). The common aromatic amino acid biosynthesis pathway is essential in *Mycobacterium tuberculosis*. *Microbiology*, Vol. 148, No.10, (Oct 2002), pp. 3069-3077. ISSN: 1350-0872.

Patel, NB., Khan, RH., Rajani, SD. (2010) Pharmacological evaluation and characterizations of newly synthesized 1,2,4-triazoles. *European Journal of Medicinal Chemistry*, Vol.45, No.9, (Jun, 2010), pp. 4293-4299, ISSN 0223-5234.

Pavelka, MS Jr., Chen, B., Kelley, CL., Collins, FM., Jacobs, Jr WR Jr. (2003). Vaccine efficacy of a lysine auxotroph of *Mycobacterium tuberculosis*. *Infection and Immunity*, Vol. 71, No.7, (Jul 2003), pp. 4190-4192. ISSN: 0019-9557.

Pavelka, MS Jr., Jacobs, WR Jr. (1999). Comparison of the construction of unmarked deletion mutations in *Mycobacterium smegmatis*, *Mycobacterium bovis* bacillus Calmette-Guérin, and *Mycobacterium tuberculosis* H37Rv by allelic exchange. *Journal of Bacteriology*, Vol. 181, No.16, (Aug 1999), pp.4780-4789. ISSN: 0021-9193.

Petrlikova, E., Waisser, K., Divisova, H., Husakova, P., Vrabcova, P., Kunes, J., Kolar, K., Stolarikova, J. (2010). Highly active antimycobacterial derivatives of benzoxazine. *Bioorganic & Medicinal Chemistry*, Vol. 18, No.23, (Oct, 2010), pp. 8178-8187, ISSN 0968-0896.

Quémard, A., Sacchettini, JC., Dessen, A., Vilcheze, C., Bittman, R., Jacobs, WR Jr., Blanchard, JS. (1995). Enzymatic characterization of the target for isoniazid in *Mycobacterium tuberculosis*. *Biochemistry*, Vol. 26, No.8243, (Jul 1995), pp. 8235-8241. ISSN: 0006-2960.

Rivers, EC., Mancera, RL. (2008). New anti-tuberculosis drugs in clinical trials with novel mechanisms of action. *Drug Discovery Today*, Vol.13, (Oct, 2008), pp. 1090-1098, ISSN 1359-6446.

Sainath, SR., Raghunathan, R., Ekambaram, R., Raghunathan, M. (2009). In vitro activities of the newly synthesised ER-2 against clinical isolates of *Mycobacterium tuberculosis* susceptible or resistant to antituberculosis drugs. *International Journal of Antimicrobial Agents*, Vol.34, No.5, (Jul, 2009), pp. 451-453, ISSN 0924-8579.

Samadhiya, P., Sharma, R., Srivastava, SK. Srivastava, SD. (2011). Synthesis and biological evaluation of 4-thiazolidinone derivatives as antitubercular and antimicrobial agents. *Arabian Journal of Chemistry*, doi: 10.1016/j.arabjc.2010.11.015, (Dec, 2010), ISSN 1878-5352.

Sankar, C., Pandiarajan, K. (2010). Synthesis and anti-tubercular and antimicrobial activities of some 2r,4c-diaryl-3-azabicyclo[3.3.1]nonan-9-one N-isonicotinylhydrazone derivatives. *European Journal of Medicinal Chemistry*, Vol.45, No.11, (Aug, 2010), pp. 5480-5485, ISSN 0223-5234.

Santos, JL., Yamasaki, PR., Chin, CM., Takashi, CH., Pava,n FR., Leite, CQF. (2009). Synthesis and in vitro anti *Mycobacterium tuberculosis* activity of a series of phthalimide derivatives. *Bioorganic & Medicinal Chemistry*, Vol.17, No.11, (May, 2009), pp. 3795-3799, ISSN 0968-0896.

Sareen, D., Newton, GL., Fahey, RC., Buchmeier, NA. (2003). Mycothiol is essential for growth of *Mycobacterium tuberculosis* Erdman. *Journal of Bacteriology*, Vol. 185, No.22, (Nov 2003), pp. 6736-6740. ISSN: 0021-9193.

Sarkar, S., Suresh, MR. (2001). An overview of tuberculosis chemotherapy - a literature review. *Journal of Pharmacy and Pharmaceutical Sciences*, Vol. 14, No.2, (Jul 2011), pp. 148-161. ISSN: 1482-1826.

Sassetti, CM., Boyd, DH., Rubin, EJ. (2003). Genes required for mycobacterial growth defined by high density mutagenesis. *Molecular Microbiology*, Vol. 48, No.1, (Apr 2003), pp. 77-84. ISSN: 0950-382X.

Savvi, S., Warner, DF., Kana, BD., McKinney, JD., Mizrahi, V., Dawes, SS. (2008). Functional characterization of a vitamin B12-dependent methylmalonyl pathway in *Mycobacterium tuberculosis*: implications for propionate metabolism during growth on fatty acids. *Journal of Bacteriology*, Vol. 190, No.11, (Jun 2008), pp. 3886-3895. ISSN: 0021-9193.

Scarsdale, JN., Kazanina, G., He, X., Reynolds, KA., Wright HT. (2001). Crystal structure of the *Mycobacterium tuberculosis* beta-ketoacyl-acyl carrier protein synthase III. *The Journal of Biological Chemistry*, Vol. 276, No.23, (Jun 2001), pp. 20516-20522. ISSN: 0021-9258.

Shi, R., Sugawara, I. (2010). Development of new anti-tuberculosis drug candidates. *The Tohoku Journal of experimental medicine*, Vol. 22, No.2, (Feb 2010), pp. 97-106. ISSN: 0040-8727

Shiradkar, M., Suresh Kumar, GV., Dasari, V., Tatikonda, S., Akula, KC., Shah, R. (2007). Clubbed triazoles: A novel approach to antitubercular drugs. *European Journal of Medicinal Chemistry*, Vol.42, No.6, (Dec, 2006), pp. 807-816, ISSN 0223-5234.

Singh, K., Singh, K., Wan, B., Franzblau, S., Chibale, K., Balzarini, J. (2011). Facile transformation of biginelli pyrimidin-2(1H)-ones to pyrimidines. In vitro evaluation as inhibitors of *Mycobacterium tuberculosis* and modulators of cytostatic activity. *European Journal of Medicinal Chemistry*, Vol.46, No.6, (Mar, 2011), pp. 2290-2294, ISSN 0223-5234.

Slayden, RA., Barry, CE 3rd. (2002). The role of KasA and KasB in the biosynthesis of meromycolic acids and isoniazid resistance in *Mycobacterium tuberculosis*. *Tuberculosis* (Edinburg, Scotland). Vol. 82, No.4, (Jan 2002), pp. 149-160. ISSN: 1472-9792.

Smith, DA., Parish, T., Stoker, NG., Bancroft, GJ. (2001). Characterization of auxotrophic mutants of *Mycobacterium tuberculosis* and their potential as vaccine candidates. *Infection and Immunity*, Vol. 69, No.2, (Feb 2001), pp. 1142-1150. ISSN: 0019-9567.

Srivastava, SK., Tripathi, RP., Ramachandran, R. (2005). NAD+-dependent DNA Ligase (Rv3014c) from *Mycobacterium tuberculosis*. Crystal structure of the adenylation domain and identification of novel inhibitors. *The Journal of Biological Chemistry*, Vol. 280, No.34, (Aug 2005), pp. 30273-30281. ISSN: 0021-9258.

Strych, U., Penland, RL., Jimenez, M., Krause, KL., Benedik, MJ. (2001). Characterization of the alanine racemases from two mycobacteria. *FEMS Microbiology Letters*, Vol. 196, No.2, (Mar 2001), pp. 93-98. ISSN: 1574-6968.

Sun, Z., Zhang, Y. (1999). Antituberculosis activity of certain antifungal and antihelmintic drugs. *Tubercle and Lung Disease*, Vol. 79, No.5, (Jan 1999), pp. 319-320. ISSN: 0962-8479.

Suresh Kumar GV., Rajendra Prasad, Y., Mallikarjuna, BP., Chandrashekar, SM. (2010). Synthesis and pharmacological evaluation of clubbed isopropylthiazole derived triazolothiadiazoles, triazolothiadiazines and mannich bases as potential antimicrobial and antitubercular agents. *European Journal of Medicinal Chemistry*, Vol.45, No.11, (Aug, 2010), pp. 5120-51299, ISSN 0223-5234.

Teo, JW., Thayalan, P., Beer, D., Yap, AS., Nanjundappa, M., Ngew, X., Duraiswamy, J., Liung, S., Dartois, V., Schreiber, M., Hasan, S., Cynamon, M., Ryder, NS., Yang, X., Weidmann, B., Bracken, K., Dick, T., Mukherjee, K. (2006). Peptide deformylase inhibitors as potent antimycobacterial agents. *Antimicrobial Agents and Chemotherapy*, Vol. 50, No.11, (Nov 2006), pp. 3665-3673. ISSN: 0066-4804.

Termentzi, A., Khouri, I., Gaslonde, T., Prado, S., Saint-Joanis, B., Bardou, F., Amanatiadou, EP., Vizirianakis, I., Kordulakova, J., Jackson, M., Brisch, R., Janin, YL., Daffe, M., Tillequin, F., Michel, S. (2010). Synthesis, biological activity and evaluation of the mode of action of novel antitubercular benzofurobenzopyrans substituted on A ring. *European Journal of Medicinal Chemistry*, Vol.45, No.12, (Oct, 2010), pp. 5833-5847, ISSN 0223-5234.

Turan-Zitouni, G., Kaplancikli, Z.A., Ozdemir, A. (2010). Synthesis and antituberculosis activity of some N-pyridyl-N-thiazolylhydrazine derivatives. *European Journal of Medicinal Chemistry*, Vol.45, No.5, (Jan, 2010), pp. 2085-2088, ISSN 0223-5234.

Turan-Zitouni, G., Ozdemir, A., Kaplancikli, Z.A., Benkli, K., Chevallet, P., Akalin, G. (2008). Synthesis and antituberculosis activity of new thiazolylhydrazone derivatives. *European Journal of Medicinal Chemistry*, Vol.43, No.5, (Jul, 2007), pp. 981-985, ISSN 0223-5234.

Vanheusden, V., Munier-Lehmann, H., Pochet, S., Herdewijn, P., Van Calenbergh, S. (2002). Synthesis and evaluation of thymidine-5'-O-monophosphate analogues as inhibitors of *Mycobacterium tuberculosis* thymidylate kinase. *Bioorganic and Medicinal Chemistry Letters*, Vol.12, No.19, (Oct 2002), pp. 2695-2698. ISSN: 0960-894X.

Vicente, E., Perez-Silanes, S., Lima, LM., Ancizu, S., Burguete, A., Solano, B., Villar, R., Aldana, I., Monge, A. (2009). Selective activity against *Mycobacterim tuberculosis* of new quinoxaline 1,4-di-N-oxides. *Bioorganic & Medicinal Chemistry*, Vol.17, No.1, (2008), pp. 385-389, ISSN 0968-0896.

Weinberg, ED., Miklossy J. (2008). Iron withholding: a defense against disease. *Journal of Alzheimer's Disease*, Vol. 13, No.4, (May 2008), pp. 451-463. ISSN: 1387-2877.

Wube, AA., Hufner, A., Thomaschitz, C., Blunder, M., Kollroser, M., Bauer, R., Bucar, F. (2011). Design, synthesis and antimycobacterial activities of 1-methyl-2-alkenyl-4(1H)-quinolones. *Bioorganic & Medicinal Chemistry*, Vol.19, No.1, (Nov, 2010), pp. 567-579, ISSN 0968-0896.

Yang, CL., Tseng, CH., Chen, YL., Lu, CM., Kao, CL., Wu, MH., Tzeng, CC. (2010). Identification of benzofuro[2,3-b]quinoline derivatives as a new class of antituberculosis agents. *European Journal of Medicinal Chemistry*, Vol.45, No.2, (Nov, 2009), pp. 602-607 ISSN 0223-5234.

Yang, F., Curran, SC., Li, LS., Avarbock, D., Graf, JD., Chua, MM., Lu, G., Salem, J., Rubin, H. (1997). Characterization of two genes encoding the *Mycobacterium tuberculosis* ribonucleotide reductase small subunit. *Journal of Bacteriology*, Vol. 179, No. 20 (Oct 1997), pp. 6408-6415. ISSN: 0021-9193.

Yang, F., Lu, G., Rubin, H. (1994). Isolation of ribonucleotide reductase from *Mycobacterium tuberculosis* and cloning, expression, and purification of the large subunit. *Journal of Bacteriology*, Vol. 176, No.21, (Nov 1994), pp. 6738-6743. ISSN: 0021-9193.

Yoya, GK., Bedos-Belval, F., Constante, P., Duran, H., Daffe, M., Balatas, M. (2009). Synthesis and evaluation of a novel series of pseudo-cinnamic derivatives as antituberculosis agents. *Bioorganic & Medicinal Chemistry Letters*, Vol.19, No.2, (Nov, 2008), pp. 341-343, ISSN 0960-894X.

Zhang, X., Hu, Y., Chen, S., Luo, R., Yue, J., Zhang, Y., Duan, W., Wang, H. (2009). Synthesis and evaluation of (S,S)-N,N'-bis[3-(2,2',6,6'-tetramethylbenzhydryloxy)-2-hydroxy-propyl]-ethylenediamine (S2824) analogs with anti-tuberculosis activity. *Bioorganic & Medicinal Chemistry Letters*, Vol.19, No.21, (Nov, 2009), pp. 6074-6077, ISSN 0960-894X.

Zhang, Y. (2004). Persistent and dormant tubercle bacilli and latent tuberculosis. *Frontiers Bioscience*, Vol. 1. No. 9, (May 2004), pp. 1136-1156. ISSN: 1093-9946.

Zhang, Y. (2005). The magic bullets and tuberculosis drug targets. *Annual Review Pharmacology and Toxicology*, Vol. 45, (Feb 2005), pp. 529-564. ISSN: 0362-1642.

Zhang, Y., Amzel, LM. (2002). Tuberculosis drug targets. *Current Drug Targets*, Vol. 3, No. 2 (Apr 2002), pp. 131-154. ISSN: 1389-4501.

Zhang, Y., Post-Martens, K., Denkin, S. (2006). New drug candidates and therapeutic targets for tuberculosis therapy. *Drug Discovery Today*, Vol. 11, No. 1, (Jan 2006), pp. 21-27. ISSN: 1359-6446.

8

Antimicrobial Peptides:
New Frontiers in the Therapy of Infections

Mario Zucca, Sara Scutera and Dianella Savoia
University of Torino
Italy

1. Introduction

The discovery of antibiotics unquestionably represents a major achievement in the treatment of infectious diseases. However, the early optimistic expectations to definitely win the war against infections have not been met, mainly because of bacterial resistance, that has evolved to each antibiotic introduced into clinical practice and complicates infections in more vulnerable individuals, such as organ transplant receivers, AIDS, hemodialysis, and cancer patients. The development of resistance is inherent to the mechanism of action of classic antibiotics, that target specific bacterial enzymes, and could be overcome by new antibiotics with different targets, but in the last 40 years very few new antibiotics have reached the market. Indeed, the great majority of antibiotics presently in use for systemic infections derives by synthetic tailoring from a limited number of dated molecular scaffolds (Fischbach & Walsh, 2009). The wide-spread use of antibiotics for both medical and non-medical purposes prompted the emergence of a number of multi-resistant bacterial strains, such as methicillin-resistant *Staphylococcus aureus* (MRSA), vancomycin-resistant *Enterococci*, *Acinetobacter baumannii*, *Escherichia coli*, carbapenem-resistant *Klebsiella pneumoniae* and *Pseudomonas aeruginosa*, *Clostridium difficile*, and *Mycobacterium tuberculosis*. Epidemic resistance to antibiotics has been described for a number of superbug pathogens, such as MRSA, *Streptococcus pneumoniae* and *Mycobacterium tuberculosis*, and multidrug- or pan-resistant gram-negative bacilli (Spellberg et al., 2008). It is estimated that infectious diseases, despite the availability of antibiotics, remain the second-leading cause of death worldwide (World Health Organization, 2004). On the other hand, the development of new drugs is considered no more fashionable by the pharmaceutical industry, due to the low probability to recover the huge investments required to license new antibacterials that will be used in a low number of selected infections. Indeed, this high cost-low revenue perspective made many large pharmaceutical companies to quit antibiotic discovery for more profitable therapeutics. That being said, let us approach the subject by reviewing the Pub-med literature regarding the up-to-date research on natural and synthetic antimicrobial molecules of proteinaceous nature, as alternatives to conventional antibiotics. Since the mid-1990s, bacterial genome sequencing was carried out with the aim to identify new bacterial targets. High-throughput target-based screening and combinatorial chemical libraries were developed, but after some time it was realized that the results were not up to the expectations, for at least three reasons: first, most enzymes essential for bacterial viability can not be easily affected by drugs; second, some of the structures that would be the best antibacterial targets (e.g. ribosomes and nascent peptidoglycan) are not accessible to *in vitro* screening; and third, chemical libraries do not have the molecular complexity of naturally produced antibiotics (Baltz, 2008). To illustrate the difficulties relative to the new targets approach, scientists at GlaxoSmithKline reviewed the outcome of an extensive program of screening chemical libraries against multiple potential Gram-positive or broad spectrum targets over a period of seven years (Payne et al., 2007). Out of the 300 genes evaluated, 160 were found to be essential for viability. The screen against 67 target proteins covering a wide range of cellular metabolic activities yielded 16 hits, but only 5 yielded leads. Of these, only two (3%) were identified as potentially new targets. The authors noted that results were unsustainably poor in relation to the effort (Baltz, 2008). Because of these difficulties, the recent trend is to look for new antimicrobials by screening natural products, that are an inexhaustible source of bioactive compounds. Technical advances in genomics, bioinformatics, microbial ecology, synthetic biology, and systems biology offer new opportunities for multidisciplinary approaches to small molecule discovery (Davies, 2011; Walsh & Fischbach, 2010). The reserve of natural molecules produced by bacteria, fungi, plants, and vertebrates can offer both novel antibiotics that work in the classic way, and new antimicrobials that being based on different molecular scaffolds will more easily bypass resistance. Most of these natural substances are of peptidic nature and work by targeting conserved mechanisms, often shared by more than one pathogen. Antimicrobials of peptidic nature can be divided into two classes: the gene-encoded, ribosomally synthesized peptides, and the non-ribosomally synthesized peptide antibiotics, typically produced by bacteria and fungi. The latter are assembled by multi-enzyme complexes, contain d-amino acids and other non-proteinogenic amino acids, and often have a cyclic or branched structure (Wiesner & Vilcinskas, 2010). Some members of this class already on the market, such as bacitracin, gramicidin S, polymyxin B, the streptogramins, vancomycin and teicoplanin have limited clinical use, mostly because of toxicity, poor solubility, or limited spectrum of activity. The ribosomally synthesized antimicrobials (none of which is yet on the market) can be subdivided into two further classes depending on their source: the term "antimicrobial peptides" (AMPs) strictly speaking indicates peptides of eukaryotic origin, whereas peptides and proteins produced by bacteria are called bacteriocins. However, considering the similarities in terms of structure and mechanism of action, in this chapter the term AMPs will be used to globally indicate members of both classes. With this premise, we can say that AMPs are widely conserved, small amphiphilic antagonistic molecules produced by both prokaryotic and eukaryotic organisms. Bacteria secrete microcins and bacteriocins that inhibit bacterial food competitors present in the same environment, whilst plants and insects, that lack the adaptive immune response, rely on AMPs for protection against infections (Scott et al., 2008). In mammals, AMPs are present in neutrophils and on skin and mucosal surfaces, where they carry out direct antimicrobial activity and participate to the innate immune response (Maroti et al., 2011). The concept of developing AMPs as potent pharmaceuticals for human therapy dates back to the 1990s (Chopra, 1993), and most research articles since then published on this topic conclude by stating that AMPs represent promising therapeutic agents against bacterial, fungal, viral and parasitic diseases. Today the issue is more relevant than ever, due to the occurrence of two concomitant factors: the emergence of multi- or pan-drug-resistant bacterial strains, and the availability of new and sophisticated technical approaches to design, engineer and optimize AMPs for every specific application. The challenge is to design synthetic mimics that maintain the potency of natural AMPs, able to kill pathogens in the low micromolar concentration range, but lose some flaws of natural molecules, such as low stability, immunogenicity, low bioavailability, and production cost (Sharma et al., 2009). According to their electrical charge, AMPs can be divided into anionic and cationic peptides. Anionic AMPs (AAMPs), found in vertebrates, invertebrates and plants, are active against bacteria, fungi, viruses, nematodes and insects. Their net negative charge ranges from -1 to -7, and their length from 5 to about 70 amino acid residues. In comparison with cationic AMPs (CAMPs), AAMPs have received little attention in the literature, and their mechanism of action so far has not been elucidated. For an outline of AAMP characteristics, the interested reader is referred to the exhaustive review by Harris et al. (2009). Vertebrate CAMPs can be also defined "host defense peptides" (HDPs), because beyond their direct antimicrobial activity, *in vivo* they often modulate the host immune response (Hölzl et al., 2008). By inducing chemokine and cytokine production, HDPs can recruit and activate immune cells, stimulate wound repair, and promote or inhibit angiogenesis (Wilmes et al., 2001). Moreover, certain CAMPs, such as amphibian temporins, neutralize bacterial endotoxins (Mangoni & Shai, 2009), and some of them, such as cecropin, buforin and magainin also exhibit selective direct cytotoxic activity against different types of human cancer cells (Schweizer, 2009). Typically, CAMPs are gene-encoded peptides derived from larger precursors by proteolytic processing, are 12-50 amino acid long with a net positive charge of +2 to +11, due to an excess of basic arginine and lysine residues, and have approximately 50% hydrophobic amino acids (Finlay & Hancock, 2004). Based on their molecular and conformational structure, CAMPs can be divided into four classes: cysteine-rich α-sheet structures stabilized by two to four disulphide bonds (human α- and β-defensins, plectasin, protegrins); linear α-helical peptides without disulphide bonds (cecropins, magainins and dermaseptins); loop-structured peptides with one disulphide bond (bactenecin, microcins from *Enterobacteriaceae*), and extended structures rich in glycine, tryptophan, proline, arginine and/or histidine (cathelicidins, indolicidin) (Hancock & Sahl, 2006). So far, more than fifteen hundreds AMPs have been identified; an updated AMP database is available on line at: http://aps.unmc.edu/AP/main.php (Wang G. et al., 2009). Positively charged CAMPs interact with the negatively charged microbial surface, and the interaction disrupts the membrane barrier function via pore-formation or unspecific membrane permeabilization. Different models, such as the toroidal pore (magainins) and barrel stave (alamethicin) models, which imply the formation of pores, or the carpet-like model (cecropins), in which the cell membrane is disintegrated and/or micellized, have been proposed to describe the structures formed between peptides and membrane phospholipids. The difference between the anionic charge of bacterial membranes and the neutral charge of mammalian cell membranes rich in zwitterionic phospholipids or cholesterol may help to explain the selectivity of action of many CAMPs (Wilmes et al., 2011). Bacterial killing is mediated by membrane disorganization, taking seconds to minutes, and/or by the binding to intracellular targets, that takes more time (3-5 hours). None mechanism is receptor-based, consistent with the finding that D-peptides are generally as active as L-peptides (Scott et al., 2008). AMPs show a highly conserved amphiphilic topology, with the hydrophilic and hydrophobic side chains segregated into distinct opposing regions or faces of the molecule. This topology is essential for insertion into and disruption of bacterial cytoplasmic membranes, and physicochemical properties, rather than any precise amino acid sequence, are responsible for AMP activity (Scott et al., 2008). Even non-peptidic compounds with amphiphilic structures, such as ceragenins, cholic acid derivatives, or polymers with phenylene ethynylene, polymethacrylate, β-lactam, or polynorbornene backbones, are effective broad spectrum antibacterials (Chin et al., 2007; Lai XZ. et al., 2008). These compounds are not currently developed, but their low cost, ease of production and non-toxicity for mammalian cells make them suitable for sterile clothing and biocompatible medical materials, such as catheters, sutures and indwelling devices (Gabriel & Tew, 2008).

2. Mammalian defensins

Defensins are the prototypic mammalian HDPs. The presence inside neutrophil granules of proteins able to kill microorganisms with an oxygen-independent mechanism has been described in the 1980s (Ganz et al., 1986). Since then, defensins have been intensively investigated, and by now the family includes many structurally related peptides found in vertebrates, fungi, plants and insects. The discovery of defensin-like peptides produced by the myxobacteria *Anaeromyxobacter dehalogenans* and *Stigmatella aurantiaca*, demonstrated by *in silico* analysis, suggests that eukaryotic defensin genes are highly conserved (Zhu, 2007). Vertebrates express three defensin mature peptide subfamilies, defined α, β, and θ, with sequences of 29–35, 35–45, and 18 amino acids, respectively. Defensins are synthesized as 'prepropeptides' which are processed to various degrees depending on the expression site. The α- and β-defensins are products of distinct gene families evolved from an ancestral α-defensin gene that is expressed in species as ancient as venomous snakes (Selsted & Ouellette, 2005). Defensins α and β show a similar tertiary structure with triple-stranded β-sheet domains, but differ by the linear spacing and disulfide pairings of their six conserved cysteine residues. The θ-defensins, first observed in *Macaca mulatta* leukocytes, are the product of a post-translational head-to-tail ligation of two truncated α-defensins, resulting in cyclized octadecapeptides stabilized by three disulfide bonds. They are the only known cyclic polypeptides of mammalian origin, and are present in several species of Old World monkeys and in orangutans but not in humans or New World primates. Although humans express mRNA encoding θ-defensin orthologs, mutations that introduce stop codons into the otherwise open reading frame of the θ-defensin precursors abolish the peptide production (Penberthy et al., 2011). Defensins are directly active against a broad spectrum of bacteria, fungi, protozoa and enveloped viruses, and indirectly concur to host defense processes such as inflammation, angiogenesis and tissue healing (Penberthy et al., 2011).

Six α-defensins encoded by five genes have been identified in humans: HNP (human neutrophil peptide)-1 to -4, and HD (human defensin)-5 and -6. HNP-2 is a truncated form of HNP-1 or HNP-3 peptides (Wiesner, 2010). HNP 1-4 are produced by neutrophils, whereas HD-5 and HD-6 are synthesized and secreted by Paneth cells, a specialized form of epithelial cells that are found at the base of the crypts of Lieberkühn in the small intestine. On stimulation through Toll-like receptor-2, -3, and -5, neutrophils and Paneth cells release stored α-defensins to the extracellular milieu, where they exert their antimicrobial activity.

At least 33 human β-defensin genes have been discovered (Schutte et al., 2002), but so far only four human β-defensins (hBD-1 to -4) have been characterized in mucosal and epithelial cells. In addition to their antimicrobial properties, β-defensins recruit immature dendritic cells and T cells, and stimulate the maturation of antigen-presenting cells (McCormick & Weinberg, 2010). The expression of hBD-2 increases upon stimulation of numerous cell types with LPS or proinflammatory cytokines, whereas hBD-1 constitutive expression is not affected (Ryan at al., 2011). Human α- and β-defensins contribute to maintain a stable commensal microbiota in the intestinal tract, preventing bacterial overgrowth. It is hypothesized that reduced defensin concentrations compromise host defense and predispose to ileal and colonic Crohn disease (CD) (Ramasundara et al., 2009). Patients with ileal CD are characterized by decreased expression of Paneth cell HD-5 and -6, whereas colonic CD is characterized by attenuated induction of β-defensins. On the contrary, in ulcerative colitis there is substantial evidence to support a significant up-regulation of the inducible β-defensins. Production difficulties, cell toxicity and concerns on the possible dysregulation of the tissue cytokine milieu have so far hindered the development of human defensins for therapeutic use (Chen H. et al., 2006; Kougias et al., 2005; Wencker & Brantly, 2005). Therefore, the defensin most promising for medical use is plectasin, a 40-amino acid peptide produced by the fungus *Pseudoplectania nigrella* (Mygind et al., 2005). Plectasin is active against *S. pneumoniae* and *S. aureus*, including penicillin-resistant strains, but weakly cytotoxic on mammalian cells. This selectivity is probably due to its recently clarified mechanism of action, that does not involve cell membrane disruption, but targets lipid II, a bacterial cell wall precursor (Schneider et al., 2010). Plectasin and one of its variants, the peptide NZ2114, are currently under development by Novozymes A/S as lead compounds to be used against vancomycin- and methicillin-resistant *S. aureus* (Brinch et al., 2010).

The presence of remarkably intact θ-defensin pseudogenes in humans, and the wide spectrum of antimicrobial activity of monkey θ-defensins, made these molecules the subject of extended research, that brought to the production of the human corresponding peptides, called "retrocyclins" (RCs), by using solid-phase synthetic approaches. RCs are synthetic, humanized θ-defensin cyclic octadecapeptides, active against HIV and herpes and influenza viruses, and able to neutralize anthrax toxin. RC-1, -2 and -3 prevent the entry of HIV-1 into target cells by blocking the virus envelope-cell membrane fusion. Studies are underway to develop RCs as local microbicides to prevent HIV-1 transmission. To this end, it has been observed that amino acid substitutions can be introduced into the RC backbone to improve the anti-HIV activity (Penberthy et al., 2011). RCs also have bactericidal activity, which makes them promising candidates for further development as topical microbicides to prevent bacterial sexually transmitted diseases. Following the observation that in eukaryotic cells aminoglycosides induce a low level of translational misreading, which suppresses the termination codon through the incorporation of an amino acid in its place, Venkataraman et al. utilized aminoglycosides to induce translational read-through of the θ-defensin pseudogene, which restored the expression of functional anti-HIV-1 retrocyclin peptides in human cervicovaginal tissue models (2009). These authors suggest that the topical application of aminoglycosides to induce the production of endogenous retrocyclins by the vaginal mucosa might soon become an effective method to combat HIV-1 sexual transmission. However, the field of RC applications is intended to widen, because it has been observed that Rhesus θ-defensin protects mice from SARS coronavirus pulmonary infection (Wohlford-Lenane et al., 2009), and that RC-2 protected both MDCK cells and chicken embryos from infection by the H5N1 avian influenza virus (Liang et al., 2010). The issue of the still prohibitive RC production cost is being addressed by Lee et al. by the use of chloroplasts as bioreactors. These authors developed a technique based on the use of chloroplast transformation vectors that allows the production of RC-101, a non-hemolytic and minimally cytotoxic RC-1 analogue with good anti-HIV-1 activity, and of protegrin-1 (a 18-residue AMP discovered in porcine leukocytes, that showed potent antimicrobial activity against bacteria, fungi and yeasts) by tobacco chloroplasts (Lee et al., 2011). The process allows the production of adequate quantities of purified peptides to be used in preclinical studies. RCs share remarkable structural and functional similarity with other small hairpin peptides of 17–18 amino acids found in diverse species. Three groups of such peptides are gomesins, protegrins and tachyplesins/polyphemusins, which were isolated from spider hemocytes (Silva et al., 2000), porcine leukocytes (Storici & Zanetti, 1993), and horseshoe crab hemocytes (Nakamura et al., 1988), respectively. Gomesins, β-hairpin peptides consisting of 18 amino acids with two disulfide bridges, are active against fungi, bacteria, protozoan parasites and tumor cells (Moreira et al., 2007; Rodrigues et al., 2008). Protegrins are cysteine-rich, 18-residue β-hairpin peptides with 2 disulfide bridges, and show potent broad-spectrum activity that targets bacteria, filamentous fungi, yeast cells, and HIV-1 (Bulet et al., 2004; Cole & Waring, 2002). Tachyplesins are 17–18 amino acid peptides with a C-terminal alpha-amide group that forms a rigid 2-stranded anti-parallel β-sheet structure connected by a β-turn. Natural tachyplesins exhibit potent antibacterial and antifungal activity and modest anti-HIV activity, but unfortunately they lyse human erythrocytes (Penberthy et al., 2011).

3. Cathelicidins

Cathelicidin discovery can be traced back to the isolation of an antimicrobial disulfide-containing cyclic dodecapeptide from bovine neutrophils (Romeo et al., 1988), soon followed by the purification of two additional peptides, designated bactenecins (after the Latin words 'bacterium necare'), and of conserved similar proteins in other species (Zanetti, 2005). The term 'cathelicidins' was proposed in 1995 to acknowledge the evolutionary relationship of the novel protein family to cathelin, a protein originally isolated from porcine neutrophils as an inhibitor of cathepsin L, and it is used to denote holoproteins containing a conserved N-terminal cathelin-like domain of 99-114 residues linked to a heterogenic C-terminal antimicrobial domain of 12-100 residues (Zhu, 2008). The C-terminal peptides exert direct and/or indirect antimicrobial activity following their cleavage from the holoprotein (Zanetti, 2005).

3.1 Mammalian cathelicidins

Cathelicidins have been found in every mammal examined, with substantial interspecies variation in the number of members. The only human cathelicidin so far identified, also defined human cationic antimicrobial peptide-18 (hCAP18), has been isolated from neutrophils in 1995, and its expression has been successively observed in skin, mucous epithelia, wound and blister fluid, and in seminal plasma (Zanetti, 2005). The coding gene is located on chromosome 3, and its expression is both constitutive (in sweat gland cells) and inducible by vitamin D3, LPS and butyric acid (in colonic epithelial cells) (White, 2010). Unlike neutrophil defensins, which are fully processed to mature peptides before storage in the azurophil granules, human cathelicidin is present as propeptide in the specific granules and is cleaved after secretion to generate the antimicrobial peptide LL-37, a cationic 37 amino acid AMP bearing tandem N-terminal leucine residues. There is evidence that within the same organism cathelicidins are processed by different proteases in different physiological contexts: in humans, the activation of neutrophil-derived hCAP18/LL-37 is carried out by the serine protease proteinase 3, whereas epididymal-derived hCAP18 in seminal plasma is cleaved by the prostate-derived protease gastricsin (pepsin C) in the presence of vaginal fluid at low pH (Zanetti, 2005). LL-37 has a stable α-helical structure and kills bacteria by cell membrane disruption. Moreover, it binds LPS with high affinity, inhibiting LPS-induced cellular responses, and prevents macrophage activation by lipoteichoic acid and lipoarabinomannan (Scott et al., 2002). LL-37 also inhibits mycobacteria and induces a Toll-like receptor-mediated killing of *M. tuberculosis* by monocytes (Méndez-Samperio, 2010). It has been shown that LL-37 is expressed by human epithelial cells in inflammatory environments such as wound healing, but it is also present in significant amounts in sweat, thus providing an innate anti-microbial defense system to the skin surface under non-inflammatory conditions (Murakami et al., 2002). LL-37 is constitutively expressed in gut epithelium and in lung alveolar macrophages and neutrophils. However, native LL-37 is hemolytic and toxic to human leukocytes. *In vivo*, LL-37 cytotoxic effects are inhibited by its binding to plasma proteins, but the binding also lowers antimicrobial efficacy (Ciornei et al., 2005). Considering LL-37 multifunctional activity, further investigation is needed to better define its biological properties and its possible therapeutic applications in the fields of immunomodulation and bacterial control. The future of cathelicidins relies on the ability to design synthetic more effective and less toxic variants (Mookherjee & Hancock, 2007). Significant achievements in this field could be not too far, considering that a synthetic 13-amino acid peptide, IDR-1, conceptually based on LL-37, with no direct antimicrobial activity, protects against bacterial infections *in vivo* by inducing chemokine production and enhancing leukocyte recruitment (Scott et al., 2007). An IDR-1 derivative, IDR-1002, showed stronger protective activity *in vitro* and in mouse models of infection with *S. aureus* and *E. coli* (Nijnik et al., 2010). Another promising new molecule currently under investigation is novicidin, a linear cationic α-helical AMP derived from ovispirin, a cationic peptide originated from the ovine cathelicidin SMAP-29 (Dorosz et al., 2010). A bovine cathelicidin with broad-spectrum activity, termed indolicidin, was originally isolated from bovine neutrophils (Selsted et al., 1992). Indolicidin is a 13-residue cationic peptide rich in tryptophan and proline, with a significant leishmanicidal activity, mediated by the disruption of *L. donovani* promastigotes and induction of autophagic cell death (Bera et al., 2003). It is also active against bacteria, fungi, and HIV, but its cytotoxicity prevents its use for therapeutic purposes (Rokitskaya et al., 2011). Less toxic derivatives such as omiganan (MBI-226), a 12-residue, indolicidin-based peptide variant, are currently under development (Rubinchik et al., 2009). This molecule, active on a wide range of bacteria and fungi, is currently undergoing confirmatory Phase III clinical trials for the prevention of infections arising from short-term central venous catheters, surgical contaminated wounds, and for the treatment of acne and rosacea (Rubinchik et al., 2009).

3.2 Avian cathelicidins
The genes of five cathelicidins termed fowlicidin-1, -2, -3, (Xiao et al., 2005), cathelicidin-B1 (Goitsuka et al., 2007), and myeloid antimicrobial peptide 27 (van Dijk et al., 2005), have been discovered by screening the chicken genome with bioinformatic methods. Functional analyses indicate that the corresponding synthesized peptides are among the most efficacious cathelicidins ever identified, with antibacterial and LPS-neutralizing activities that make them attractive candidates as antimicrobial and anti-sepsis agents. Fowlidicin-1, -2 and -3, are highly active against both Gram-negative and Gram-positive bacteria including MRSA, even in the presence of salts, whilst many AMPs, as for example LL37, are inactivated by high salt concentrations. These features could be useful in the treatment of

cystic fibrosis and Crohn's disease, both of which are related with aberrant local expression or inactivation of antimicrobial peptides (Saravanan & Bhattacharjya, 2011). Starting from the consideration that fowlicidin-1 is active against bacteria in the 1 to 2 μM concentration range, has potent LPS-neutralizing activity, but is hemolytic and toxic to epithelial cells, a fowlicidin-1 analog denominated fowl-1(6-26), is currently being developed. It maintains the full-length peptide antibacterial and LPS-neutralizing efficacy, but following carboxyl-terminal amidation it is more stable in serum. The resulting peptide, fowl-1(6-26)-NH2, reduced bacterial titers in the peritoneal fluid and spleen and improved the survival of mice by 50% in MRSA-induced lethal infections, which makes it an excellent drug candidate against infections and sepsis induced by drug-resistant bacteria (Bommineni et al., 2010). In comparison with fowlicidin-1, fowlicidin-2 exhibits similar antibacterial efficacy but lower cell toxicity. To further reduce fowlicidin-2 toxicity several deletion analogs were designed and analyzed for their antibacterial, cytotoxic, membrane permeabilizing and LPS-neutralizing activities. This work brought to the identification of 2 short peptide analogs, fowlicidin-2(1–18) and fowlicidin-2(15–31), which maintained the antibacterial and LPS-neutralizing activities, but showed a significantly reduced cytotoxicity (Xiao et al., 2009).

3.3 Snake cathelicidins

Snake venoms are composed of active substances endowed with a wide array of neurotoxic, myotoxic, cardiotoxic, hemorrhagic, pro- and anticoagulant, antiparasitic and antibacterial effects. The whole venom of *Bothrops marajoensis*, a snake of the *Viperidae* family, as well as one of its purified components, i.e. L-amino acid oxidase, exhibits a strong inhibition on the growth of a wide range of microorganisms, such as *S. aureus, C. albicans, P. aeruginosa*, and *Leishmania* species (Costa Torres et al., 2009). The opportunities offered by the recent development of bioinformatic techniques have been exploited to identify the genes with AMP-related sequences expressed in venom gland tissues. Three cathelicidins from the elapid species *Naja atra* (Chinese cobra), *Bungarus fasciatus* (banded krait) and *Ophiophagus hannah* (king cobra) have been identified by molecular cloning (Zhao et al., 2008). Phylogenetic analysis suggests that snake cathelicidins are closely related to rodent neutrophilic granule proteins, avian fowlicidins and chicken myeloid antimicrobial peptide 27. Unlike the highly divergent mammalian cathelicidins, the nucleotide and deduced protein sequences of the three cloned elapid cathelicidins are remarkably conserved. Each of them has a 22 amino acid residue signal peptide, a conserved cathelin domain of 135 amino acids and a mature antimicrobial peptide of 34 amino acids. In order to explore the structure–function relationships relative to the bactericidal and hemolytic activities, king cobra cathelicidin (OH-CATH) has been used as a molecular template to develop shorter synthetic analogs. Among OH-CATH and its analogs, OH-CATH(5–34) has the lowest hemolytic activity but maintains a strong antimicrobial activity. To evaluate its potential clinic values, the biological activities of OH-CATH(5–34) have been compared with those of pexiganan, a well-known phase III AMP derived from magainin. The bactericidal activity of OH-CATH(5–34) against 5 different species of bacteria (*E. coli, P. aeruginosa, S. aureus, Enterobacter aerogenes* and *E. cloacae*) was 2–4 times stronger than that of pexiganan. Hemolytic activity of OH-CATH(5–34) against human erythrocytes was 0.69% while that of pexiganan was 16.5% at the dosage of 200 μg/ml. The intravenous LD_{50} value of OH-CATH(5–34) on mice was 7-fold higher than that of pexiganan (175 mg/kg vs 25 mg/kg). Taken together, these results suggest that OH-CATH(5–34) can be considered an excellent candidate for developing therapeutic drugs (Zhang et al., 2010).

4. Epithelial host defense peptides

Healthy intact skin controls microbial growth by the combined action of complementary systems. The stratum corneum layer, with its lipid-rich matrix and protective low pH, constitutes a physical and chemical barrier further supported by bacterial nutrient limitation and physical removal by desquamation. A wide array of bacteriostatic and bactericidal compounds belonging to the HDP family concurs to the prevention of skin infections by inhibiting potentially invading microorganisms and maintaining a balanced commensal flora on the skin. Once this biochemical barrier is disturbed, bacteria or bacterial factors have access to living epidermal keratinocytes and stimulate the innate immune response that goes under the name of inflammation (Meyer-Hoffert et al., 2011). In human skin HDPs are mainly produced by keratinocytes, neutrophils, sebocytes or sweat glands and are either expressed constitutively or following an inflammatory stimulus. The relevance of HDPs in the skin physiology and pathology is underlined by the fact that in several human skin diseases there is an inverse correlation between severity of the disease and the level of HDP production. Decreased HDP levels are associated with burns, chronic wounds, and atopic dermatitis. In contrast, in some cases HDP over-expression is believed to lead to increased protection against skin infections as seen in patients with psoriasis and rosacea, whose lesions rarely result in bacterial superinfection. In skin infections, such as *acne vulgaris*, increased levels of HDPs can be found in inflamed tissues, indicating a role of these peptides in the immune reaction to infection. The broad spectrum of antimicrobial activity, the low incidence of bacterial resistance and the immunomodulatory function are attractive features that suggest a high HDP potential as topical anti-infective drugs in several skin diseases (Schittek et al., 2008). The best studied among skin-related antibacterials are some members of the already treated defensin (hBD-1-3) and cathelicidin (LL-37) families, and a number of heterogeneous factors, such as psoriasin, dermcidin, RNase 7, and peptidoglycan recognition proteins.

4.1 Psoriasin

Psoriasin is a low molecular weight protein that owes its name to the fact of being intensely expressed by the keratinocytes of patients with psoriasis (Madsen et al., 1991). After cloning of the cDNA, the 11,457 kDa protein was classified in the S100 protein family, that so far includes 21 low molecular weight (9–13 kDa) calcium-binding proteins characterized by the solubility in 100 % ammonium sulphate, from which is derived the name of the family. S100 proteins regulate many epithelial cell functions such as intracellular Ca^{2+} signaling, differentiation, cell-cycle progression, cytoskeletal membrane interactions, and leukocyte chemotaxis (McCormick & Weinberg, 2010). Psoriasin antibacterial activity was discovered in 2005 (Glaser et al., 2005). The abundance of psoriasin on human skin together with its high antimicrobial activity against *E. coli* suggest that psoriasin may be an important factor in controlling *E. coli* growth on the skin surface. The physiological role of psoriasin in protecting the skin against *E. coli* colonization and infection has been confirmed by *in vivo* experiments with neutralizing antibodies. These experiments performed on the skin of various healthy people identified psoriasin as a principal *E. coli*–killing factor. Subsequent studies in cultured human keratinocytes identified flagellin, a Toll-like receptor-5 ligand, as the *E. coli* "pathogen-associated molecular pattern" responsible for the expression of psoriasin mRNA and protein. It has been observed that the production of psoriasin in human skin can also be induced by *P. aeruginosa* flagellin and rhamnolipids (Meyer-Hoffert et al., 2011). Indeed, *P. aeruginosa* is another ubiquitous bacterium that is however not usually present on healthy skin. These studies suggest that human skin might control the microflora to prevent colonization of the skin surface by unwanted microbes. Psoriasin is a metal ion-binding protein with a Ca^{2+} and Zn^{2+} binding capacity. Experiments aimed to clarify the mechanism of its antibacterial action demonstrated that in low concentrations (0.5 µM) psoriasin kills 90 % of all exposed *E. coli*. In higher doses (> 30 µM) psoriasin is bactericidal against *P. aeruginosa* and *S. aureus*, also. It seems that the mechanism of antibacterial action is mediated by zinc deprivation, zinc being an essential trace element for bacterial metabolism. Correspondingly, mutation experiments with recombinant psoriasin confirmed that zinc but not calcium binding is of significance for antibacterial activity (Glaser et al., 2005). Further, it was recently reported that psoriasin at pH values under 6 can also induce the formation of pores in the bacterial membrane (Glaser et al., 2011). The production by normal human keratinocytes of antimicrobial peptides, such as β-defensin-2 and -3, RNase 7, and psoriasin may be induced by ultraviolet radiation (Glaser et al., 2009). It is known that exposure to UV rays, especially of the B-waveband (UV-B, 280–315 nm), may suppress both systemic and local immune responses to a variety of antigens, and to several microorganisms (Termorshuizen et al., 2002). These findings suggest that UV-B irradiation suppresses T-cell–mediated immune responses but up-regulates the innate immune response by inducing the release of antimicrobial peptides.

4.2 Dermcidin

Dermcidin (DCD) is a human HDP isolated from sweat in 2001 (Schittek et al., 2001). It participates in the defense of the cutaneous surface, being constitutively secreted by eccrine sweat glands, but its expression has not been observed in epidermal keratinocytes of healthy skin, and it is not inducible by skin injury or inflammation. To date, DCD gene and mature peptide have been identified in humans only, and they show no homology to other known AMPs. Full length DCD consists of 110 amino acid residues with an N-terminal 19 amino acids signal peptide that is the hallmark of secreted proteins. In the sweat fluid, the DCD protein is cleaved by means of a post-secretory cathepsin D-mediated proteolytic process, giving rise to anionic and cationic peptides, two of which are recognized as the real effectors of the antimicrobial activity. A C-terminal 47 amino acid peptide corresponding to aa 63-109 of the originally translated product, named DCD-1, and a related peptide, DCD-1L, consisting of DCD-1 plus the last leucine (L) residue of the original precursor protein, have been identified in the sweat (Lai YP. et al., 2005). These peptides possess a potent and wide-spectrum antimicrobial activity against *S. aureus, E. coli, Enterococcus faecalis, Listeria monocytogenes, Salmonellae, Pseudomonas* and *Candida albicans* (Hata & Gallo, 2008; Pathak et al., 2009). By means of nuclear magnetic resonance it has been established that DCD-1 has an α-helical structure with a helix-hinge-helix motif, which is a common molecular fold among antimicrobial peptides (Jung et al., 2010). It seems that the affinity with which DCD-1 binds to bacterial-mimetic membranes is primarily dependent on its amphipathic α-helical structure and its length (>30 residues), whereas its negative net charge and acidic isoelectric point have little effect on binding. These findings suggest that the DCD mode of action is similar to that of other membrane-targeting antimicrobial peptides, though the details of its antimicrobial action remain to be determined. Using immune electron microscopy, it has been shown that DCD-1 antimicrobial activity originates with its binding to the bacterial membrane, and that the molecule effectively kills *S. epidermidis*. DCD-1L shows stronger antimicrobial activity than the parent peptide, and it is highly effective against drug-resistant *S. aureus*, as well as other Gram-positive and Gram-negative bacterial strains (Jung et al., 2010). The mechanisms by which DCD-derived peptides kill bacteria are still unclear. Bactericidal activity is time-dependent and induce bacterial membrane depolarization. However, these molecules do not induce pore formation in the membranes of Gram-negative and Gram-positive bacteria. Interestingly, LL-37, as well as DCD-derived peptides, inhibit bacterial macromolecular synthesis, especially RNA and protein synthesis, without binding to microbial DNA or RNA. Binding studies indicate that DCD-derived peptides bind to the bacterial envelope but show only a weak binding to lipopolysaccharide from Gram-negative bacteria or to peptidoglycan, lipoteichoic acid, and wall teichoic acid, isolated from *S. aureus*. In contrast, LL-37 binds strongly in a dose-dependent fashion to these components. These data indicate that the mode of action of DCD-derived peptides is different from that of the cathelicidin LL-37 and that components of the bacterial membranes play a role in the antimicrobial activity of DCD (Senyurek et al., 2009). Being a non-inducible factor, DCD contributes to the epithelial defense by modulating the surface colonization rather than by responding to injury and inflammation as is the case of the inducible peptides hBD-2 and -3, or LL-37 and psoriasin. Modulation and control of the skin-resident flora may be achieved by two types of effects: the non-specific prevention of microbial overgrowth on the skin surface, and the more specific prevention of skin colonization by pathogenic microorganisms, thereby establishing a host-friendly resident flora (Rieg et al., 2004). It appears that DCD could be the first of a new class of potential broad-spectrum antimicrobial drugs. In order to obtain large quantities of highly purified peptide for experimental use, it has been developed a method for the production of recombinant DCD-1L, in which it is expressed as a fusion protein, followed by enzymatic cleavage to release the active peptide. Recombinant DCD-1L is not cytotoxic against erythrocytes when assayed in PBS. This is supposed to be due to the presence of negatively charged sialic acid on the erythrocytes, that would electrostatically repel DCD-1L, which also has a net negative charge. This favorable condition suggests that it is of noteworthy potential as a therapeutic substance in clinical settings (Lai YP. et al., 2005).

4.3 Ribonuclease 7

RNase 7 was discovered as part of a broad screening protocol aimed at identifying antimicrobial agents in human skin (Harder & Schroder, 2002). Successively, it has been discovered that it is also expressed by various epithelial tissues, especially in the respiratory and genitourinary tract. It is a highly cationic protein that shares a potent antibacterial activity with another member of the human RNase A superfamily, the eosinophil-derived RNase denominated ECP (eosinophil cationic protein/RNase 3). ECP possesses bactericidal, antiviral and antiparasitic activities and inhibits mammalian cell growth. Its ribonucleolytic activity with common RNA substrates is low and does not appear to be necessary for the antibacterial capacity. The finding that RNase 7 exhibited both antimicrobial and ribonuclease activity gave rise to the speculation that the enzymatic activity is involved in microbial killing. However, although the mechanisms involved in the antimicrobial properties of RNase 7 are not completely understood, its bactericidal activity has been linked to its capacity to permeate and disrupt the bacterial membrane, independent of its RNase activity (Spencer, 2011). RNase 7 is currently considered a major component of the antimicrobial protein and peptide group that constitutes the biochemical skin barrier (Boix & Nogués, 2007), being active in the low micromolar concentration range against *S. aureus*, *P. aeruginosa*, *Propionibacterium acnes*, and *C. albicans* (Spencer, 2011). The hypothesis that RNase 7 may play an important role in the cutaneous antimicrobial defense system is further supported by the observation that contact of keratinocytes with bacteria induces RNase 7 gene expression, a finding that is in agreement with what is known for other epithelial antimicrobial proteins like the human defensins hBD-2, hBD-3, and hBD-4. Of particular interest is RNase 7 activity against vancomycin-resistant *Enterococcus faecium*. This potent antimicrobial activity supports the idea that RNase 7 might be a useful agent to treat the emerging infections caused by this and other multiresistant bacteria.

4.4 Peptidoglycan recognition proteins

The definition "peptidoglycan recognition protein"(PGRP) was first introduced in 1996 to indicate a 19 kDa protein, present in the hemolymph and cuticle of a silkworm (*Bombyx mori*), that binds the peptidoglycan of Gram-positive bacteria and activates the prophenoloxidase cascade which generates melanin (Yoshida et al., 1996). Subsequently, many other similar molecules have been identified and added to the PGRP group, that includes conserved lectin-like proteins present in insects, mollusks, echinoderms, and vertebrates, but not in nematodes or plants. Mammals express a family of 4 PGRPs, which were initially named PGRP-S, PGRP-L, PGRP-I-α and PGRP-I-β (for short, long and intermediate-α and -β transcripts, respectively), analogous to insect PGRPs. These names were changed by the Human Genome Organization Gene Nomenclature Committee to PGLYRP-1, PGLYRP-2, PGLYRP-3, and PGLYRP-4, respectively. This terminology is also used for mouse PGRPs, and is now in use to selectively indicate vertebrate PGRPs. Both invertebrate and vertebrate PGRPs function as pattern recognition and effector molecules in innate immunity. All PGRP proteins have at least one C-terminal PGRP domain about 165 amino-acid residues long, that is homologous to the bacteriophage and bacterial type 2 amidases. This homology indicates that PGRPs and prokaryotic type 2 amidases might have evolved from a common primordial ancestor gene. Almost all PGRPs have two closely spaced, conserved Cys residues in the centre of the PGRP domain that form a disulphide bond, which is required for PGRP structural integrity and activity. Mammalian PGLYRPs are differentially expressed in various organs and tissues and perform both amidase and antibacterial activity. PGLYRP-1 is present in the granules of the polymorphonuclear leukocytes, and contributes to the killing of phagocytosed bacteria. PGLYRP-2, which is constitutively produced in the liver and secreted into the blood, is also induced in the skin and intestines. It is an *N*-acetylmuramoyl-L-alanine amidase that hydrolyzes peptidoglycan reducing its proinflammatory activity. PGLYRP-3 has direct bactericidal activity and is expressed in the skin, eyes, tongue, esophagus, stomach, and intestines. PGLYRP-4 and the PGLYRP-3:4 dimer also have direct bactericidal activity in the same tissues; PGLYRP-4 is also expressed in the salivary gland, mucus-secreting glands in the throat and in saliva (Dziarski & Gupta, 2006). It has been demonstrated that the bactericidal activity of human PGLYRP-1, PGLYRP-3, PGLYRP-4, and PGLYRP-3:4 against both Gram-positive and Gram-negative bacteria requires zinc (Wang M. et al., 2007). A previously unknown mechanism of bacterial killing by PGRPs has been recently elucidated by Kashyap et al., (2011). In Gram-positive bacteria, to perform their action PGRPs need to pass through the thick cell wall and bind peptidoglycan near the cell membrane. This can be accomplished only at the separation sites of newly formed daughter cells during cell division. The binding induces the activation of the bacterial CssR-CssS two-component system, which triggers bacterial killing by inducing membrane depolarization and the production of toxic [OH]• in the cytoplasm. This process is accompanied by the cessation of all major intracellular biosynthetic reactions, probably because of the lack of membrane potential–dependent generation of energy. Due to the different external structure of Gram-negative bacteria, in which a thin peptidoglycan layer is covered by a lipopolysaccharide-containing outer membrane, the initial interaction of PGRPs with Gram-negative bacteria is different. The analysis of the localization of PGRPs in *E. coli* by immunofluorescence and confocal microscopy demonstrated that the entire *E. coli* outer membrane uniformly binds PGRPs at all stages of growth, in contrast to the described selective localization of PGRPs to cell separation sites in Gram-positive bacteria. Following the binding to the outer membrane, the CpxA-CpxR two-component system, functionally homologous to the CssR-CssS system of Gram-positive bacteria, is activated. The CssR-CssS and CpxA-CpxR systems are designed to detect and dispose of extracellular misfolded bacterial proteins at the cell membrane–cell wall interface, after these proteins have been exported from the cell, and in Gram-negative bacteria CpxA-CpxR also detects proteins in the outer membrane. Notwithstanding the difference between the initial interaction mechanism, the killing mechanism of PGRPs seems common for all bacteria and depends on the activation of the protein-sensing two-component systems. These two-component systems can therefore be considered appealing targets for the development of new antibacterial therapies. PGRPs could be used as a basis for the design of shorter molecules that would maintain the broad-spectrum bactericidal activity of natural factors, but would be more convenient in terms of immunogenicity and production costs.

5. Amphibian host defense peptides

The skin of amphibia Anura (frogs and toads) is one of the richest reservoir of biologically active peptides. These HDPs are produced by dermal glands, stored within granules and released on the skin surface upon stress, injury, or electrical or norepinephrine stimulation. Their synthesis is induced by contact with microorganisms and is transcriptionally regulated by the NF-jB/IjBa machinery (Mangoni & Shai, 2011). These peptides constitute a rich arsenal of broad-spectrum, cytolytic AMPs characterized by highly variable sequences (Vanhoye et al., 2003). It is estimated that there may be as many as 10^5 different peptides produced by the known 5000 species of anuran amphibians, and more than 400 have been already identified from South American *Hylidae* or European, Asian or North American *Ranidae* amphibians (Nicolas & El Amri, 2008). Therefore, the main work still concerns the screening and identification of the most useful factors. The structural characteristics of some amphibian peptides are interesting for their potential implications in the mechanism of antimicrobial activity. A class of structurally unique molecules, still in the characterization phase, contains an intermolecular disulphide bridge in the C-terminal portion of the peptide that creates a 7–9 residue macrocyclic region, sometimes referred to as the "Rana box". Many of these peptides originate from frogs belonging to the *Rana* genus and examples include esculentins, brevinins, ranacyclins, ranalexins, gaegurins, ranateurins and nigrocins (Haney et al., 2009). Here we focus on four families that include some of the better known and most representative peptides, namely magainins, dermaseptins, bombinins and temporins.

5.1 Magainins and magainin-related peptides

Magainin-1 and -2 are the first AMPs isolated from the skin of the African clawed frog *Xenopus laevis* (Zasloff et al., 1987). Because they were among the first identified antimicrobial peptides, there has been considerable research associated with magainin structure and mechanism of action. Magainins are 23 amino acid peptides with α-helical structure. Following the observation that magainin-2 possesses broad spectrum antibacterial and antifungal activity, many synthetic analogs have been developed in order to maximize the antimicrobial effects and minimize cytotoxicity. Magainin-A, a magainin-2 analog, underwent preclinical evaluation studies on *Macaca radiata* monkeys as local contraceptive, showing good spermicidal, antibacterial and antifungal activity (Clara et al., 2004), but has not been further developed. An extensive structure-activity investigation on magainin 2, performed by Zasloff and co-workers of Magainin Pharmaceuticals, resulted in the development of MSI-78 or pexiganan, a molecule that entered clinical trials for topical treatment of diabetic foot ulcers. In 1999 the FDA denied approval of pexiganan after completion of two phase III clinical trials, in which pexiganan resulted no more effective than already approved treatments for diabetic foot ulcers, and required addition clinical trials for consideration. Following successive acquisitions, pexiganan is by now being developed by Access Pharmaceuticals Inc. Improvements in clinical trial design, greater understanding of diabetic foot ulcers and topical anti-infective treatments, and advances in peptide manufacturing keep hopes alive regarding the potential FDA approval of pexiganan (Gottler & Ramamoorthy, 2009).

A new peptide that is not a magainin, but is often included in the magainin family, is peptidyl-glycine-leucine-carboxyamide (PGLa), whose existence was predicted through the screening of a c-DNA library for clones encoding the precursor of caerulein (Hoffmann et al., 1983), when searching in amphibian skin secretions for peptides closely related to mammalian hormones and neurotransmitters. In this study it was concluded that this peptide could form a membrane-active amphipathic helix similar to peptides with bacteriostatic, cytotoxic and/or lytic properties. The natural PGLa counterpart was isolated two years later from the skin secretions of *X. laevis* by the same group (Andreu et al., 1985). At neutral pH this peptide has a positive net charge of 5 because of the four lysine residues and the amino group at the N-terminal glycine. It also has an amidated C-terminus that provides good resistance to proteases (Lohner & Prossnigg, 2009). PGLa showed good *in vitro* activity against *E. coli*, *S. aureus*, and *S. pyogenes* in the concentration range of 10-50 μg/ml, and was also active, but at higher concentrations, against *P. aeruginosa* (200-500 μg/ml), *Saccharomyces cerevisiae* (100-200 μg/ml), and *C. albicans* (100-200 μg/ml) (Soravia et al., 1988). PGLa activity has been also tested *in vitro* against *Plasmodium falciparum*, at a concentration range of 20-60 μM (Boman et al., 1989). However, the peptide with the greatest potential for development into a therapeutically valuable anti-infective agent is by some considered the caerulein precursor fragment B1 (CPF-B1) (Mechkarska et al., 2010). Caerulein is a short peptide whose amino acid sequence shows a close resemblance to the mammalian gastrointestinal hormone gastrin. It was originally isolated from the skin of the Australian frog *Hyla caerulea* (De Caro et al., 1967). The structure of the caerulein precursor extracted from the *X. laevis* skin has been determined in 1985 (Wakabayashi et al., 1985). CPF-B1 is one of four CPF fragments (CPF-B1 -B4) that can be found in the skin secretions obtained from the norepinephrine-stimulated skin of the tetraploid frog *Xenopus borealis* (*Pipidae*). CPF-B1 is the most abundant fragment and is active against clinical isolates of the nosocomial pathogen MRSA and multidrug-resistant *Acinetobacter baumannii* with MIC values in the range 4–8 µM. It is also active against *E. coli* (MIC=5 µM) and *C. albicans* (MIC=25 µM), and shows low hemolytic activity on human erythrocytes. The high potency of CPF-B1 against MRSA and multidrug-resistant *A. baumannii*, together with its low toxicity suggest that the peptide could be used for the topical treatment of skin infections caused by these pathogens and in therapeutic regimes to promote wound healing (Mechkarska et al., 2010).

5.2 Dermaseptins

Dermaseptins are genetically related α-helical amphipathic AMPs 28-34 amino acid-long, with 3-6 lysine residues, and a highly conserved tryptophan residue in the third position from the C-terminus residue (Zairi et al., 2007). Dermaseptins are present in the skin of *Hylidae* and *Ranidae* frogs. They show a remarkable identity in the signal sequences of their preproforms, but have clearly diverged to yield several families of microbicidal cationic peptides that are structurally distinct (Amiche & Galanth, 2011). Dermaseptin S1, the first member of the dermaseptin family to be discovered, was isolated from an extract of dried skin of *Phyllomedusa sauvagei* in the early 1990s (Mor et al., 1991). It was followed by the isolation of dermaseptin B2, also denominated adenoregulin for its ability to interact with the adenosine receptor, from the skin of the arboreal frog *P. bicolor* (Daly et al., 1992). Subsequently, dermaseptin B1, a 27-residue peptide, was also isolated from *P. bicolor* skin (Mor et al., 1994). These last 2 peptides were thought to be unrelated until attempts to clone their precursor polypeptides revealed the presence of a common preproregion and 5′- and 3′-UTRs (Amiche et al., 1993). Since then, additional dermaseptins were rapidly identified in various South American species and now constitute the dermaseptin super-family. Basic research on dermaseptins is of relevance because genetic studies on the evolution and diversity of frog skin AMPs may lead to the identification of new peptides with alternative targets. In addition, the discovery of new isoforms with novel structural and biochemical properties may also shed light on the exact roles of various parameters, such as net charge, percent of α-helical/β-sheet structure, amphipathy and conformational flexibility, on the ability of antimicrobial peptides to bind to and disrupt bacterial membranes (Nicolas & El Amri, 2008). Dermaseptin antimicrobial activity is currently being characterized and analogs are being developed. Dermaseptin S4 analogs are active against *Neisseria gonorrhoeae* (Zairi et al., 2007) and 15 analogs of dermaseptin S1, synthesized by our group, showed variable activity against *Trichomonas vaginalis*, *Herpes simplex virus-1* and human *Papillomavirus 16* (Savoia et al., 2008, 2010). These properties, coupled with the already demonstrated spermicidal activity of dermaseptins S, suggest that dermaseptins, as well as magainins, alone or even better in combination, could be used as topical contraceptives and microbicides to contemporarily prevent unwanted conceptions and sexually transmitted diseases.

5.2.1 Plasticins

Plasticins constitute a family of orthologous peptides with antimicrobial activity classified in the dermaseptin superfamily. They are quite similar as far as amino acid sequence, hydrophobicity, and amphipathicity are concerned, but differ markedly in their conformational plasticity and spectrum of activity (Vanhoye et al., 2003). The plasticins from phyllomedusid frogs of the *Hylidae* family may be divided into two classes on the basis of their cytolytic activities: the strongly cationic peptides plasticin-B1 (from *P. bicolor*) and -S1 (from *P. sauvagei*) that contain lysine residues and show potent, broad spectrum antimicrobial activity and hemolytic activity; and the weakly cationic or neutral plasticins (plasticin-A1, from *Agalychnis annae*, plasticin -C1 and -C2 from *A. callidryas*, and plasticin-DA1 from *Pachymedusa danicolor*), that are hemolytic but devoid of antibacterial activity (Conlon et al., 2009). Plasticin-L1, more recently isolated from the South American frog *Leptodactylus laticeps*, falls into the second category and is devoid of cytolytic activity against Gram-positive and Gram-negative bacteria. However, in contrast to the other plasticins, it does not produce lysis of human erythrocytes at concentrations up to 500 µM (Conlon et al., 2009). The plasticin peptide family constitutes a good model to address the relationships between structural polymorphism, membrane-interacting property, and biological activity of antimicrobial, cell-penetrating, and viral fusion peptides (El Amri & Nicolas, 2008). Unlike amphipathic helical dermaseptins, plasticins display considerable conformational flexibility and polymorphism that modulate their ability to bind to and disrupt the bilayer membranes of prokaryotic and eukaryotic cells, and/or to reach intracellular targets (Nicolas & El Amri, 2008).

5.3 Bombinins and temporins
In the 1960s, Csordas and Michl published a series of papers that culminated in 1970 with a report on the characterization of a hemolytic and antibacterial peptide 24 amino acid long, isolated from the European toad *Bombina variegata* (Csordás & Michl, 1970). This peptide, called "bombinin," shares many of its general structural features with the larger group of magainins. A series of peptides from the skin of a closely related amphibian, *Bombina orientalis* (or Asian toad) has been subsequently isolated and characterized (Zangger et al., 2008). These peptides share considerable homology with bombinin and are called bombinin-like peptides, or BLPs, and were found to possess potent antibacterial activities but, unlike bombinin, lack any appreciable hemolytic activity. Other peptides, structurally unrelated with previously discovered bombinins and containing a D-amino acid as the second residue, are the bombinins H, endowed with both antibacterial and hemolytic properties (hence the final –H) that were isolated from *B. variegata* skin (Mignogna et al. 1993). The expression of the genes encoding the common precursor for bombinins and bombinin H has been shown to be induced by bacterial infection *in vivo* as well as *in vitro* (Miele et al., 1998). Remarkably, after processing of the precursor, bombinin H is further modified by a recently characterized peptidyl-aminoacyl-L/D-isomerase that catalyses the inversion of the stereochemistry of the second amino terminal residue (Jilek et al., 2011; Zangger et al., 2008).

The first molecule belonging to the temporin family was identified in methanol extracts of the skin of the Asian frog *Rana erythraea*. In the early 1990s, Simmaco et al. identified a family of similar peptides with antibacterial and antifungal properties from the skin secretion of the European red frog *Rana temporaria* and termed them temporins (Mahalka et al., 2009; Simmaco et al., 1996). Subsequently, many other temporins have been isolated from the secretions of other ranid frogs of both North American and Euroasian origin. At present, the temporin family includes more than 100 members, which share a number of unique properties, such as: i) a short amino acid sequence, that favors cost-efficient chemical synthesis: most temporins are 10–14 amino acid long, with a few 16–17 amino acids exceptions, and an ultrashort temporin of only eight amino acid residues, that represents the smallest naturally occurring linear AMP so far identified, has been isolated from the skin of the frog *Phelophylax saharica* (Abbassi et al., 2010); ii) a low positive charge ranging from +2 to +3 at neutral pH (in contrast with most AMPs belonging to other families, which usually have a higher net positive charge); iii) high efficiency against a wide range of pathogens, that is retained in serum, and concomitant low or null toxicity to mammalian cells; iv) at least in some cases, immuno-modulatory and/or antiendotoxin activity (Mangoni & Shai, 2011). Temporins exhibit antibacterial, antifungal, antiviral and antiprotozoan activities. Their potent action against Gram-positive bacteria, including methicillin-resistant strains, is of particular interest, because a synergistic action of the temporin A-methicillin association has been observed in a rat model of infection with methicillin-resistant *S. epidermidis* (Ghiselli et al., 2002). Temporin-1Tl has a higher and broader spectrum of activity than the other isoforms, being active against fungi and Gram-negative bacteria such as *P. aeruginosa* and *E. coli*, but it disrupts human erythrocytes at microbicidal concentrations (Mangoni et al., 2011). Temporins-1Ta, Tb, and Tl have been shown to neutralize the toxic effect of LPS derived from various species of *E. coli*, by complexing with it and making it unavailable for interaction with macrophage receptors to stimulate the production of TNF-α, considered a primary mediator of endotoxemia (Mangoni & Shai, 2008). Owing to their characteristics, temporins are considered worth of further development. In this perspective, by studying the structure-activity relationship of a library of Tl derivatives, Mangoni and co-workers identified novel analogues with better properties that could be used for future developments (Mangoni et al., 2011).

6. Insect host defense peptides: Defensins and cecropins

Insects such as moths, flies and bees rely on a wide array of humoral peptidic factors to defend themselves against potential pathogens. A recently identified family of peptides isolated from the *Apis mellifera* royal jelly is represented by the jelleins. These are composed of 8–9 amino acids, are amidated at the C-terminus and bear a +2 charge (Romanelli et al., 2010). While these molecules are still in the characterization phase, the research on insect defensin went a little further. The core structure of invertebrate defensins is composed of an α-helical domain linked to a two-stranded antiparallel β-sheet with three or four disulphide bonds forming the so-called cysteine-stabilized α-helix β-sheet motif. Some antifungal peptides like drosomycin from *Drosophila melanogaster* contain an additional short N-terminal β-strand, so presenting a βαββ-scaffold that is similar to that of antifungal plant defensins (Wilmes et al., 2011). Royalisin, an insect defensin isolated from the royal jelly of *A. mellifera* (Fujiwara et al., 1990), consists of 51 amino acids, in which six cysteine residues form three disulfide bonds that give the molecule a compact globular structure. Royalisin inhibits the growth of Gram-positive bacteria and fungi and is particularly active against the honeybee pathogen *Paenibacillus larvae larvae*, that causes American foulbrood, a serious disease found in honeybee larvae (Bilikova et al., 2001). Recombinant and functionally active royalisin has been recently obtained with a yield of the final purified product in the range of 0.192 mg/L of bacterial cell culture. Considering that the substance shows antibacterial activity at the 1–27 μg/ml concentration range, this breakthrough makes it possible to proceed to an extensive characterization of royalisin for both beekeeping and human therapeutic purposes (Tseng et al., 2011).

6.1 Cecropins

Cecropins are lytic peptides that possess antibacterial activity *in vitro*, originally isolated from the hemolymph of the giant silk moth *Hyalophora cecropia* (Hultmark et al., 1980). The killing is mediated by membrane permeabilization, with a detergent-like effect accompanied by pore formation (Bechinger & Lohner, 2006). Cecropin specificity of action relies upon the differences in the composition and physicochemical properties of germ and host cell membranes. Pore formation is easily achieved in bacterial membranes rich in anionic phospholipids, but not in animal cell membranes, rich in neutral phospholipids and further stabilized by cholesterol. Cecropins are considered worth of further development because they show a well demonstrated biological activity and consist of a single polypeptide chain well suited for economical production through recombinant DNA technology or peptide synthesis. Cecropin-like peptides are currently being developed following different strategies to improve antimicrobial and anticancer activity and diminish cytotoxicity (Plunkett et al., 2009; Wu et al., 2009). Based on the assumption that lysozyme is inactive on Gram-negative bacteria because it cannot reach the peptidoglycan layer, and that cecropin may disrupt the outer membrane of Gram-negatives, giving the enzyme access to peptidoglycan, a novel hybrid protein combining *Musca domestica* cecropin with human lysozyme has been expressed in *E. coli*. This chimeric protein showed an improvement of antibacterial activity and spectrum compared to its single original components (Lu et al., 2010). Another chimera, the cecropin AD peptide, composed by the first 11 residues of *H. cecropia* cecropin A and the last 26 residues of *H. cecropia* cecropin D, has been produced in a *Bacillus subtilis* expression system (Chen X. et al., 2009). The potent antimicrobial activity against *S. aureus* and *E. coli* of the recombinant product, and the low cost of the production process, with a yield of 30.6 mg of pure recombinant protein obtained from 1 liter of culture supernatant, make this molecule a suitable option for veterinary and medical applications. Cecropins have properties similar to those of melittin, a peptide that is the major component of the *A. mellifera* venom (Pandey et al., 2010). Some melittin analogues showed a drastic cytotoxicity reduction though maintaining comparable bactericidal activity. Two recombinant cecropin A- and cecropin B-melittin hybrid peptides CA(1-7)-M(4-11) and CB(1-7)-M(4-11) have been expressed in the yeast *Pichia pastoris*. Both chimeric peptides showed strong antibacterial activity against *E. coli, S. aureus, P. aeruginosa, Klebsiella pneumoniae, Bacillus subtilis, B. thuringiensis*, and *Salmonella derby* (Cao et al., 2010). The efficacy of a cecropin A-melittin hybrid peptide CA(1-8)M(1-18) and shorter derivatives against pan-resistant *Acinetobacter baumannii* has been tested both *in vitro* and in a mouse sepsis model. The peptide showed an *in vitro* good activity, that was not affected by the presence of capsule (Rodríguez-Hernández et al., 2006). However, *in vivo* the peptides showed bacteriostatic activity only, and PD_{50} was not achieved with non-toxic doses (López-Rojas et al., 2011). The antifungal and anti-inflammatory effects of a cecropin A(1-8)–magainin 2(1-12) hybrid peptide analog (P5) have been tested on *Malassezia furfur* and human keratinocytes. The minimal inhibitory concentration of P5 against *M. furfur* was 0.39 µM, making it 3-4 times more potent than commonly used antifungal agents such as ketoconazole (1.5 µM) or itraconazole (1.14 µM). P5 efficiently inhibited the expression of IL-8 and Toll-like receptor 2 in *M. furfur*-infected human keratinocytes without eukaryotic cytotoxicity at its fungicidal concentration. Moreover, P5 significantly down-regulated NF-kB activation and intracellular calcium fluctuation, which are closely related with enhanced responses of keratinocyte inflammation induced by *M. furfur* infection. Taken together, these observations suggest that P5 may be a potential therapeutic agent for *M. furfur*-associated human skin diseases because of its distinct antifungal and anti-inflammatory action (Ryu et al., 2011).

7. Bacterial antimicrobial peptides

A wide array of proteinaceous molecules is produced by Gram-positive and Gram-negative bacteria to counteract the proliferation of closely related microorganisms competing for limited resources within the same ecological niche (Héchard & Sahl, 2002). The first description of antagonistic interactions between different *Staphylococcus* strains was made in 1855 by Babes, who with Cornil co-authored the first text on bacteriology. The same phenomenon was described by Pasteur, who noted the inhibitory effect of common bacteria from urine on *Bacillus anthracis* (Pasteur & Joubert, 1877). However, the first clear documentation of an antibiotic agent produced by *E. coli* was provided by Gratia, who in 1925 demonstrated that in liquid media strain V (for virulence) produced a dialyzable and heat-stable substance (later referred to as colicin V) that even in high dilutions inhibited the growth of *E. coli* strain φ (Gratia, 1925). Subsequently, a number of colicins produced by *E. coli* and closely related members of the *Enterobacteriaceae* were discovered. Following the discovery that antibiotic substances of the colicin type are also produced by non-coliform bacteria, the more general term "bacteriocin" was coined (Jacob et al., 1953), to define proteinaceous antibiotics of the colicin type, characterized by predominant intra-specific killing activity, and adsorption to specific receptors on the surface of sensitive cells (Jack et al., 1995; Tagg et al., 1976). Bacteriocins produced by Gram-positive bacteria differ in many characteristics from those produced by Gram-negative bacteria: the former are initially produced as propeptides, which are subsequently separated from a leader peptide to form the biologically active molecule. In some cases, such as the lantibiotics, post-translational modifications are introduced into the propeptide region of the precursor molecule prior to cleavage of the leader component (Cotter et al., 2005a). In contrast, Gram-negative bacteriocins (colicins) are generally high-molecular-mass (29- to 90-kDa) proteins that contain characteristic domains specifying either attachment specificity, translocation, or killing activity. Similar domain constructs have been found in some of the pyocins produced by *P. aeruginosa* (Jack et al., 1995).

7.1 Gram-positive bacteriocins

Although there is not a definitive classification for bacteriocins from Gram-positive bacteria, it is generally accepted the division into class I, composed by post-translationally modified peptides containing lanthionine or methyl-lanthionine; class II, or heat-stable non-lanthionine-containing bacteriocins, which are small thermostable, non-modified proteins (with the exception of disulfide bridges linkage), with or without leader peptide; and class III, which includes secreted heat-labile, cell wall-degrading enzymes. A family of circular, post-translationally modified bacteriocins has been recently grouped to form a new class of bacteriocins, class IV, that encompasses globular, thermostable, helical, and post-translationally modified proteins, ranging between 35 and 70 amino acids, with the N- and C-termini linked by a peptide bond (Sanchez-Hidalgo et al., 2011).

7.1.1 Class I bacteriocins: Lantibiotics

Class I bacteriocins produced by lactic acid bacteria are the most widely investigated: they are small, heat-stable post-translationally modified peptides commonly called lantibiotics, that naturally occur in food and in the gastro-enteric tract of mammals. Some of them, such as nisin and lacticin, are widely used as antibacterial agents by the food and agricultural industry of more than 50 countries (Chatterjee et al., 2005; Cotter et al., 2005b). Lantibiotics are ribosomally synthesized as precursor peptides, and post-translationally modified by the dehydration of serine and threonine residues and subsequent intramolecular addition of cysteine, resulting in the formation of (β-methyl) lanthionine thioether bridges, that characterizes the group (Abriouel et al., 2010). A N-terminal leader sequence is believed to keep the peptides inactive while inside the producing cell. To further protect themselves from the action of secreted lantibiotics, the lantibiotic-producing bacteria have evolved self-protection mechanisms that consist of individual immunity proteins (generically termed the LanI proteins), or of highly conserved ATP-binding cassette transporter (ABC-transporter) proteins, usually composed of two or three subunits, generically termed LanFE(G) (Draper et al., 2008). Many lantibiotics are extremely potent antibacterial agents with minimum inhibitory concentrations in the nanomolar range (Ross & Vederas, 2011). Lantibiotics are active against several very common food spoilage organisms (for example, *Listeria monocytogenes* and *Clostridium botulinum*) and show very promising activity against resistant *S. aureus* and enterococcal infections (Cotter et al., 2005a). In the last few years some bacteriocins have been considered for human health and medical purposes: nisin A, the prototype lantibiotic produced by *Lactococcus lactis*, is highly efficient against Gram-positive bacteria and has no human toxicity. It was discovered in 1928 and has been accepted by the Food and Drug Administration as a food additive in 1988. Its 34-amino acid residue structure contains five macrocyclic rings stabilized by thioether bonds (Turpin et al., 2010). Nisin inhibits the growth of vegetative Gram-positive bacteria by binding to lipid II, so disrupting cell wall biosynthesis and facilitating pore formation. Nisin also inhibits the outgrowth of bacterial spores, including *Bacillus anthracis* spores (Gut et al., 2011). However, natural nisin A is unsuitable for medical uses, being unstable and poorly soluble in neutral or basic conditions and easily inactivated by thiols such as cysteine and glutathione (Rollema et al., 1995). Nisin A derivatives obtained by amino acid substitution are being developed and evaluated as anti-mycobacterial drugs (Carroll et al., 2010). Lacticin 3147, another lantibiotic produced by lactic acid bacteria, is more stable than nisin and is active against MRSA and VRE at nanomolar concentrations (Piper et a., 2009). Lacticin 3147 consists of a 2-peptide (lacticin A1 and A2) system: lacticin A1 binds lipid II, and the complex binds lacticin A2, that induces pore formation in the bacterial membrane. To the class I bacteriocins also belongs thuricin CD, another 2-component peptide system produced by *Bacillus thuringiensis* and selectively active against *Clostridium difficile*. A problem inherent the current antibiotic treatment of *C. difficile*-associated bowel disease is that large-spectrum antibiotics can perturb the gut flora to the point to interfere with recovery and in same cases even to promote recurrences. These problems could be avoided by the use of thuricin CD that, according to extensive tests against a broad range of Gram-positive and Gram-negative bacteria, targets a restricted spectrum of spore-forming Gram-positive bacteria (Rea et al., 2010).

7.1.2 Class II bacteriocins

Class II bacteriocins include class IIa one-peptide pediocin-like bacteriocins and class-IIb, that are two-peptide bacteriocins (Nissen-Meyer et al., 2010). Pediocin PA-1 is a representative member of the class IIa bacteriocins, i.e. low molecular weight, plasmid-encoded peptides, with marked antilisterial activity, produced by *Pediococcus acidilactici*

(Devi & Halami, 2011). It is currently investigated as a useful tool to control *Listeria monocytogenes* in food (Hartmann et al., 2011). At least 15 two-peptide members of the class-IIb bacteriocins have been isolated and characterized since the first isolation of lactococcin G (Nissen-Meyer et al., 1992). Like lacticins, these bacteriocins consist of two different peptides, and optimal antibacterial activity requires the presence of both peptides in about equal amounts. The two peptides are synthesized as preforms that contain a 15–30 residue N-terminal leader sequence that apparently facilitates interaction with the dedicated ABC-transporter membrane protein and might possibly also function to keep the bacteriocin inactive until it has been secreted. The genes encoding the preforms of the two peptides are always found next to each other in the same operon along with the gene that encodes the immunity protein. Class IIb bacteriocins are still in the characterization phase, in order to develop variants useful for medical and biotechnological applications, such as infection treatment and food and animal feed preservation (Nissen-Meyer et al., 2010). Class III bacteriocins, like enterolysin A, are large antibacterial proteins with enzymatic activity (Nilsen et al., 2003), that for their structure are not considered suitable for drug development. On the contrary, low-molecular weight, circular class IV bacteriocins possess some interesting features: the joining of the ends protects from degradation by exopeptidase enzymes, increasing stability and making the molecules highly resistant to a wide range of pH and temperatures. A representative member of class IV bacteriocins is AS-48, that is the first reported circular bacteriocin and whose structure and genetic regulation have been elucidated. It can be considered a good starting point to develop analogs with new and/or improved features for practical chemical, pharmaceutical and agricultural applications. (Sanchez-Hidalgo et al., 2011).

7.2 Gram-negative bacteriocins

Enterobacteria can secrete colicins and microcins, both encoded by gene clusters that codify for their production, export and self-immunity. To date, all colicins and microcins found are plasmid-encoded, except class IIb microcins, that are chromosome-encoded. Colicin gene clusters are highly conserved, but simpler than microcin gene clusters. In contrast to microcins, the production of colicins is mainly induced *via* the DNA repair network, called the SOS response, that can be activated by an environmental stress, such as UV irradiation, exposure to DNA damaging agents, or cell starvation. The major differences between microcins and colicins, besides the molecular mass, lie in their structure and in the fact that contrary to most microcins, colicins are not post-translationally modified.

7.2.1 Colicins

Colicins are large proteins organized in three functional domains: a central receptor binding domain, an N-terminal translocation domain and a C-terminal catalytic domain. These domains, which are common to all colicins, ensure every common step of the colicin mechanisms of action, *i.e.* i) recognition by a specific receptor at the outer membrane, ii) translocation across the outer membrane and iii) lethal interaction with a specific cellular target. The ability of an *E. coli* strain to kill neighboring strains by releasing colicins into the surroundings has been known since the 1920s (Gratia, 1925). However, the mechanism by which colicins reach the target cell cytoplasm, crossing the outer membrane, the peptidoglycan layer and the inner membrane, has only recently begun to be unraveled at the molecular level. It seems that the penetration mechanism is similar, even though different colicins parasitize different protein systems and kill cells by different mechanisms (Cascales et al., 2007). Colicins are not considered for development into suitable antibacterial drugs, mainly because of their high molecular weight, but their study has significantly contributed to the progress of basic research in a number of fields, such as the bacterial outer membrane protein receptors, and the proteins of the translocation machinery.

7.2.2 Microcins

The name microcin was introduced to distinguish the class of antibacterial peptides with molecular mass below 10 kDa, from the higher molecular mass colicins (Asensio et al., 1976). Whereas many antimicrobial peptides of bacterial origin are produced by large multi-domain enzyme complexes termed peptide synthetases, microcins are typically produced as ribosomally synthesized precursors, similar to the bacteriocins from Gram-positive bacteria. Microcins are encoded by plasmid- or chromosome-located gene clusters, which typically include open reading frames encoding the microcin precursor, self-immunity factors, secretion proteins and modification enzymes, giving rise to an amazing diversity of microcin structures and mechanisms of action (Duquesne et al., 2007). Microcins are secreted by enterobacteria (mostly *E. coli*) under conditions of nutrient depletion, and are involved in the regulation of microbial competition within the intestinal microbiota. They are generally hydrophobic, highly resistant to heat, extreme pH and proteases, and exert potent antibacterial activity in nanomolar concentrations, usually against a narrow spectrum of closely related species. Their mechanism of action has been defined as a "Trojan horse" behavior: they are recognized as siderophores by the outer membrane receptors of susceptible bacteria, and as such internalized; once inside they bind essential enzymes or interact with the inner membrane killing the bacterium (Duquesne et al., 2007). At present microcins are still into the characterization phase, and despite their potent antibacterial activity, they are not being developed as antibacterials (Corsini et al., 2010). Microcin E492, a pore-forming molecule produced by *Klebsiella pneumoniae*, beyond exerting antibacterial activity on related strains, has been shown to induce apoptosis of malignant human cell lines (Lagos et al., 2009). Microcin B17, produced by various *E. coli* strains harboring the 70-kb single-copy, conjugative pMccB17 plasmid, is a potent inhibitor of DNA gyrase, whereas microcin J25, the best-studied member of the lasso peptides, inhibits RNA polymerase (Oman & van der Donk, 2010).

8. Lipopeptides and lipoglycopeptides

Antimicrobial lipopeptides (LiPs) are non-ribosomally produced by bacteria and fungi during cultivation on various carbon sources. They are a class of antibiotics highly active against multidrug-resistant bacteria. Most native LiPs consist of a short (six to seven amino acids) linear or cyclic peptide sequence, either positively or negatively charged, with a fatty acid moiety covalently attached to the N-terminus. (Mangoni & Shai, 2011). Both the composition of the peptide moiety and the type of the lipophilic part are sensitive to modifications. In general, native LiPs are non-cell-selective and therefore quite toxic to mammalian cells. Despite toxicity, in 2003 a member of this family, daptomycin, which is active only toward Gram-positive bacteria, has been approved by the FDA in an injection formulation for the treatment of complicated skin and skin structure infections (SSSI) caused by susceptible strains of the following species: *S. aureus* (including methicillin-resistant strains), *Streptococcus pyogenes*, *S. agalactiae*, *S. dysgalactiae* subspecies *equisimilis*, and *Enterococcus faecalis* (vancomycin-susceptible strains only). This example confirms the growing opinion that peptide-based antibiotics will be among the next generation of anti-infective therapy (Mangoni & Shai, 2011). Dalbavancin, oritavancin and telavancin are semisynthetic lipoglycopeptides active against multidrug-resistant Gram-positive pathogens (Zhanel et al., 2010). These molecules share a heptapeptide core that affects cell wall synthesis by inhibiting transglycosilation and transpeptidation, and contain lipophilic side chains that facilitate binding to cell membranes and increase antibacterial activity. Lipophilic residues also prolong *in vivo* half life, that is of 147-258 h for dalbavancin, of 393 h for oritavancin and of 12-24 h for telavancin. These drugs must be administered i.v. and are indicated for patients with complicated SSSI resistant to vancomycin. Telavancin has been approved for SSSI therapy by the FDA in September 2009. Dalbavancin, a teicoplanin derivative, has a long half life that allows for once weekly dosing. In published clinical trials, a dose on day 1 and 8 of treatment provided 14 days of antimicrobial activity, and demonstrated non-inferiority as measured by safety and efficacy for the treatment of uncomplicated SSSI, catheter-related bloodstream infections, and complicated SSSI (Welte & Pletz, 2010).

9. Bacteriophage endolysins

Since the pioneer work of d'Herelle, several studies demonstrated that bacteriophages can be successfully used in the therapy of animal and human bacterial infections (Harper & Enright, 2011; Verma et al., 2009). Phages are already used in the agricultural, food-processing and fishery industries, and for the treatment of human bacterial infections in Georgia and Eastern Europe (Housby & Mann, 2009). Recent experiments performed by Fu et al. on the efficacy of a bacteriophage cocktail to prevent the formation of *P. aeruginosa* biofilms on catheters in an *in vitro* model showed a 99.9% reduction of the number of bacteria (Fu et al., 2010). The human use of phages in Western countries has been hindered so far by cost, safety concerns about phage injection into the bloodstream, and by the sometimes inconsistent outcome of the treatments, due to the poor characterization of bacteriophage preparations. Moreover, the *in vivo* pharmacokinetics of phages are complex, being influenced by the host immune system-mediated phage clearance rate and by the possible insurgence of bacterial resistance due to lysogeny or mutations concerning metabolic steps or surface receptors (Payne &Jansen, 2003). However, phage therapy is considered a potential treatment for some selected infections, such as multidrug resistant *P. aeruginosa* lung infection in cystic fibrosis patients (Morello et al., 2011), and chronic otitis (Wright et al., 2009). A different approach overcoming some of the above-mentioned problems involves the use of purified phage products as anti-infective agents. Double-stranded DNA phages naturally produce endolysins, i.e. mureine-degrading enzymes, that have been originally studied and developed to control mucous membrane infections (Borysowski et al., 2006), and are also denominated "enzybiotics" (Briers et al., 2011). They only work on Gram-positive bacteria because the outer membrane of Gram-negative bacteria prevents direct lysin-peptidoglycan interaction (Fischetti, 2010). To this end, the paper from Briers et al. reports that the use of endolysins in conjunction with outer membrane permeabilizers resulted in strong lytic activity against *P. aeruginosa*, with a reduction of more than four log units of viable bacteria in 30 min. Endolysins, some of which have been found active against *B. anthracis* (Schuch et al., 2002), *S. pneumoniae* (Jado et al., 2003) and *S. agalactiae* (Cheng et al., 2005), alone or in combination with conventional antibiotics or lysozyme, have a short half-life (15-20 min), but their action is so rapid that nanogram quantities kill sensitive Gram-positive bacteria in seconds after contact (Loeffler et al., 2001). Moreover, they are *per se* non toxic and, unexpectedly, not easily inactivated by antibodies (Fischetti, 2008). Considering that the endolysin target, peptidoglycan, is not present in eukaryotic cells, it can be anticipated that they will also be well tolerated by humans. Experiments performed on a murine model of pneumococcal pneumonia showed that an endolysin with muramidase activity, Cpl-1, protected 100% of mice when administered by intraperitoneal injections starting 24 hours after pulmonary infection (Witzenrath et al., 2009). These results suggest that Cpl-1 and related molecules could provide a new therapeutic option for pneumococcal pneumonia. The issue of the possible toxic effect due to the massive release of pro-inflammatory molecules by lysed bacteria has also been addressed. Circulating endotoxin, teichoic and lipoteichoic acids, and peptidoglycan could result in septic shock and multiple organ failure, but so far no side-effects related to lysin-induced bacteriolysis have been reported (Borysowski et al., 2006). According to experiments performed on a murine model, lysins may also cure already established infections (Witzenrath et al., 2009). More predictable endolysin applications include the elimination of bacteria from mucous membranes, the treatment of bacterial infections, and the biocontrol of bacteria in food.

10. Conclusions

Modern antibiotics are or derive from natural molecules isolated during the "golden age" of antibiotic discovery, i.e. the period between the1940s and the 1970s. Even those currently under development are nothing more than new, improved versions of these old natural products, because the chemical modification of existing molecules remains the most cost-efficient way to develop novel drugs active against resistant strains. As examples, we can cite the cephalosporin ceftaroline (Corey et al., 2010), the tetracycline amadacycline (PTK0796), the streptogramin NXL-103 (Politano & Sawyer, 2010) and the macrolide CEM-101 (Woosley et al., 2010). However, the perspective that these agents, new but based on old molecular scaffolds, will in their turn face the development of bacterial resistance, prompted both the academic community and the biotech/pharmaceutical companies to look for alternative strategies. In this scenario, the low molecular weight, broad-spectrum activity and rapid mode of action of AMPs make them promising drug candidates. Among potential advantages of some AMPs we can add the endotoxin-neutralizing ability and the capacity to modulate the host immune response. Moreover, they are usually unaffected by classic antibiotic resistance mechanisms (Zasloff, 2002). In this regard, however, concerns have been raised by the finding that some microorganisms are able to thwart AMP effects: *C. albicans* is sensitive to histatin-5, the most potent antifungal peptide present in human saliva (Edgerton & Koshlukova, 2000), but it produces aspartyl proteases that target this molecule, and in the presence of low histatin levels, as those occurring in AIDS patients, the yeast turns from a harmless commensal to a disease-causing pathogen (Meiller et al., 2009). Moreover, taking for granted that acquired resistance to AMPs is less likely to occur as compared to the traditional antibiotics, it has been observed that some Gram-negative bacteria can utilize various enzymes to reduce their surface net negative charge, so evading the action of cationic peptides (Roy et al., 2009). Several other bacterial strategies have been described that can result in decreased susceptibility to AMPs, such as secretion of inactivating proteins or exportation via efflux pumps. Therefore, the onset of resistance in microbial populations consistently exposed to AMPs cannot be excluded (Peters et al., 2010), and a theoretical concern about the pharmacological use of AMPs closely related to human ones is that long term selection could generate organisms with unpredictable virulence potential (Fernebro, 2011). In addition to these (for now) theoretical concerns, we must recognize that some more practical AMP flaws, such as the high production cost and the susceptibility to proteolytic degradation, have until now effectively prevented AMPs from entering the market. Most AMPs today in preclinical and clinical trials have been developed for topical applications (Hancock & Sahl, 2006). Examples of indications are catheter site infections, cystic fibrosis, acne and wound healing. For complicated wounds and ulcers caused by multidrug-resistant bacteria, phage therapy, although the available literature is in many ways unsatisfactory, could be an option. In the EU, it has been proposed that specific sections concerning phage therapy should be included in the Advanced Therapy Medicinal Product Regulation to make it easier to get approval for clinical trials involving such therapy (Verbeken et al., 2007). For practical and economical reasons it could be easier to market purified lysins for which, so far, resistance development has not been observed. However, most lysins are endowed with short *in vivo* half-life (Loeffler et al., 2003), an issue that has to be solved before they enter clinical use. Another relevant issue is the possibility to use narrow spectrum AMPs, such as microcins. Conceptually, a broad spectrum antibiotic is not always the best choice, especially when considering its effects on the commensal flora and the risk of inducing opportunistic infections. However, the use of narrow spectrum antibiotics should be supported by diagnostics faster and more accurate than those in use today. The development of new antimicrobials is a formidable challenge, and out of this concern, in 2009 the U.S. and European Community presidencies established a Transatlantic Task Force, and the Infectious Diseases Society of America called for a global commitment to develop 10 novel antimicrobials by 2020 (Gwinn et al., 2010). In our view, the achievement of badly needed good results relies on a balanced interaction between well funded academic laboratories and the lead discovery departments of private companies, to make the most of existent and future techniques.

11. References

Abbassi, F., Lequin, O., Piesse, C., Goasdoué, N., Foulon, T., Nicolas, P., & Ladram, A. (2010). Temporin-SHf, a new type of phe-rich and hydrophobic ultrashort antimicrobial peptide. *The Journal of Biological Chemistry*, Vol.285, No. 22, (May 28), pp. 16880-16892, ISSN 0021-9258

Abriouel, H., Franz, CM., Ben Omar, N., & Gálvez, A. (2011). Diversity and applications of Bacillus bacteriocins. *FEMS Microbiology Reviews*, Vol. 35, No. 1, pp. 201-232, ISSN 0168-6445

Amiche, M., Ducancel, F., Lajeunesse, E., Boulain, JC., Ménez, A., & Nicolas, P. (1993). Molecular cloning of a cDNA encoding the precursor of adenoregulin from frog skin. Relationships with the vertebrate defensive peptides, dermaseptins. *Biochemical and Biophysical Research Communications*, Vol. 191, No. 3, (Mar 31), pp. 983-990, ISSN 0006-291X

Amiche, M., & Galanth, C. (2011). Dermaseptins as models for the elucidation of membrane-acting helical amphipathic antimicrobial peptides. *Current pharmaceutical biotechnology*, Vol. 12, No. 8, (Aug 1), pp. 1184-1193, ISSN 1389-2010

Andreu, D., Aschauer, H., Kreil, G., & Merrifield, RB. (1985). Solid-phase synthesis of PYLa and isolation of its natural counterpart, PGLa [PYLa-(4-24)] from skin secretion of *Xenopus laevis*. *European Journal of Biochemistry*, Vol. 149, pp. 531–535, ISSN 0014-2956

Asensio, C., & Pérez-Díaz, JC. (1976). A new family of low molecular weight antibiotics from enterobacteria. *Biochemical and Biophysical Research Communications*, Vol. 69, No. 1, (Mar 8), pp. 7-14, ISSN 0006-291X

Baltz, RH. (2008). Renaissance in antibacterial discovery from actinomycetes. *Current Opinion in Pharmacology*, Vol. 8, No. 5, pp. 557-63, ISSN 1471-4892

Bechinger, B., & Lohner, K. (2006). Detergent-like actions of linear amphipathic cationic antimicrobial peptides. *Biochimica et Biophysica Acta*, Vol. 1758, No. 9, 1529-1539, ISSN 0006-3002

Bera, A., Singh, S., Nagaraj, R., & Vaidya, T. (2003). Induction of autophagic cell death in *Leishmania donovani* by antimicrobial peptides. *Molecular and Biochemical Parasitology*, Vol. 127, No. 1, pp. 23-35, ISSN 0166-6851

Bilikova, K., Gusui, W., & Simuth, J. (2001). Isolation of a peptide fraction from honeybee royal jelly as a potential antifoulbrood factor. *Apidologie*, Vol. 32, pp. 275–283, ISSN 0044-8435

Boix, E., & Nogués, MV. (2007). Mammalian antimicrobial proteins and peptides: overview on the RNase A superfamily members involved in innate host defence. *Molecular BioSystems*, Vol. 3, No. 5, pp. 317-335, ISSN 1742-206X

Bommineni, YR., Dai, H., Gong, YX., Soulages, JL., Fernando, SC., Desilva, U., Prakash, O., & Zhang, G. (2007). Fowlicidin-3 is an alpha-helical cationic host defense peptide with potent antibacterial and lipopolysaccharide-neutralizing activities. *FEBS Journal*, Vol. 274, No. 2, pp. 418-428, ISSN 1432-1033

Borysowski, J., Weber-Dabrowska, B., & Górski, A. (2006). Bacteriophage endolysins as a novel class of antibacterial agents. *Experimental Biology and Medicine (Maywood)*, Vol. 231, No. 4, pp. 366-377, ISSN 1535-3702

Briers, Y., Walmagh, M., & Lavigne, R. (2011). Use of bacteriophage endolysin EL188 and outer membrane permeabilizers against *Pseudomonas aeruginosa*. *Journal of Applied Microbiology*, Vol. 110, No. 3, pp. 778-785, ISSN 1364-5072

Brinch, KS., Tulkens, PM., Van Bambeke, F., Frimodt-Møller, N., Høiby, N., & Kristensen, HH. (2010). Intracellular activity of the peptide antibiotic NZ2114: studies with *Staphylococcus aureus* and human THP-1 monocytes, and comparison with daptomycin and vancomycin. *Journal of Antimicrobial Chemotherapy*, Vol. 65, No. 8, pp. 1720-1724, ISSN 0305-7453

Bulet, P., Stöcklin, R., & Menin, L. (2004). Anti-microbial peptides: from invertebrates to vertebrates. *Immunology Reviews*, Vol. 198, pp.169-184, ISSN 0105-2896

Cao, Y., Yu, RQ., Liu, Y., Zhou, HX., Song, LL., Cao, Y., & Qiao, DR. (2010). Design, recombinant expression, and antibacterial activity of the cecropins-melittin hybrid antimicrobial peptides. *Current Microbiology*, Vol. 61, No. 3, pp. 169-175, ISSN 0343-8651

Carroll, J., Field, D., O'Connor, PM., Cotter, PD., Coffey, A., Hill, C., Ross, RP., & O'Mahony, J. (2010). Gene encoded antimicrobial peptides, a template for the design of novel anti-mycobacterial drugs. *Bioengineered Bugs*, Vol 1, No. 6, pp. 408-412, ISSN 1949-1018

Cascales, E., Buchanan, SK., Duché, D., Kleanthous, C., Lloubès, R., Postle, K., Riley, M., Slatin, S., & Cavard, D. (2007). Colicin biology. *Microbiology and Molecular Biology Reviews*, Vol. 71, No. 1, pp. 158-229, ISSN 0005-3678

Chatterjee, C., Paul, M., Xie, L., & van der Donk, WA. (2005). Biosynthesis and mode of action of lantibiotics. *Chemical Reviews*, Vol. 105, No. 2, pp. 633-684, ISSN 0009-2665

Chen, H., Xu, Z., Peng, L., Fang, X., Yin, X., Xu, N., & Cen, P. (2006). Recent advances in the research and development of human defensins. *Peptides*, Vol. 27, No. 4, pp. 931-940, ISSN 0196-9781

Chen, X.,; Zhu, F., Cao, Y., & Qiao, S. (2009). Novel expression vector for secretion of cecropin AD in *Bacillus subtilis* with enhanced antimicrobial activity. *Antimicrobial Agents and Chemotherapy*, Vol. 53, No. 9, pp. 3683-3689, ISSN 0066-4804

Cheng, Q., Nelson, D., Zhu, S., & Fischetti, VA. (2005). Removal of group B streptococci colonizing the vagina and oropharynx of mice with a bacteriophage lytic enzyme. *Antimicrobial Agents and Chemotherapy*, Vol. 49, No. 1, pp. 111-117, ISSN 0066-4804

Chin, JN., Rybak, MJ., Cheung, CM., & Savage, PB. (2007). Antimicrobial activities of ceragenins against clinical isolates of resistant *Staphylococcus aureus*. *Antimicrobial Agents and Chemotherapy*, Vol. 51, pp. 1268–1273, ISSN 0066-4804

Chopra, I. (1993). The magainins: antimicrobial peptides with potential for topical application. *The Journal of Antimicrobial Chemotherapy*, Vol. 32, No. 3, pp. 351-353, ISSN 0305-7453

Ciornei, CD., Sigurdardóttir, T., Schmidtchen, A., & Bodelsson, M. (2005). Antimicrobial and chemoattractant activity, lipopolysaccharide neutralization, cytotoxicity, and inhibition by serum of analogs of human cathelicidin LL-37. *Antimicrobial Agents and Chemotherapy*, Vol. 49, No. 7, pp. 2845-2850, ISSN 0066-4804

Clara, A., Manjramkar, DD., & Reddy, VK. (2004). Preclinical evaluation of magainin-A as a contraceptive antimicrobial agent. *Fertility and Sterility*, Vol. 81, No. 5, pp. 1357-1365, ISSN 0015-0282.

Cole, AM., & Waring, AJ. (2002). The role of defensins in lung biology and therapy. *American Journal of Respiratory and Critical Care Medicine*, Vol. 1, No. 4, pp. 249-59, ISSN 1073-449X

Conlon, JM., Abdel-Wahab, YH., Flatt, PR., Leprince, J., Vaudry, H., Jouenne , T., & Condamine, E. (2009). A glycine-leucine-rich peptide structurally related to the plasticins from skin secretions of the frog *Leptodactylus laticeps (Leptodactylidae)*. *Peptides*, Vol. 30, No. 5, pp. 888-892, ISSN: 0196-9781

Corey, GR., Wilcox, M., Talbot, GH., Friedland, HD., Baculik, T., Witherell, GW., Critchley, I., Das, AF., & Thye, D. (2010). Integrated Analysis of CANVAS 1 and 2: Phase 3, Multicenter, Randomized, Double-Blind Studies to Evaluate the Safety and Efficacy of Ceftaroline versus Vancomycin plus Aztreonam in Complicated Skin and Skin-Structure Infection. *Clinical Infectious Diseases*, Vol. 51, pp. 641–650, ISSN 1058-4838

Corsini, G., Karahanian, E., Tello, M., Fernandez, K., Rivero, D., Saavedra, JM., & Ferrer, A. (2010). Purification and characterization of the antimicrobial peptide microcin N. *FEMS Microbiology Letters*, Vol. 312, No. 2, pp.119-125, ISSN 0378-1097

Costa Torres, AF., Dantas, RT., Toyama, MH., Diz Filho, E., Zara, FJ., Rodrigues de Queiroz, MG., Pinto Nogueira, NA., Rosa de Oliveira, M., de Oliveira Toyama, D., Monteiro, HS., & Martins, AM. (2010). Antibacterial and antiparasitic effects of *Bothrops marajoensis* venom and its fractions: Phospholipase A2 and L-amino acid oxidase. *Toxicon*, Vol. 55, No. 4, (Apr 1), pp. 795-804, ISSN 0041-0101

Cotter, PD., Hill, C., & Ross, RP. (2005a). Bacterial lantibiotics: strategies to improve therapeutic potential. *Current Protein & Peptide Science*, Vol. 6, No. 1, pp. 61-75, ISSN 1389-2037

Cotter, PD., Hill, C., & Ross, RP. (2005b) Bacteriocins: developing innate immunity for food. *Nature Reviews Microbiology*, Vol. 3, No. 10, pp. 777-788, ISSN 1740-1526

Csordás, A., & Michl H. (1970). Isolation and structure of a haemolytic polypeptide from the defensive secretion of European Bombina species. *Monatshefte fur Chemie*. Vol. 101, pp. 182–189, ISSN 1434-4475

Daly, JW., Caceres, J., Moni, RW., Gusovsky, F., Moos, M. Jr., Seamon, KB., Milton, K., & Myers, CW. (1992). Frog secretions and hunting magic in the upper Amazon: identification of a peptide that interacts with an adenosine receptor. *Proceedings of the National Academy of Sciences USA*, Vol. 89, No. 22, (Nov 15), pp. 10960-10963, ISSN 0027-8424

Davies, J. (2011). How to discover new antibiotics: harvesting the parvome. *Current Opinion in Chemical Biology*, Vol. 15, No. 1, pp. 5-10, ISSN 1367-5931

De Caro, G., Endean, R., Erspamer, V., & Roseghini, M. (1968). Occurrence of caerulein in extracts of the skin of *Hyla caerulea* and other Australian hylids. *British Journal of Pharmacology and Chemotherapy*, Vol. 33, No. 1, pp. 48-58, ISSN 0366-0826

Devi, SM., & Halami, PM. (2011). Detection and Characterization of Pediocin PA-1/AcH like Bacteriocin Producing Lactic Acid Bacteria. *Current Microbiology*, Vol. 63, No. 2, pp. 181-185, ISSN 0343-8651

Dorosz, J., Gofman, Y., Kolusheva, S., Otzen, D., Ben-Tal, N., Nielsen, NC., & Jelinek, R. (2010). Membrane interactions of novicidin, a novel antimicrobial peptide: phosphatidylglycerol promotes bilayer insertion. *The Journal of Physical Chemistry B*, Vol. 114, No. 34, pp. 11053-11060, ISSN 1089-5647

Draper, LA., Ross, RP., Hill, C., & Cotter, PD. (2008). Lantibiotic immunity. *Current Protein & Peptide Science*, Vol. 9, No. 1, pp. 39-49, ISSN 1389-2037

Duquesne, S., Petit, V., Peduzzi, J., & Rebuffat, S. (2007). Structural and functional diversity of microcins, gene-encoded antibacterial peptides from enterobacteria. *Journal of Molecular Microbiology and Biotechnology*, Vol. 13, No. 4, pp. 200-209, ISSN 1464-1801

Dziarski, R., & Gupta, D. (2006). The peptidoglycan recognition proteins (PGRPs). *Genome Biology*, Vol. 7, No. 8, p. 232, ISSN 1465-6906

Edgerton, M., & Koshlukova, SE. (2000). Salivary histatin 5 and its similarities to the other antimicrobial proteins in human saliva. *Advances in Dental Research*, Vol. 14, pp. 16-21, ISSN 0895-9374

El Amri, C., & Nicolas, P. (2008). Plasticins: membrane-damaging peptides with 'chameleon-like' properties. *Cellular and Molecular Life Sciences*, Vol. 65, No. 6, pp. 895-909, ISSN 1420-682X

Fernebro, J. (2011). Fighting bacterial infections-future treatment options. *Drug Resistance Updates*, Vol. 14, No. 2, pp. 125-139, ISSN 1368-7646

Finlay, BB., & Hancock, RE. (2004). Can innate immunity be enhanced to treat microbial infections? *Nature Reviews Microbiology*, Vol. 2, No. 6, pp. 497-504, ISSN 1740-1526

Fischbach, MA., & Walsh, CT. (2009). Antibiotics for emerging pathogens. *Science*, Vol. 325, No. 5944, pp. 1089-1093, ISSN 0036-8075

Fischetti, VA. (2008). Bacteriophage lysins as effective antibacterials. *Current Opinion in Microbiology*, Vol. 11, No. 5, pp. 393-400, ISSN 1369-5274

Fischetti, VA. (2010). Bacteriophage endolysins: a novel anti-infective to control Gram-positive pathogens. *International Journal of Medical Microbiology*, Vol. 300, No. 6, 357-362, ISSN 1438-4221

Fu, W., Forster, T., Mayer, O., Curtin, JJ., Lehman, SM., & Donlan, RM. (2010). Bacteriophage cocktail for the prevention of biofilm formation by *Pseudomonas aeruginosa* on catheters in an in vitro model system. *Antimicrobial Agents and Chemotherapy*, Vol. 54, No. 1, pp. 397-404, ISSN 0066-4804

Fujiwara, S., Imai, J., Fujiwara, M., Yaeshima, T., Kawashima, T., & Kobayashi, K. (1990). A potent antibacterial protein in royal jelly. *The Journal of Biological Chemistry*, Vol. 265, pp. 11333–11337, ISSN 0021-9258

Gabriel, GJ., & Tew, GN. (2008). Conformationally rigid proteomimetics: a case study in designing antimicrobial aryl oligomers. *Organic and Biomolecular Chemistry*, Vol. 6, No. 3, pp. 417-423, ISSN 1477-0520

Ganz, T., Selsted, ME., & Lehrer, RI. (1986). Antimicrobial activity of phagocyte granule proteins. *Seminars in Respiratory Infections*, Vol. 1, No. 2, pp. 107-117, ISSN 0882-0546

Ghiselli, R., Giacometti, A., Cirioni, O., Mocchegiani, F., Orlando, F., Kamysz, W., Del Prete, MS., Lukasiak, J., Scalise, G., & Saba, V. (2002). Temporin A as a prophylactic agent against methicillin sodium-susceptible and methicillin sodium-resistant *Staphylococcus epidermidis* vascular graft infection. *Journal of Vascular Surgery*, Vol. 36, No. 5, pp. 1027-1030, ISSN 0741-5214

Gläser, R., Harder, J., Lange, H., Bartels, J., Christophers, E., & Schröder, JM. (2005). Antimicrobial psoriasin (S100A7) protects human skin from *Escherichia coli* infection. *Nature Immunology*, Vol. 6, No. 1, pp. 57-64, ISSN 1529-2908

Gläser, R., Navid, F., Schuller, W., Jantschitsch, C., Harder, J., Schröder, JM., Schwarz, A., & Schwarz, T. (2009). UV-B radiation induces the expression of antimicrobial peptides in human keratinocytes in vitro and in vivo. *Journal of Allergy and Clinical Immunology*, Vol. 123, pp. 1117–1123, ISSN 0091-6749

Gläser, R. (2011). Research in practice: Antimicrobial peptides of the skin. *Journal der Deutschen Dermatologischen Gesellschaft*. May. 25. doi: 10.1111/j.1610-0387.2011.07708.x. [Epub ahead of print], ISSN 1610-0379

Goitsuka, R., Chen, CL., Benyon, L., Asano, Y., Kitamura, D., & Cooper, MD. (2007). Chicken cathelicidin-B1, an antimicrobial guardian at the mucosal M cell gateway. *Proceedings of the National Academy of Sciences USA*, Vol. 104, No. 38, (Sep 18), pp. 15063-15068, ISSN 0027-8424

Gottler, LM., & Ramamoorthy, A. (2009). Structure, membrane orientation, mechanism, and function of pexiganan--a highly potent antimicrobial peptide designed from magainin. *Biochimica et Biophysica Acta*, Vol. 1788, No. 8, pp. 1680-1686, ISSN 0006-3002

Gratia, A. (1925). Sur un remarquable exemple d'antagonisme entre deux souches de colibacille. *Comptes Rendus des Séances et Mémoires de la Société de Biologie*, Vol. 93, pp. 1040-1041, ISSN 0037-9026

Gut, IM., Blanke, SR., & van der Donk, WA. (2011). Mechanism of Inhibition of *Bacillus anthracis* Spore Outgrowth by the Lantibiotic Nisin. *ACS Chemical Biology*, E pub. April 26, ISSN 1554-8929

Gwynn, MN., Portnoy, A., Rittenhouse, SF., & Payne, DJ. (2010). Challenges of antibacterial discovery revisited. *Annals of the New York Academy of Sciences*, Vol. 1213, pp. 5-19, ISSN 0077-8923

Hancock, RE., & Sahl, HG. (2006). Antimicrobial and host-defense peptides as new anti-infective therapeutic strategies. *Nature Biotechnology*, Vol. 24, No. 12, pp. 1551-1557, ISSN 1087-0156

Haney, EF., Hunter, HN., Matsuzaki, K., & Vogel, HJ. (2009). Solution NMR studies of amphibian antimicrobial peptides: linking structure to function? *Biochimica et Biophysica Acta*, Vol. 1788, No. 8. pp. 1639-1655, ISSN 0006-3002

Harder, J., & Schroder, JM. (2002). RNase 7, a novel innate immune defense antimicrobial protein of healthy human skin. *The Journal of Biological Chemistry*, Vol. 277, No. 48, (Nov 29), pp. 46779-46784, ISSN 0021-9258

Harper, DR., & Enright, MC. (2011). Bacteriophages for the treatment of *Pseudomonas aeruginosa* infections. *Journal of Applied Microbiology*, Mar 16 Epub ahead of print. Online ISSN 1365-2672

Harris, F., Dennison, SR., & Phoenix, DA. (2009). Anionic antimicrobial peptides from eukaryotic organisms. *Current Protein & Peptide Science*, Vol. 10, No. 6, pp. 585-606, ISSN 1389-2037

Hartmann, HA., Wilke, T., & Erdmann, R. (2011). Efficacy of bacteriocin-containing cell-free culture supernatants from lactic acid bacteria to control *Listeria monocytogenes* in food. *International Journal of Food Microbiology*, Vol. 146, No. 2, (Mar 30), pp. 192-199, ISSN 0168-1605

Hata, TR., & Gallo, RL. (2008). Antimicrobial peptides, skin infections, and atopic dermatitis. *Seminars in Cutaneous Medicine and Surgery*, Vol. 27, No. 2, pp. 144-150, ISSN 1085-5629

Héchard, Y., & Sahl, HG. (2002). Mode of action of modified and unmodified bacteriocins from Gram-positive bacteria. *Biochimie*, Vol. 84, No. 5-6, pp. 545-557, ISSN 0300-9084

Hoffmann, W., Richter, K., & Kreil, G. (1983). A novel peptide designated PYLa and its precursor as predicted from cloned mRNA of *Xenopus laevis* skin. *EMBO Journal*, Vol. 2, pp. 711-714, ISSN 0261-4189

Hölzl, MA., Hofer, J., Steinberger, P., Pfistershammer, K., & Zlabinger, GJ. (2008). Host antimicrobial proteins as endogenous immunomodulators. *Immunology Letters*, Vol. 119, No. 1-2, pp. 4-11, ISSN 0165-2478

Housby, JN., & Mann, NH. (2009). Phage therapy. *Drug Discovery Today*, Vol. 14, No. 11-12, pp. 536-540, ISSN 1359-6446

Hultmark, D., Steiner, H., Rasmuson, T., & Boman, HG. (1980). Insect immunity. Purification and properties of three inducible bactericidal proteins from hemolymph of immunized pupae of *Hyalophora cecropia*. *European Journal of Biochemistry*, Vol. 106, No. 1, pp. 7-16, ISSN 0014-2956

Jack, RW., Tagg, JR., & Ray, B. (1995). Bacteriocins of gram-positive bacteria. *Microbiological Reviews*. Vol. 59, No. 2, pp. 171-200, ISSN 0146-0749

Jacob, F., Lwoff, A., Siminovitch, A., & Wollman, E. (1953). Definition de quelques termes relatifs a la lysogenie. *Annales de l'Institut Pasteur*, Vol. 84, pp. 222-224, ISSN 0924-4204

Jado, I., López, R., García, E., Fenoll, A., Casal, J., & García, P. (2003). Spanish Pneumococcal Infection Study Network. Phage lytic enzymes as therapy for antibiotic-resistant *Streptococcus pneumoniae* infection in a murine sepsis model. *Journal of Antimicrobial Chemotherapy*, Vol. 52, No. 6, pp. 967-973, ISSN 0305-7453

Jilek, A., Mollay, C., Lohner, K., & Kreil, G. (2011). Substrate specificity of a peptidyl-aminoacyl-L: /D: -isomerase from frog skin. *Amino Acids*, Mar 22. Epub ahead of print, ISSN 0939-4451

Jung, HH., Yang, ST., Sim, JY., Lee, S., Lee, JY., Kim, HH., Shin, SY, & Kim, JI. (2010). Analysis of the solution structure of the human antibiotic peptide dermcidin and its interaction with phospholipid vesicles. *Biochemistry and Molecular Biology Reports*, Vol. 43, No. 5, pp. 362-368, ISSN 1976-6696

Kashyap, DR., Wang, M., Liu, LH., Boons, GJ., Gupta, D., & Dziarski, R. (2011). Peptidoglycan recognition proteins kill bacteria by activating protein-sensing two-component systems. *Nature Medicine*, Vol. 17, No. 6, pp. 676-683, ISSN 1078-8956

Kougias, P., Chai, H., Lin, PH., Yao, Q., Lumsden, AB., & Chen, C. (2005). Defensins and cathelicidins: neutrophil peptides with roles in inflammation, hyperlipidemia and atherosclerosis. *Journal of Cellular and Molecular Medicine*, Vol. 9, No. 1, pp. 3-10, ISSN 1582-1838

Lagos, R., Tello, M., Mercado, G., García, V., & Monasterio, O. (2009). Antibacterial and antitumorigenic properties of microcin E492, a pore-forming bacteriocin. *Current Pharmaceutical Biotechnology*, Vol. 10, No. 1, pp. 74-85, ISSN 1389-2010

Lai, XZ., Feng, Y., Pollard, J., Chin, JN., Rybak, MJ., Bucki, R., Epand, RF., Epand, RM., & Savage, PB. (2008). Ceragenins: cholic acid-based mimics of antimicrobial peptides. *Accounts of Chemical Research*, Vol. 41, No. 10, pp. 1233-1240, ISSN 0001-4842

Lai, YP., Peng, YF., Zuo, Y., Li, J., Huang, J., Wang, LF., & Wu, ZR. (2005). Functional and structural characterization of recombinant dermcidin-1L, a human antimicrobial peptide. *Biochemical and Biophysical Research Communications*, Vol. 328, No. 1, (Mar 4), pp. 243-250, ISSN 0006-291X

Lee, SB., Li, B., Jin, S., & Daniell, H. (2011). Expression and characterization of antimicrobial peptides Retrocyclin-101 and Protegrin-1 in chloroplasts to control viral and bacterial infections. *Plant Biotechnology Journal*, Vol. 9, No. 1, pp. 100-115, ISSN 1863-5466

Liang, QL., Zhou, K., & He, HX. (2010). Retrocyclin 2: a new therapy against avian influenza H5N1 virus in vivo and vitro. *Biotechnology Letters*, Vol. 32, No. 3, pp. 387-392, ISSN 0141-5492

Loeffler, JM., Nelson, D., & Fischetti, VA. (2001). Rapid killing of *Streptococcus pneumoniae* with a bacteriophage cell wall hydrolase. *Science*, Vol. 294, No. 5549, pp. 2170-2172, ISSN 0036-8075

Loeffler, JM., Djurkovic, S., Fischetti, VA. (2003). Phage lytic enzyme Cpl-1 as a novel antimicrobial for pneumococcal bacteremia. *Infection and Immunity*, Vol. 71, pp. 6199-6204, ISSN 0019-9567

Lohner, K, & Prossnigg, F. (2009). Biological activity and structural aspects of PGLa interaction with membrane mimetic systems. *Biochimica et Biophysica Acta*, Vol. 788, No. 8, pp. 1656-1666, ISSN 0006-3002

López-Rojas, R., Docobo-Pérez, F., Pachón-Ibáñez, ME., de la Torre, BG., Fernández-Reyes, M., March, C., Bengoechea, JA., Andreu, D., Rivas, L., & Pachón, J. (2011). Efficacy of cecropin A-melittin peptides on a sepsis model of infection by pan-resistant *Acinetobacter baumannii*. *European Journal of Clinical Microbiology and Infectious Diseases*, Apr 12. Epub ahead of print, ISSN 0934-9723

Lu, XM., Jin, XB., Zhu, JY., Mei, H,F., Ma, Y., Chu, FJ., Wang, Y., & Li, XB. (2010). Expression of the antimicrobial peptide cecropin fused with human lysozyme in *Escherichia coli*. *Applied Microbiology and Biotechnology*, Vol. 87, No. 6, pp. 2169-2176, ISSN 0175-7598

Madsen, P., Rasmussen, HH., Leffers, H., Honore, B., Dejgaard, K., Olsen, E., Kiil, J., Walbum, E., Andersen, AH., Basse, B., Lauridsen, JB., Ratz, GP., Celis, A., Vandekerckhove, J., & Celis, JE. (1991). Molecular cloning, occurrence, and expression of a novel partially secreted protein "psoriasin" that is highly up-regulated in psoriatic skin. *Journal of Investigative Dermatology*, Vol. 97, pp. 701–712, ISSN 0022-202X

Mahalka, AK., & Kinnunen, PK. (2009). Binding of amphipathic alpha-helical antimicrobial peptides to lipid membranes: lessons from temporins B and L. *Biochimica et Biophysica Acta*, Vol. 1788, No. 8, pp. 1600-1609, ISSN 0006-3002

Mangoni, ML., & Shai, Y. (2009). Temporins and their synergism against Gram-negative bacteria and in lipopolysaccharide detoxification. *Biochimica et Biophysica Acta*, Vol. 1788, No. 8, pp. 1610-1619, ISSN 0006-3002

Mangoni, ML., & Shai, Y. (2011). Short native antimicrobial peptides and engineered ultrashort lipopeptides: similarities and differences in cell specificities and modes of action. *Cellular and Molecular Life Sciences*, Vol. 68, No. 13, pp. 2267-2280, ISSN 1420-682X

Mangoni, ML., Carotenuto, A., Auriemma, L., Saviello, MR., Campiglia, P., Gomez-Monterrey, I., Malfi, S., Marcellini, L., Barra, D., Novellino, E., & Grieco, P. (2011). Structure-activity relationship, conformational and biological studies of temporin L analogues. *Journal of Medicinal Chemistry*, Vol. 54, No. 5, pp. 1298-1307, ISSN 0022-2623

Maróti, G., Kereszt, A., Kondorosi, E., & Mergaert, P. (2011). Natural roles of antimicrobial peptides in microbes, plants and animals. *Research in Microbiology*, Vol. 162, No. 4, pp. 363-374, ISSN 0923-2508

McCormick, TS., & Weinberg, A. (2010). Epithelial cell-derived antimicrobial peptides are multifunctional agents that bridge innate and adaptive immunity. *Periodontology 2000*, Vol. 54, No. 1, pp. 195-206, ISSN 0906-6713

Mechkarska, M., Ahmed, E., Coquet, L., Leprince, J., Jouenne, T., Vaudry, H., King, JD., & Conlon, JM. (2010). Antimicrobial peptides with therapeutic potential from skin secretions of the Marsabit clawed frog *Xenopus borealis* (Pipidae). *Comparative biochemistry and physiology. Toxicology & pharmacology*, Vol. 152, No. 4, pp. 467-472, ISSN 1532-0456

Meiller, TF., Hube, B., Schild, L., Shirtliff, ME., Scheper, MA., Winkler R, Ton., A, & Jabra-Rizk, MA. (2009). A novel immune evasion strategy of *Candida albicans*: proteolytic cleavage of a salivary antimicrobial peptide. *PLoS One*, Vol. 4, No. 4, e5039, ISSN 1932-6203

Méndez-Samperio, P. (2010). The human cathelicidin hCAP18/LL-37: a multifunctional peptide involved in mycobacterial infections. *Peptides*, Vol. 31, No. 9, pp. 1791-1798, ISSN 0196-9781

Meyer-Hoffert, U., Zimmermann, A., Czapp, M., Bartels, J., Koblyakova, Y., Gläser, R., Schröder, JM., & Gerstel, U. (2011). Flagellin delivery by *Pseudomonas aeruginosa* rhamnolipids induces the antimicrobial protein psoriasin in human skin. *PLoS One*, Vol. 6, No. 1, e16433, ISSN 1932-6203

Miele, R., Ponti, D., Boman, HG., Barra, D., & Simmaco, M. (1998). Molecular cloning of a bombinin gene from *Bombina orientalis*: detection of NF-kappaB and NF-IL6 binding sites in its promoter. *FEBS Letters*, Vol. 431, No. 1, (Jul 10), pp. 23-28, ISSN 0014-5793

Mignogna, G., Simmaco, M., Kreil, G., & Barra, D. (1993). Antibacterial and haemolytic peptides containing D-alloisoleucine from the skin of *Bombina variegata*. *EMBO Journal*, Vol. 12, No. 12, pp. 4829-4832, ISSN 0261-4189

Mookherjee, N., & Hancock, RE. (2007). Cationic host defence peptides: innate immune regulatory peptides as a novel approach for treating infections. *Cellular and Molecular Life Sciences*, Vol. 64, No. 7-8, pp. 922-933, ISSN 1420-682X

Mor, A., Nguyen, VH., Delfour, A., Migliore-Samour, D., Nicolas, P. (1991). Isolation, amino acid sequence, and synthesis of dermaseptin, a novel antimicrobial peptide of amphibian skin. *Biochemistry*, Vol. 30; No. 36, (Sep 10), pp. 8824-8830, ISSN 0006-2960

Mor, A., Hani, K., & Nicolas, P. (1994). The vertebrate peptide antibiotics dermaseptins have overlapping structural features but target specific microorganisms. *The Journal of Biological Chemistry*, Vol. 269, No. 50, (Dec 16), pp. 31635-31641, ISSN 0021-9258

Moreira, CK., Rodrigues, FG., Ghosh, A., Varotti, Fde P., Mirando, A., Daffare, S., Jacobs-Lorena, M., & Moreira, LA. (2007). Effect of the antimicrobial peptide gomesin against different life stages of Plasmodium spp. *Experimental Parasitology*, Vol. 116, No. 4, pp. 346-353, ISSN 0014-4894

Morello, E., Saussereau, E., Maura, D., Huerre, M., Touqui, L., & Debarbieux, L. (2011). Pulmonary bacteriophage therapy on *Pseudomonas aeruginosa* cystic fibrosis strains: first steps towards treatment and prevention. *PLoS One*, Vol. 6, No. 2, e16963, ISSN 1932-6203

Murakami, M., Ohtake, T., Dorschner, RA., Schittek, B., Garbe, C., & Gallo, RL. (2002). Cathelicidin anti-microbial peptide expression in sweat, an innate defense system for the skin. *Journal of Investigative Dermatology*, Vol. 119, No. 5, pp. 1090-1095, ISSN 0022-202X

Mygind, PH., Fischer, RL., Schnorr, KM., Hansen, MT., Sönksen, CP., Ludvigsen, S., Raventós, D., Buskov, S., Christensen, B., De Maria, L., Taboureau, O.,, Yaver, D., Elvig-Jørgensen, SG., Sørensen, MV., Christensen, BE., Kjaerulff, S., Frimodt-Moller, N., Lehrer, RI., Zasloff, M., & Kristensen, HH. (2005). Plectasin is a peptide antibiotic with therapeutic potential from a saprophytic fungus. *Nature*, Vol. 437, pp. 975-980, ISSN 0028-0836

Nakamura, T., Furunaka, H., Miyata, T., Tokunaga, F., Muta, T., Iwanaga, S., Niwa, M., Takao, T., & Shimonishi, Y. (1988). Tachyplesin, a class of antimicrobial peptide from the hemocytes of the horseshoe crab (*Tachypleus tridentatus*). Isolation and chemical structure. *The Journal of Biological Chemistry*, Vol. 263, No. 32, (Nov 15), pp. 16709-11673, ISSN 0021-9258

Nicolas, P., & El Amri, C. (2009). The dermaseptin superfamily: a gene-based combinatorial library of antimicrobial peptides. *Biochimica et Biophysica Acta*, Vol. 1788, No. 8, pp. 1537-1550, ISSN 0006-3002

Nijnik, A., Madera, L., Ma, S., Waldbrook, M., Elliott, MR., Easton, DM., Mayer, ML., Mullaly, SC., Kindrachuk, J., Jenssen, H., & Hancock, R.E. (2010). Synthetic cationic peptide IDR-1002 provides protection against bacterial infections through chemokine induction and enhanced leukocyte recruitment. *The Journal of Immunology*, Vol. 184, No. 5, pp. 2539-2550, ISSN 0022-1767

Nilsen, T., Nes, IF., & Holo, H. (2003). Enterolysin A, a cell wall-degrading bacteriocin from *Enterococcus faecalis* LMG 2333. *Applied and Environmental Microbiology*, Vol. 69, No. 5, pp. 2975-2984, ISSN 0099-2240

Nissen-Meyer, J., Holo, H., Håvarstein, LS., Sletten, K., Nes, IF. (1992). A novel lactococcal bacteriocin whose activity depends on the complementary action of two peptides. *The Journal of Bacteriology*, Vol. 174, No. 17, pp. 5686-5692, ISSN 0021-9193

Nissen-Meyer, J., Oppegård, C., Rogne, P., Haugen, HS., Kristiansen, PE. (2010). Structure and Mode-of-Action of the Two-Peptide (Class-IIb) Bacteriocins. *Probiotics and Antimicrobial Proteins*, Vol. 2, No. 1, pp. 52-60, ISSN 1867-1306

Oman, T.J., & van der Donk, WA. (2010). Follow the leader: the use of leader peptides to guide natural product biosynthesis. *Nature Chemical Biology*, Vol. 6, No. 1, pp. 9-18, ISSN 1552-4450

Pandey, BK., Ahmad, A., Asthana, N., Azmi, S., Srivastava, RM., Srivastava, S., Verma, R., Vishwakarma, AL., & Ghosh, JK. (2010). Cell-selective lysis by novel analogues of melittin against human red blood cells and *Escherichia coli*. *Biochemistry*, Vol. 49, No. 36, pp. 7920-7929, ISSN 0006-2960

Pasteur, L., & Joubert, JF. (1877). Charbon et septicemie. *Comptes Rendus des Séances et Mémoires de la Société de Biologie*, Vol. 85, pp. 101–115, ISSN 0037-9026

Pathak, S., De Souza, GA., Salte, T., Wiker, HG., & Asjö, B. (2009). HIV induces both a down-regulation of IRAK-4 that impairs TLR signalling and an up-regulation of the antibiotic peptide dermcidin in monocytic cells. *Scandinavian Journal of Immunology*, Vol. 70, No. 3, pp. 264-276, ISSN 0300-9475

Payne, RJ., & Jansen, VA. (2003). Pharmacokinetic principles of bacteriophage therapy. *Clinical Pharmacokinetics*, Vol. 42, No. 4, pp. 315-325, ISSN 0312-5963

Payne, DJ., Gwynn, MN., Holmes, DJ., & Pompliano DL. (2007). Drugs for bad bugs: confronting the challenges of antibacterial discovery. *Nature Review of Drug Discovery*, Vol. 6, No. 1, pp. 29-40, ISSN 1474-1776

Penberthy, WT., Chari, S., Cole, AL., & Cole, AM. (2011). Retrocyclins and their activity against HIV-1. *Cellular and Molecular Life Sciences*, Vol. 68, No. 13, pp. 2231-2242, ISSN 1420-682X

Peters, BM., Shirtliff, ME., & Jabra-Rizk, MA. (2010). Antimicrobial peptides: primeval molecules or future drugs? *PLoS Pathogens*, Vol. 6, No. 10 (Oct 28), e1001067, ISSN 1553-7374

Piper, C., Draper, LA., Cotter, PD., Ross, RP., & Hill, C. (2009). A comparison of the activities of lacticin 3147 and nisin against drug-resistant *Staphylococcus aureus* and

Enterococcus species. *Journal of Antimicrobial Chemotherapy*, Vol. 64, No. 3, pp. 546-551, ISSN 0305-7453

Plunkett, RM., Murray, SI., & Lowenberger, CA. (2009). Generation and characterization of the antibacterial activity of a novel hybrid antimicrobial peptide comprising functional domains from different insect cecropins. *Canadian Journal of Microbiology*, Vol. 55, No. 5, pp. 520-528, ISSN 0008-4166

Politano, AD., & Sawyer, RG. (2010). NXL-103, a combination of flopristin and linopristin, for the potential treatment of bacterial infections including community-acquired pneumonia and MRSA. *Current Opinion in Investigational Drugs*, Vol. 11, pp. 225-236, ISSN 1472-4472

Ramasundara, M., Leach, ST., Lemberg, DA., & Day, AS. (2009). Defensins and inflammation: the role of defensins in inflammatory bowel disease. *Journal of Gastroenterology and Hepatology*, Vol. 24, No. 2, pp. 202-208, ISSN 0815-9319

Rea, MC., Sit, CS., Clayton, E., O'Connor, PM., Whittal, RM., Zheng, J., Vederas, JC., Ross, RP., & Hill, C. (2010). Thuricin CD, a posttranslationally modified bacteriocin with a narrow spectrum of activity against *Clostridium difficile*. *Proceedings of the National Academy of Sciences U S A*, Vol. 107, No. 20, pp. 9352-9357, ISSN 0027-8424

Rieg, S., Garbe, C., Sauer, B., Kalbacher, H., & Schittek, B. (2004). Dermcidin is constitutively produced by eccrine sweat glands and is not induced in epidermal cells under inflammatory skin conditions. *British Journal of Dermatology*, Vol. 151, No. 3, pp. 534-539, ISSN 0007-0963

Rodrigues, EG., Dobroff, AS., Cavarsan, CF., Paschoalin, T., Nimrichter, L., Mortara, RA., Santos, EL., Fázio, MA., Miranda, A., Daffre, S., & Travassos, LR. (2008). Effective topical treatment of subcutaneous murine B16F10-Nex2 melanoma by the antimicrobial peptide gomesin. *Neoplasia*, Vol. 10, No. 1, pp. 61-68, ISSN 1522-8002

Rodríguez-Hernández, MJ., Saugar, J., Docobo-Pérez, F., de la Torre, BG., Pachón-Ibáñez, ME., García-Curiel, A., Fernández-Cuenca, F., Andreu D., Rivas, L., & Pachón, J. (2006). Studies on the antimicrobial activity of cecropin A-melittin hybrid peptides in colistin-resistant clinical isolates of *Acinetobacter baumannii*. *Journal of Antimicrobial Chemotherapy*, Vol. 58, No. 1, pp. 95-100, ISSN 0305-7453

Rokitskaya, TI., Kolodkin, NI., Kotova, EA., & Antonenko, YN. (2011). Indolicidin action on membrane permeability: Carrier mechanism versus pore formation. *Biochimica et Biophysica Acta*, Vol. 1808, No. 1, pp. 91-97, ISSN 0006-3002

Rollema, HS., Kuipers, OP., Both, P., de Vos, WM., & Siezen, RJ. (1995). Improvement of solubility and stability of the antimicrobial peptide nisin by protein engineering. *Applied and Environmental Microbiology*, Vol. 61, No. 8, pp. 2873-2878, ISSN 0099-2240

Romanelli, A., Moggio, L., Montella, RC., Campiglia, P., Iannaccone, M., Capuano, F., Pedone, C., & Capparelli, R. (2011). Peptides from Royal Jelly: studies on the antimicrobial activity of jelleins, jelleins analogs and synergy with temporins. *Journal of Peptide Science*, Vol. 17, No. 5, pp. 348-352, ISSN 1075-2617

Romeo, D., Skerlavaj, B., Bolognesi, M., & Gennaro, R. (1988). Structure and bactericidal activity of an antibiotic dodecapeptide purified from bovine neutrophils. *The Journal of Biological Chemistry*, Vol. 263, No. 20, (Jul 15), pp. 9573-9575, ISSN 0021-9258

Ross, AC.; & Vederas, JC. (2011). Fundamental functionality: recent developments in understanding the structure-activity relationships of lantibiotic peptides. *The Journal of Antibiotics*, Vol. 64, No. 1, pp. 27-34, ISSN 0021-8820

Roy, H., Dare, K., & Ibba, M. Adaptation of the bacterial membrane to changing environments using aminoacylated phospholipids. *Molecular Microbiology*. (2009) Vol. 71, No. 3, pp. 547-550, ISSN 0950-382X

Rubinchik, E., Dugourd, D., Algara, T., Pasetka, C., & Friedland, HD. (2009). Antimicrobial and antifungal activities of a novel cationic antimicrobial peptide, omiganan, in experimental skin colonisation models. *International Journal of Antimicrobial Agents*, Vol. 34, No. 5, pp. 457-461, ISSN 0924-8579

Ryan, LK., Dai J., Yin, Z., Megjugorac, N., Uhlhorn, V., Yim, S., Schwartz, KD., Abrahams, JM., Diamond, G., & Fitzgerald-Bocarsly, P. (2011). Modulation of human {beta}-defensin-1 (hBD-1) in plasmacytoid dendritic cells (PDC), monocytes, and epithelial cells by influenza virus, Herpes simplex virus, and Sendai virus and its possible role in innate immunity. *Journal of Leukocyte Biology*, May 6, Epub ahead of print, ISSN 0741-5400

Ryu, S., Choi, SY., Acharya, S., Chun, YJ., Gurley, C., Park, Y., Armstrong, CA., Song, PI., Kim, BJ. (2011). Antimicrobial and Anti-Inflammatory Effects of Cecropin A(1-8)-Magainin2(1-12) Hybrid Peptide Analog P5 against *Malassezia furfur* Infection in Human Keratinocytes. *Journal of Investigative Dermatology*, Vol. 131, No. 8, pp. 1677-1683, ISSN 0022-202X

Sánchez-Hidalgo, M., Montalbán-López, M., Cebrián, R., Valdivia, E., Martínez-Bueno, M., Maqueda, M. (2011). AS-48 bacteriocin: close to perfection. *Cellular and Molecular Life Sciences*. May 17, Epub ahead of print, ISSN 1420-682X

Saravanan, R., & Bhattacharjya, S. (2011). Oligomeric structure of a cathelicidin antimicrobial peptide in dodecylphosphocholine micelle determined by NMR spectroscopy. *Biochimica et Biophysica Acta*, Vol. 1808, No. 1, pp. 369-381, ISSN 0006-3002

Savoia, D., Guerrini, R., Marzola, E., & Salvadori, S. (2008). Synthesis and antimicrobial activity of dermaseptin S1 analogues. *Bioorganic & Medicinal Chemistry*, Vol. 16, No. 17, pp. 8205-8209, ISSN 0968-0896

Savoia, D., Donalisio, M., Civra, A., Salvadori, S., & Guerrini, R. (2010). In vitro activity of dermaseptin S1 derivatives against genital pathogens. *Acta Pathologica, Microbiologica et Immunologica Scandinavica*, Vol. 118, No. 9, pp. 674-680, ISSN 0903-4641

Schittek, B., Hipfel, R., Sauer, B., Bauer, J., Kalbacher, H., Stevanovic, S., Schirle, M., Schroeder, K., Blin, N., Meier, F., Rassner, G., & Garbe, C. (2001). Dermcidin: a novel human antibiotic peptide secreted by sweat glands. *Nature Immunology*, Vol. 2, No. 12, pp. 1133-1137, ISSN 1529-2908

Schittek, B., Paulmann, M., Senyürek, I., & Steffen, H. (2008). The role of antimicrobial peptides in human skin and in skin infectious diseases. *Infectious Disorders Drug Targets*, Vol. 8, No. 3, pp. 135-143, ISSN 1871-5265

Schneider, T., Kruse, T., Wimmer, R., Wiedemann, I., Sass, V., Pag, U., Jansen, A., Nielsen, AK., Mygind, PH.; Raventós, DS., Neve, S., Ravn, B., Bonvin, AM., De Maria, L., Andersen, A.S., Gammelgaard, LK., Sahl, HG., & Kristensen, HH. (2010). Plectasin, a fungal defensin, targets the bacterial cell wall precursor Lipid II. *Science*, Vol. 328, No. 5982, pp. 1168-1172, ISSN 0036-8075

Schuch, R., Nelson, D., & Fischetti, VA. (2002). A bacteriolytic agent that detects and kills *Bacillus anthracis*. *Nature*, Vol. 418, No. 6900, pp. 884-889, ISSN 0028-0836

Schutte, BC., Mitros, JP., Bartlett, JA., Walters, JD., Jia, HP., Welsh, MJ., Casavant, TL., & McCray, PB. Jr. (2002). Discovery of five conserved beta -defensin gene clusters using a computational search strategy. *Proceedings of the National Academy of Sciences USA*, Vol. 99, No. 4, (Feb 19), pp. 2129-2133, ISSN 0027-8424

Schweizer, F. (2009). Cationic amphiphilic peptides with cancer-selective toxicity. *European Journal of Pharmacology*, Vol. 625, No. 1-3, (Dec 25), pp. 190-194, ISSN 0014-2999

Scott, MG., Davidson, DJ., Gold, MR., Bowdish, D., & Hancock, RE. (2002). The human antimicrobial peptide LL-37 is a multifunctional modulator of innate immune responses. *The Journal of Immunology*, Vol. 169, No. 7, pp. 3883-3891, ISSN 0022-1767

Scott, MG., Dullaghan, E., Mookherjee, N., Glavas, N., Waldbrook, M., Thompson, A., Wang, A., Lee, K., Doria, S., Hamill, P., Yu, JJ., Li, Y., Donini, O., Guarna, MM., Finlay, BB., North, JR., & Hancock, RE. (2007). An anti-infective peptide that selectively modulates the innate immune response. *Nature Biotechnology*, Vol. 25, No. 4, pp. 465-472, ISSN 1087-0156

Scott, RW., DeGrado, WF., & Tew, GN. (2008). De novo designed synthetic mimics of antimicrobial peptides. *Current Opinion in Biotechnology*, Vol. 19, No. 6, pp. 620-627, ISSN 0958-1669

Selsted, ME., Novotny, MJ., Morris, WL., Tang, YQ., Smith, W., & Cullor, JS. (1992). Indolicidin, a novel bactericidal tridecapeptide amide from neutrophils. *The Journal of Biological Chemistry*, Vol. 267, No. 7, (Mar 5), pp. 4292-4295, ISSN 0021-9258.

Selsted, ME., & Ouellette, AJ. (2005). Mammalian defensins in the antimicrobial immune response. *Nature Immunology*, Vol. 6, No. 6, pp. 551-557, ISSN 1529-2908

Senyürek, I., Paulmann, M., Sinnberg, T., Kalbacher, H., Deeg, M., Gutsmann, T., Hermes, M., Kohler, T., Götz, F., Wolz, C., Peschel, A., & Schittek, B. (2009). Dermcidin-derived peptides show a different mode of action than the cathelicidin LL-37 against *Staphylococcus aureus*. *Antimicrobial Agents and Chemotherapy*, Vol. 53, No. 6, pp. 2499-2509, ISSN 0066-4804

Sharma, KR., Reddy, PR., Tegge, W., & Jain, R. (2009). Discovery of Trp-His and His-Arg analogues as new structural classes of short antimicrobial peptides. *The Journal of Medicinal Chemistry*, Vol. 52, pp. 7421-7431, ISSN 0022-2623

Silva, PI. Jr., Daffre, S., & Bulet, P. (2000). Isolation and characterization of gomesin, an 18-residue cysteine-rich defense peptide from the spider *Acanthoscurria gomesiana* hemocytes with sequence similarities to horseshoe crab antimicrobial peptides of the tachyplesin family. *The Journal of Biological Chemistry*, Vol. 275, No. 43, (Oct 27), pp. 33464-33470, ISSN 0021-9258

Simmaco, M., Mignogna, G., Canofeni, S., Miele, R., Mangoni, ML., & Barra, D. (1996). Temporins, antimicrobial peptides from the European red frog *Rana temporaria*. *European Journal of Biochemistry*, Vol. 242, No. 3, pp. 788-792, ISSN 0014-2956

Soravia, E., Martini, G., & Zasloff, M. (1988). Antimicrobial properties of peptides from Xenopus granular gland secretions. *FEBS Letters*, Vol. 228, pp. 337–340, ISSN 0014-5793.

Spellberg, B., Guidos, R., Gilbert, D., Bradley, J., Boucher, HW., Scheld, WM., Bartlett, JG. & Edwards J. Jr. (2008). Infectious Diseases Society of America. The epidemic of antibiotic-resistant infections: a call to action for the medical community from the Infectious Diseases Society of America. *Clinical Infectious Diseases*, Vol. 46, No. 2, (Jan 15), pp. 155-164, ISSN 1058-4838

Spencer, JD., Schwaderer, AL., Dirosario, JD., McHugh, KM., McGillivary, G., Justice, SS., Carpenter, AR., Baker, PB., Harder, J., & Hains, DS. (2011). Ribonuclease 7 is a potent antimicrobial peptide within the human urinary tract. *Kidney International*, Vol. 80, No. 2, pp. 174-180, ISSN 0085-2538

Storici, P., & Zanetti, M. (1993). A cDNA derived from pig bone marrow cells predicts a sequence identical to the intestinal antibacterial peptide PR-39. *Biochemical and Biophysical Research Communications*, Vol. 196, No. 3, (Nov 15), pp. 1058-65, ISSN 0006-291X

Tagg, JR., Dajani, AS., & Wannamaker, LW. (1976). Bacteriocins of gram-positive bacteria. *Bacteriological Reviews*, Vol. 40, No. 3, pp. 722-756, ISSN 0005-3678

Termorshuizen, F., Garssen, J., Norval, M., Koulu, L., Laihia, J., Leino, L., Jansen, CT., De Gruijl, F., Gibbs, NK., De Simone, C., & Van Loveren, H. (2002). A review of studies on the effects of ultraviolet irradiation on the resistance to infections: evidence from rodent infection models and verification by experimental and observational human studies. *International Immunopharmacology*, Vol. 2, No. 2-3, pp. 263-275, ISSN 1567-5769

Tseng, JM., Huang, JR., Huang, HC., Tzen, JT., Chou, WM., & Peng, CC. (2011). Facilitative production of an antimicrobial peptide royalisin and its antibody via an artificial oil-body system. *Biotechnology Progress*, Vol. 27, No. 1, pp. 153-161, ISSN 8756-7938

Turpin, ER., Bonev, BB., & Hirst, JD. (2010). Stereoselective disulfide formation stabilizes the local peptide conformation in nisin mimics. *Biochemistry*, Vol. 49, No. 44, pp. 9594-9603, ISSN 0006-2960

van Dijk, A., Veldhuizen, EJ., van Asten, AJ., & Haagsman, HP. (2005). CMAP27, a novel chicken cathelicidin-like antimicrobial protein. *Veterinary Immunology and Immunopathology*, Vol. 106, No. 3-4, (Jul 15), pp. 321-327, ISSN 0165-2427

Vanhoye, D., Bruston, F., Nicolas, P., & Amiche, M. (2003). Antimicrobial peptides from hylid and ranin frogs originated from a 150-million-year-old ancestral precursor with a conserved signal peptide but a hypermutable antimicrobial domain. *European Journal of Biochemistry*, Vol. 270, No. 9, pp. 2068-2081, ISSN 0014-2956

Venkataraman, N., Cole, AL., Ruchala, P., Waring, AJ., Lehrer, RI., Stuchlik, O., Pohl, J., & Cole, AM. (2009). Reawakening retrocyclins: ancestral human defensins active against HIV-1: *PLoS Biology*, Vol. 7, No. 4, e95, ISSN 1932-6203

Verbeken, G., De Vos, D., Vaneechoutte, M., Merabishvili, M., Zizi, M., & Pirnay, J.P. (2007). European regulatory conundrum of phage therapy. *Future Microbiology*, Vol. 2, pp. 485-491, ISSN 1746-0913

Verma, V., Harjai, K., & Chhibber, S. (2009). Characterization of a T7-like lytic bacteriophage of *Klebsiella pneumoniae* B5055: a potential therapeutic agent. *Current Microbiology*, Vol. 59, No. 3, pp. 274-281, ISSN 0343-8651

Wakabayashi, T., Kato, H., & Tachibana, S. (1985). Complete nucleotide sequence of mRNA for caerulein precursor from Xenopus skin: the mRNA contains an unusual repetitive structure. *Nucleic Acids Research*, Vol. 13, No. 6, (Mar 25), pp. 1817-28, ISSN 0305-1048

Walsh, CT., & Fischbach, MA. (2010). Natural products version 2.0: connecting genes to molecules. *Journal of the American Chemical Society*, Vol. 132, No. 8, (Mar 3), pp. 2469-93, ISSN 0002-7863

Wang, G., Li, X., & Wang, Z. (2009). APD2: the updated antimicrobial peptide database and its application in peptide design. *Nucleic Acids Research*, Vol. 37, (Database issue), pp. D933-D937, ISSN 0305-1048

Wang, M., Liu, LH., Wang, S., Li, X., Lu, X., Gupta, D, & Dziarski, R. (2007). Human peptidoglycan recognition proteins require zinc to kill both gram-positive and gram-negative bacteria and are synergistic with antibacterial peptides. *The Journal of Immunology*, Vol. 178, No. 5, (Mar 1), pp. 3116-3125, ISSN 0022-1767

Welte, T., & Pletz, MW. (2010). Antimicrobial treatment of nosocomial meticillin-resistant *Staphylococcus aureus* (MRSA) pneumonia: current and future options. *International Journal of Antimicrobial Agents*, Vol. 36, No. 5, pp. 391-400, ISSN 0924-8579

Wencker, M., & Brantly, ML. (2005). Cytotoxic concentrations of alpha-defensins in the lungs of individuals with alpha 1-antitrypsin deficiency and moderate to severe lung disease. *Cytokine*, Vol. 32, No. 1, pp. 1-6, ISSN 1043-4666

White, JH. (2010). Vitamin D as an inducer of cathelicidin antimicrobial peptide expression: past, present and future. *The Journal of Steroid Biochemistry and Molecular Biology*, Vol. 121, No. 1-2, pp. 234-238, ISSN 0960-0760.

Wiesner, J., & Vilcinskas, A. (2010). Antimicrobial peptides: the ancient arm of the human immune system. *Virulence*, Vol. 1, No. 5, pp. 440-464, ISSN 2150-5594

Wilmes, M., Cammue, BP., Sahl, HG., & Thevissen, K. (2011). Antibiotic activities of host defense peptides: more to it than lipid bilayer perturbation. *Natural Products Reports*, May 27, Epub ahead of print, ISSN 0265-0568

Witzenrath, M., Schmeck, B., Doehn, JM., Tschernig, T., Zahlten, J., Loeffler, JM., Zemlin, M., Müller, H., Gutbier, B., Schütte, H., Hippenstiel, S., Fischetti, VA.; Suttorp, N., & Rosseau, S. (2009). Systemic use of the endolysin Cpl-1 rescues mice with fatal pneumococcal pneumonia. *Critical Care Medicine*, Vol. 37, No. 2, pp. 642-649, ISSN 0090-3493

Wohlford-Lenane, CL., Meyerholz, DK., Perlman, S., Zhou, H., Tran, D., Selsted, ME., & McCray, PB. Jr. (2009). Rhesus theta-defensin prevents death in a mouse model of severe acute respiratory syndrome coronavirus pulmonary disease. *The Journal of Virology*, Vol. 83, No. 21, pp. 11385-11390, ISSN 0022-538X

Woosley, LN., Castanheira, M., & Jones, RN. (2010). CEM-101 activity against Grampositive organisms. *Antimicrobial Agents and Chemotherapy*, Vol. 54, pp. 2182-2187, ISSN 0066-4804

World Health Organization. (2004). Deaths by cause, sex and mortality stratum in WHO regions, estimates for 2002: *World Health Report – 2004*. Geneva: World Health Organization.

Wright, A., Hawkins, CH., Anggård, EE., & Harper, DR. (2009). A controlled clinical trial of a therapeutic bacteriophage preparation in chronic otitis due to antibiotic-resistant *Pseudomonas aeruginosa*; a preliminary report of efficacy. *Clinical Otolaryngology*, Vol. 34, No. 4, pp. 349-357, ISSN 0307-7772

Wu, JM., Jan, PS., Yu, HC., Haung, HY., Fang, HJ., Chang, YI., Cheng, JW., & Chen, HM. (2009). Structure and function of a custom anticancer peptide, CB1a. *Peptides*, Vol. 30, No. 5, pp. 839-848, ISSN 0196-9781

Xiao, Y., Cai, Y., Bommineni, YR., Fernando, SC., Prakash, O., Gilliland, SE., & Zhang, G. (2006). Identification and functional characterization of three chicken cathelicidins with potent antimicrobial activity. *The Journal of Biological Chemistry*, Vol. 281, No. 5, (Feb 3), pp. 2858-2867, ISSN 0021-9258

Xiao, Y., Herrera, AI., Bommineni, YR., Soulages, JL., Prakash, O., & Zhang, G. (2009). The central kink region of fowlicidin-2, an alpha-helical host defense peptide, is critically involved in bacterial killing and endotoxin neutralization. *Journal of Innate Immunity*, Vol. 1, No. 3, pp. 268-280, ISSN 1662-811X

Yoshida, H., Kinoshita, K., & Ashida, M. (1996). Purification of a peptidoglycan recognition protein from hemolymph of the silkworm, Bombyx mori. *The Journal of Biological Chemistry*, Vol. 271, No. 23, (Jun 7), pp. 13854-13860, ISSN 0021-9258

Zairi, A., Tangy, F., Ducos-Galand, M., Alonso, JM., & Hani, K. (2007). Susceptibility of *Neisseria gonorrhoeae* to antimicrobial peptides from amphibian skin, dermaseptin, and derivatives. *Diagnostic Microbiology and Infectious Diseases*, Vol. 57, No. 3, pp. 319-324, ISSN 0732-8893

Zanetti, M. (2005). The role of cathelicidins in the innate host defenses of mammals. *Current Issues in Molecular Biology*, Vol. 7, No. 2, pp. 179-196, ISSN 1467-3037

Zangger, K., Gössler, R., Khatai, L., Lohner, K., & Jilek, A. (2008). Structures of the glycine-rich diastereomeric peptides bombinin H2 and H4. *Toxicon*, Vol. 52, No. 2, (Aug 1), pp. 246-254, ISSN 0041-0101

Zasloff, M. (1987). Magainins, a class of antimicrobial peptides from Xenopus skin: isolation, characterization of two active forms, and partial cDNA sequence of a precursor. *Proceedings of the National Academy of Sciences USA*, Vol. 84, No. 15, pp. 5449-53, ISSN 0027-8424

Zasloff, M. (2002). Antimicrobial peptides of multicellular organisms. *Nature*, Vol. 415, pp. 389-395, ISSN 0028-0836

Zhanel, GG., Calic, D., Schweizer, F., Zelenitsky, S., Adam, H., Lagacé-Wiens, PR., Rubinstein, E., Gin, AS., Hoban, DJ., & Karlowsky, JA. (2010). New lipoglycopeptides: a comparative review of dalbavancin, oritavancin and telavancin. *Drugs*, Vol. 70, No. 7, pp. 859-886, ISSN 0012-6667

Zhang, Y., Zhao, H., Yu, G.Y., Liu, X.D., Shen, J.H., Lee, W.H., & Zhang Y. (2010). Structure-function relationship of king cobra cathelicidin. *Peptides*, Vol. 31, No. 8, pp. 1488-1493, ISSN 0196-9781

Zhao, H., Gan, TX., Liu, XD., Jin, Y., Lee, WH., Shen, JH., & Zhang, Y. (2008). Identification and characterization of novel reptile cathelicidins from elapid snakes. *Peptides*, Vol. 29, No. 10, pp. 1685-1691, ISSN 0196-9781

Zhu, S. (2007). Evidence for myxobacterial origin of eukaryotic defensins. *Immunogenetics*, Vol. 59, No. 12, pp. 949-954, ISSN 0093-7711

Zhu, S. (2008). Did cathelicidins, a family of multifunctional host-defense peptides, arise from a cysteine protease inhibitor? *Trends in Microbiology*, Vol. 16, No. 8, pp. 353-360, ISSN 0966-842X

9

Potentiation of Available Antibiotics by Targeting Resistance – An Emerging Trend in Tuberculosis Drug Development

Kerstin A. Wolff[*], Marissa Sherman[*] and Liem Nguyen[**]
Case Western Reserve University School of Medicine, Cleveland, Ohio
United States of America

1. Introduction

Mycobacterial infections are one of the leading causes of death through disease world-wide (World Health Organization, 2010), encompassing infections such as tuberculosis (TB), leprosy, Buruli ulcers, and opportunistic non-tuberculosis mycobacterial (NTM) infections in immune-compromised individuals, especially patients with acquired immune deficiency syndrome (AIDS). The World Health Organization has estimated that one third of the world's population is currently infected with *Mycobacterium tuberculosis*, the causative agent of TB, although only ten percent of those infected will develop active disease (World Health Organization, 2010). Highest TB incidences are located in sub-Saharan Africa and Southeast Asia, coinciding with human immunodeficiency virus (HIV) hot spots (World Health Organization, 2010).

The extremely high level of intrinsic resistance to most antimicrobial drug classes exhibited by *M. tuberculosis* has left us with a very limited arsenal of useful anti-TB drugs (Nguyen & Thompson, 2006). The five available first-line drugs, isoniazid (INH), rifampicin (RIF), ethambutol (EMB), pyrazinamide, and streptomycin, are all more than sixty years old (Nguyen & Pieters, 2009, Nguyen & Thompson, 2006). Furthermore, the current standard regimen (DOTS) for TB is comprised of six to nine months of daily antibiotic treatment with a combination of four out of these five drugs, often leading to poor patient adherence and incomplete courses of treatment. The rapid rate of mutations occurring in bacteria in general, together with the frequent exposure of *M. tuberculosis* to sub-optimal doses of drugs, have granted ample opportunity for this pathogen to acquire additional resistance by amassing sequential mutations in drug-target encoding genes (Nguyen & Pieters, 2009, Nguyen & Thompson, 2006). Accordingly, we now face the problem of multiple drug resistant (MDR) and extensively drug resistant (XDR) *M. tuberculosis* strains. MDR strains exhibit resistance to at least the two most potent first-line drugs (RIF and INH). Besides RIF and INH, XDR strains are resistant to any fluoroquinolones and to at least one of the three injectable second-line drugs (capreomycin, kanamycin, and amikacin) (World Health Organization, 2006). Infections with such strains require further prolonged and aggressive treatment courses employing

[*] Both authors contributed equally to this work.
[**]Correspondence: liem.nguyen@case.edu

combinations of numerous second-line drugs that often exhibit toxic side effects and are expensive to administer (Dye, 2000, Nguyen & Thompson, 2006). Moreover, the spread of these infections is diminishing our already limited arsenal of effective antibiotics even further with which some XDR *M. tuberculosis* strains have become virtually untreatable with current medicines (Gandhi *et al.*, 2006, Jassal & Bishai, 2009, LoBue, 2009).

The current prevalence of drug-resistant strains poses a dire need for alternative TB therapies. Development of completely new TB drugs is both time-intensive and costly. Although a few compounds have made their way into pre-clinical or clinical stages, this approach thus far has provided us with no newly approved anti-TB drugs. On average, it takes twelve to fifteen years and US $500 million to get a new drug from the laboratory to the market (Bolten & DeGregorio, 2002). Clearly, the possibility that new resistant strains may rapidly occur and diminish the utility of a new drug after approval represents a significant risk factor for the development of anti-infective drugs. An alternative approach to this pathway is presented by the concept of "targeting resistance". This drug potentiation approach, which uses knowledge of resistance mechanisms to (re)sensitize pathogenic bacteria to already available drugs, may become an important trend in the new era of drug development for infectious diseases. The coadministration of existing drugs and inhibitors that suppress resistance mechanisms allows ineffective drugs to (re)gain their antimicrobial activity (Wright, 2000, Wright & Sutherland, 2007) (Figure 1). In the case of *M. tuberculosis*, this approach could be used to rescue and extend the utility of current TB drugs, or make use of other available drugs that are currently inactive against the bacillus. The extended lifespan of valuable approved antibiotics of known pharmacology, toxicology, and treatment schedule, represents a unique advantage of the drug potentiation approach.

This chapter will explore recent findings that suggest several available drugs as promising candidates for resistance-targeted potentiation. Future directions regarding this approach in TB-drug development will also be discussed.

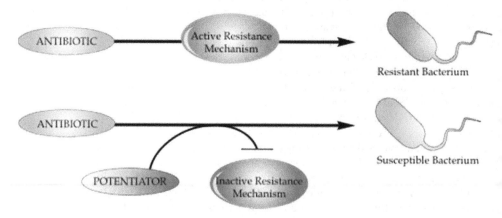

Fig. 1. Concept of drug potentiation by targeting resistance. An active resistance mechanism allows survival of bacterial pathogens in the face of an antibiotic(s). A potentiator that inhibits the resistance mechanism would (re)sensitize the bacteria to the antibiotic(s), thus enhancing antibacterial activity.

2. β–Lactams

The most widely used group of antibiotics today is the β–lactams, a broad class of drugs including penicillin and penicillin derivatives, cephalosporins, monobactams and carbapenems (Figure 2 A), that target bacterial cell wall synthesis at the peptidoglycan layer (Koch, 2003, Waxman *et al.*, 1980). Peptidoglycan is the major component of the cell wall in both Gram-positive and Gram-negative bacteria and is extensively cross-linked by penicillin-binding proteins (PBPs), lending it stability (Koch, 2003, Waxman *et al.*, 1980). β–lactam antibiotics are cyclic amides containing a hetero-atomic ring consisting of three carbon atoms, and one nitrogen atom (Figure 2 A), mimicking certain precursors of peptidoglycan (Koch, 2003, Waxman *et al.*, 1980). When PBPs mistakenly use β–lactams as their substrate rather than peptidoglycan precursors, the antibiotics are incorporated irreversibly into the PBP structure, inhibiting cross-linking activity (Koch, 2003, Waxman *et al.*, 1980), leading to consequent cell lysis in hypotonic environments (Beveridge, 1999, Lee *et al.*, 2001, Severin *et al.*, 1997).

Although serving as the only successful clinical example of potentiation through targeting resistance, inhibitors of β–lactamases have prolonged the life of β–lactams for more than thirty years (Drawz & Bonomo, 2010). Without these potentiators, many β–lactams would have long become useless against multiple bacterial pathogens. β–lactams such as penicillin are now commonly coadministered with β–lactamase inhibitors such as clavulanic acid, sulbactam, or tazobactam that prevent degradation of β–lactams, thus sustaining bacterial susceptibility to β–lactams.

2.1 β–Lactam resistance mechanisms in *Mycobacterium tuberculosis*

In the case of mycobacteria, resistance to β–lactams involves three main components: permeability of the mycobacterial cell wall (Chambers *et al.*, 1995, Jarlier *et al.*, 1991, Jarlier & Nikaido, 1990, Kasik & Peacham, 1968), affinity of the drugs to their target PBPs (Chambers *et al.*, 1995, Mukherjee *et al.*, 1996), and degradation by β–lactamase activity (Jarlier *et al.*, 1991, Quinting *et al.*, 1997). In addition, since *M. tuberculosis* is an intracellular pathogen, an effective TB drug must be able to penetrate the macrophage and phagosomal membranes to reach the bacilli residing within.

Although mycobacteria are classified as Gram-positive bacteria, their cell wall is extremely thick and multi-layered with varied hydrophobicity, posing an effective obstacle for the entry of most chemical compounds. The peptidoglycan network is covered by an arabinogalactan layer, both of which are hydrophilic and likely limit penetration of hydrophobic compounds (Brennan & Nikaido, 1995). On top of these aforementioned layers is another layer consisting of mycolic acids linked to acyl lipids, which forms a waxy, non-fluid barrier restricting transport of both hydrophobic and hydrophilic molecules (Liu *et al.*, 1995). Penetration by diffusion of β–lactams through the mycobacterial cell wall is hundreds of times slower than that of *Escherichia coli* (Chambers *et al.*, 1995, Kasik & Peacham, 1968). However, because of the extremely long generation time of *M. tuberculosis*, the slow rate of drug penetration is enough to allow for half-equilibration over the membrane well before the cell divides, making cell wall permeability and therefore drug penetration important but not a major determinant of β–lactam resistance (Chambers *et al.*, 1995, Quinting *et al.*, 1997). As for drug target affinity, four major PBPs have been identified in *M. tuberculosis*, all of which bind β–lactams at therapeutically achievable concentrations (Chambers *et al.*, 1995). The 49-kDa PBP from *M. smegmatis* is also sensitive to several β–lactams at similar concentrations (Mukherjee *et al.*, 1996). Therefore, target affinity does not significantly contribute to the mycobacterial β–lactam resistance. Cell division in *M. tuberculosis* is extremely slow, only occurring every 15-20 hours. This slow growth contributes both negatively and positively to drug resistance. Carbapenem antibiotics, which seem to be the most effective β–lactam with antimycobacterial activity, are relatively unstable and lose activity much faster than the mycobacterial growth rate (Watt *et al.*, 1992). It has however been shown that a daily antibiotic regimen can compensate for loss of activity and markedly increase growth inhibitions *in vitro* (Watt *et al.*, 1992).

With drug penetration and target affinity being negligible for β–lactam resistance in mycobacteria, degradation by β–lactamases constitutes the principal resistance mechanism. β–lactamase activity has been reported in all known mycobacterial species (Kasik, 1979), except the non-pathogenic *M. fallax*, which exhibits hypersusceptibility to β–lactams (Quinting *et al.*, 1997). Mycobacteria, including *M. tuberculosis*, export β–lactamases to the cell wall via the twin-arginine translocation (Tat) pathway (McDonough *et al.*, 2005, Voladri *et al.*, 1998), thus disruption of the Tat transporter leads to lower β–lactamase activity in *M. smegmatis* culture filtrates and increased β–lactam susceptibility (McDonough *et al.*, 2005). The major β–lactamase in *M. tuberculosis*, BlaC, is a member of the Ambler Class-A β–lactamases and exhibits broad substrate specificity, catalysing hydrolysis of both cephalosporins and penicillins (Voladri *et al.*, 1998, Wang *et al.*, 2006). This broad substrate specificity is attributed to the large and flexible substrate-binding site of this particular β–lactamase (Wang *et al.*, 2006). Two additional β–lactamase-like proteins, encoded by the *rv0406c* and *rv3677c* genes, have been identified to provide *M. tuberculosis* H37Rv with a lower β–lactamase activity (Nampoothiri *et al.*, 2008). Expression of these proteins in *E. coli* confers significant resistance to β–lactam antibiotics (Nampoothiri *et al.*, 2008).

In general, mycobacterial β–lactamases exhibit low-level activity compared to those of other pathogenic bacteria. However, because of the slow equilibration of β–lactams across the thick cell wall, this low β–lactamase activity is effective enough to provide protection to mycobacteria from β–lactam action (Jarlier *et al.*, 1991). When *M. fallax in trans* expresses the β–lactamase from *M. fortuitum*, MICs for β–lactams increase dramatically, indicating that β–lactamase-mediated degradation is the critical contributor to β–lactam resistance in mycobacteria (Quinting *et al.*, 1997). For most bacterial β–lactamases, β–lactams of the carbapenem subgroup are highly resistant to hydrolysis. Unfortunately, *M. tuberculosis* BlaC shows measurable activity with carbapenem compounds including imipenem, ertapenem, doripenem and meropenem, even though imipenem and meropenem seem somewhat more effective than other carbapenems and penicillins in antimycobacterial activity (Hugonnet & Blanchard, 2007, Tremblay *et al.*, 2010).

Interestingly, BlaC production in *M. tuberculosis* is β–lactam inducible, and controlled by a regulatory network that is also present in other Gram-positive bacteria (Sala *et al.*, 2009). The transcriptional repressor BlaI, a winged helix regulator, forms homodimers that bind DNA at specific recognition sites in the absence of β–lactam antibiotics (Sala *et al.*, 2009). BlaC is the only β–lactamase in *M. tuberculosis* whose gene is among the BlaI regulon (Sala *et al.*, 2009). Exposure to β–lactams dissociates BlaI from its DNA binding site, lifting its suppression on *blaC* transcription thus allowing the production of BlaC β–lactamase activity (Sala *et al.*, 2009).

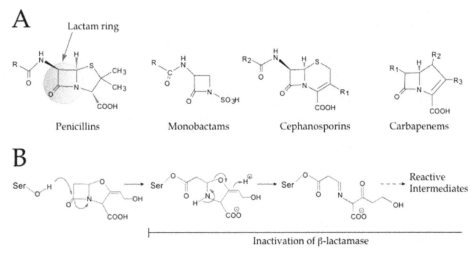

Fig. 2. (A) Structures of β–lactams. The β–lactam ring structure constitutes the base of all β–lactams while the secondary ring structure determines the class. (B) Mechanism of reaction between β–lactamase and clavulanate. The serine residue of the reactive site of β–lactamase reacts with the carbonyl group of clavulanate, followed by breakage of the amide bond that results in acylation. The acylation step is followed by the formation of an imine and secondary ring opening. Note that the ring opening step does not occur with all β–lactamase inhibitors.

2.2 Potentiation of β–lactams in mycobacteria

Attempts to promote the utility of β–lactams to treat TB and other mycobacterial infections have been continuously explored by many laboratories. Rather than ignoring these antibiotics, their antimycobacterial activity could be potentiated by coadministration with β–lactamase inhibitors, as routinely practiced for other bacterial infections. As mycobacterial susceptibility to β–lactams is quite high in the absence of β–lactamase activity (Flores *et al.*, 2005, Quinting *et al.*, 1997), effective chemical inactivation of β–lactamases should similarly increase β–lactam sensitivity in these bacteria. In fact, *in vitro* studies first showed that three FDA-approved inhibitors, sulbactam, tazobactam, and clavulanate, effectively inhibit nitrocefin degradation by purified BlaC protein (Hugonnet & Blanchard, 2007, Tremblay *et al.*, 2008). While sulbactam inhibits BlaC competitively and reversibly, tazobactam inhibits BlaC in a time-dependent manner with reappearing enzyme activity. Interestingly, clavulanate forms hydrolytically stable, inactive forms of the enzyme, completely and irreversibly inhibiting BlaC in a mechanism in which after acylation of clavulanate, a secondary ring-opening leads to reactive intermediates that occupy the active site of the enzyme (Figure 2 B) (Hugonnet and Blanchard 2007; Tremblay *et al.* 2008). Hence, clavulanate provides a potential lead for the development of effective β–lactam potentiators for TB.

Whereas data obtained from the aforementioned *in vitro* studies are promising, drugs used for TB must be able to penetrate the mycobacterial cell wall in order to exert their activity. A later *in vitro* study showed that meropenem/clavulanate combination is very effective in killing both aerobically and anaerobically grown *M. tuberculosis* (Hugonnet *et al.*, 2009).

More importantly, the drug combination is also effective against thirteen tested XDR *M. tuberculosis* strains (Hugonnet *et al.*, 2009). Furthermore, studies using mouse peritoneal macrophages infected with *M. tuberculosis* indicated that penetration through neither host macrophage nor phagosomal membranes appears to be a problem for β–lactams and/or β–lactamase inhibitors (Chambers *et al.*, 1995, Prabhakaran *et al.*, 1999). Significant reduction of mycobacterial counts in mouse macrophages upon treatment with various combinations of β–lactams and β–lactamase inhibitors within clinically achievable doses has been demonstrated (Chambers *et al.*, 1995, Prabhakaran *et al.*, 1999). Encouraging results were also reported in animal models. Although less effective than the first-line anti-TB drug INH, imipenem significantly reduced *M. tuberculosis* counts in the lungs and spleens of infected mice (Chambers *et al.*, 2005). As a result, imipenem doubled the survival rate of infected mice (35% mortality vs. 70%). While only a very few cases in which TB patients treated with β–lactams in conjunction with or without potentiators have been reported, the results were always promising. One study using imipenem alone in MDR-TB patients with poor predicted outcomes achieved a 70% cure rate (Chambers *et al.*, 2005). Another study showed that treatment of TB patients with an amoxicillin/clavulanate combination significantly reduced *M. tuberculosis* counts with early bactericidal activity comparable to patients treated with the frontline drug INH (Chambers *et al.*, 1998). Importantly, a case report recently described the successful recovery of an advanced XDR-TB patient treated with meropenem/clavulanate in conjunction with other drugs (Dauby *et al.*, 2011).

In summary, evidence obtained from numerous studies performed *in vitro*, in animals, and in humans, all support that β–lactams potentiated by β–lactamase inhibitors could provide an effective addition to the treatment of drug resistant TB.

2.3 Future perspectives

Much work remains to be done in potentiating β–lactams for the treatment of mycobacterial infections. More existing carbapenems should be tested in combination with various β–lactamase inhibitors. With crystal structures and kinetic data now available (Hugonnet & Blanchard, 2007, Hugonnet *et al.*, 2009, Tremblay *et al.*, 2010, Tremblay *et al.*, 2008), rational design or high throughput screening should be done to identify better inhibitors that specifically target BlaC or the other β–lactamases of *M. tuberculosis*. Similarly, sensitization of *M. tuberculosis* to β–lactams could be achieved by preventing dissociation of BlaI from its binding site on the *blaC* promoter, thereby repressing the expression of this major β–lactamase in the face of β–lactam exposure. In other bacteria, BlaI homologs are inactivated by proteolytic cleavage at a highly conserved Asparagine-Phenylalanine bond located in helix α5, which is also present in *M. tuberculosis* BlaI (Sala *et al.*, 2009). Although it has not been identified yet, the most likely candidate for the inactivating protease is predicted to be Rv1845c, a zinc metalloprotease encoded by a gene located adjacent to *blaI* (Sala *et al.*, 2009). If proteolysis of BlaI could be prevented by targeting Rv1845c with protease inhitors, the BlaI-mediated repression of *blaC* could be promoted to render the bacilli more susceptible to β–lactams. Similarly, inhibition of β–lactamase translocation by targeting the Tat transpoter system may also represent a novel strategy for β–lactam potentiation.

Since very promising results have been obtained with *in vitro* studies of MDR and XDR *M. tuberculosis* using β–lactamase inhibitors, more comprehensive and well-structured clinical trials with human MDR and XDR TB need to be done in order to affirm the efficacy of these agents for TB treatment. Currently, a phase II clinical trial in 100 TB patients utilizing meropenem potentiated by clavulanate is being planned in South Korea (Drug Information Online, 2011, Science Centric, 2009). In addition, frequency of dosing will need to be determined to improve and maintain effective doses over longer periods of time. One of the major obstacles to the effective use of β–lactams in long course regimens is that currently used carbapenems have to be administered intravenously, leading to high costs of treatment due to necessary supervision by health care professionals as well as complicating patient compliance over the entire course of treatment.

3. Ethionamide

Ethionamide (ETH, 2-ethylthioisonicotinamide, or Trecator SC, Figure 3 A) is an important component of most current drug regimens used in the treatment of MDR-TB. While an effective drug against more than 80% of MDR-TB clinical strains, ETH has a low therapeutic index, or margin of safety, characterized by a narrow therapeutic effective concentration range (Sood & Panchagnula, 2003, Zimmerman et al., 1984). In other words, it is more difficult to prescribe ETH treatment doses that ensure effective treatment outcomes and yet avoid toxic side effects (Burns, 1999). The lowest dose of ETH required to inhibit M. tuberculosis growth has been shown to elicit adverse side effects such as hepatitis and gastrointestinal ailments (Flipo et al., 2011). Discovered in 1956, ETH is a structural thioamide analogue of INH and must be metabolically activated in order to form adducts with nicotinamide adenine dinucleotide (NAD). The ETH-NAD adducts subsequently inhibit InhA, the NADH-dependent enoyl-ACP reductase of the fatty acid biosynthesis type II system, allowing ETH to exert its activity against the synthesis of mycolic acids, the major component of the tubercle bacilli cell wall (Brossier et al., 2011, Morlock et al., 2003, Vannelli et al., 2002, Vilcheze et al., 2008, Zhang, 2005).

3.1 Ethionamide resistance mechanisms in mycobacteria

ETH activation requires an NADPH-specific FAD-containing monooxygenase, encoded by ethA, which oxidizes ETH to form the covalent ETH-NAD adducts. The active ETH-NAD adducts tightly bind to and inhibit InhA activity (Figure 3 A) (Brossier et al., 2011, DeBarber et al., 2000, Frenois et al., 2004, Morlock et al., 2003, Wang et al., 2007). EthA was shown to catalyze the conversion of ketones to esters, suggesting its physiological function in mycolic acid metabolism of M. tuberculosis (Fraaije et al., 2004). In the majority of ETH resistant M. tuberculosis isolates, mutations have been mapped to four principal catagories: (i) mutations that alter activity of EthA, (ii) mutations in ethR, the gene located adjacent to ethA, (iii) mutations in InhA that prevent binding of the activated drug, and (iv) mutations in the inhA promoter region that lead to InhA overexpression, (Banerjee et al., 1994, Baulard et al., 2000, Brossier et al., 2011, DeBarber et al., 2000, Morlock et al., 2003). Besides these four main catagories, several additional genes (ndh, mshA, and dfrA) might also be involved in ETH resistance. For example, mutations in ndh, which encodes a NADH dehydrogenase, may result in an increased intracellular concentration of NADH that competitively inhibits the binding of ETH-NAD adducts to InhA (Vilcheze et al., 2005). While the connection of ndh mutations and ETH resistance has been demonstrated in M. bovis BCG and M. smegmatis, it has not been observed in M. tuberculosis (Brossier et al., 2011). mshA encodes a glycosyltransferase involved in the biosynthesis of mycothiol that may enhance the ETH activation by EthA (Brossier et al., 2011, Vilcheze et al., 2008, Xu et al., 2011). Whereas mshA mutations might be readily identified *in vitro* under ETH selection pressure, mutations in *mshA* only represent a minority among ETH resistant *M. tuberculosis* clinical isolates (Brossier *et al.*, 2011). Lastly, *dfrA* encodes the dihydrofolate reductase activity involved in folate biosynthesis. As it was suggested that dihydrofolate reductase is inhibited by INH adducts (Argyrou *et al.*, 2006), this enzyme may also be targeted by the adducts of ETH. Thus far, mutations in *dfrA* have not been identified among ETH resistant clinical isolates (Brossier *et al.*, 2011).

In summary, the reduced EthA-mediated activation of ETH represents the principal molecular mechanism contributing to ETH resistance. Indeed, *in trans* overexpression of the prodrug activator EthA in *M. smegmatis* leads to increased ETH sensitivity and inhibition of mycolic acid synthesis (Morlock *et al.*, 2003, Willand *et al.*, 2009) whereas attempts to overexpress EthA in *M. tuberculosis* have been unsuccessful (DeBarber *et al.*, 2000, Morlock *et al.*, 2003). In recent studies, it has been clarified that the production of EthA is negatively controlled by the transcriptional regulator EthR, encoded by an adjacent gene (Figure 3B) (Baulard *et al.*, 2000, Morlock *et al.*, 2003). *In trans* overexpression of *ethR* causes strong inhibition of *ethA* expression, whereas chromosomal inactivation of *ethR* stimulates ETH hypersensitivity (Dover *et al.*, 2004, Engohang-Ndong *et al.*, 2004). Furthermore, electrophoretic mobility shift assays and DNA footprinting analysis indicate direct interaction of EthR with the *ethA* promoter (Dover *et al.*, 2004, Engohang-Ndong *et al.*, 2004). EthR is a member of the TetR/CamR family of repressors that is suggested to sterically inhibit the interaction between RNA polymerase and the affected promoter (Engohang-Ndong *et al.*, 2004, Frenois *et al.*, 2004, Willand *et al.*, 2009). In fact, *M. tuberculosis* EthR was shown to cooperatively multimerize on a 55-bp operator, O_{ethR}, located within the *ethA* promotor, thereby repressing *ethA* expression (Frenois *et al.*, 2004, Vannelli *et al.*, 2002, Weber *et al.*, 2008).

Similar to other TetR/CamR repressors, recent X-ray crystallographic structures revealed that EthR exists as a homodimer organized by two functional domains, each composed of nine α-helices (Dover *et al.*, 2004, Frenois *et al.*, 2004, Willand *et al.*, 2009). The amino terminus of each DNA binding domain consists of a classical helix-turn-helix motif formed by α1, 2, and 3. The remaining six α-helices comprise the carboxy-terminus, which contains the ligand-binding site responsible for controlling the conformational changes that prevent binding of EthR to O_{ethR}. Interactions between α-helices of each monomer form a four-helix bundle resulting in dimerization of the repressor. The crystal structures also revealed a ligand cocrystallized with EthR (Frenois *et al.*, 2006, Frenois *et al.*, 2004). This ligand, hexadecyl octanoate (HexOc), occupies the hydrophobic tunnel of each monomer by means of hydrophobic interactions and hydrogen bonds (Willand *et al.*, 2009). In the presence of HexOc, the distance between the two DNA binding domains in the EthR structure is augmented by 18 Å. As a result, the conformational change impairs the ability of EthR to bind to its operator (Frenois *et al.*, 2006, Frenois *et al.*, 2004, Willand *et al.*, 2009). The ligand-binding domain, embedded in the core domain of each monomer, is characterized as a narrow hydrophobic tunnel rich in aromatic residues (Dover *et al.*, 2004, Willand *et al.*, 2009). More recently, two ETH resistant isolates expressing two unique mutations in EthR, Phenylalanine 110 changed to Leucine and Alanine 95 changed to Threonine, further illuminated the derepression mechanism of EthR. Both Phenylalanine 110 (located within the α5 helix) and Alanine 95 (located within the vicinity of helices α4 and α5) contribute to the ligand-binding domain (Brossier *et al.*, 2011). Based on this wealth of knowledge, recent efforts are being made to develop compounds that could potentially interfere with EthR repressor function. Such inhibitors could therefore potentiate the antimycobacterial efficacy of ETH and possibly reduce its adverse side effects by allowing lower prescribed doses (Flipo *et al.*, 2011).

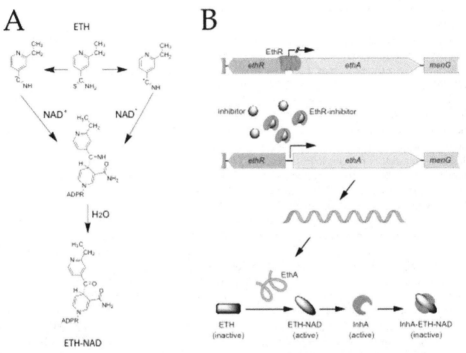

Fig. 3. Ethionamide activation and potentiation. (A) Model of ETH activation by EthA. ETH is first oxidized by EthA to a corresponding thioamide S-oxide that is further oxidized to form the final cytotoxic species. Although the latter oxidation steps remain unclear, it is postulated that thioamide S-oxide is converted to an imidoyl radical (right), which attacks NAD⁺. Following hydrolysis and release of the amine group, the final ETH-NAD adducts are formed. Alternatively, the amidoyl anion (left) can serve as the intermediate before the NAD attack. Scheme redrawn from (Wang *et al.*, 2007). (B) Potentiation of ETH by targeting EthR. Binding of inhibitors releases EthR from its interaction with the *ethA* promoter. This allows for derepression of EthA expression, which is responsible for converting ETH to its active form ETH-NAD. The activated drug then binds to InhA and inhibits its activity in mycolate biosynthesis. EthR inhibitors could thereby function as ETH potentiators.

3.2 Potentiation of ethionamide in mycobacteria

Since ligand binding was shown to affect EthR function in repressing *ethA* expression, and increase susceptibility of *M. tuberculosis* to ETH (Flipo *et al.*, 2011, Frenois *et al.*, 2006, Frenois *et al.*, 2004, Willand *et al.*, 2009), much interest has been invested in determining whether synthetic compounds could be utilized to regulate DNA-binding activity of EthR (Weber *et al.*, 2008, Willand *et al.*, 2009). Since the DNA-binding domain of EthR is able to accommodate a hydrophobic ester such as HexOc, initial attempts were made using several ketones to assay their ability to function as EthR ligands as well as to increase mycobacterial ETH sensitivity (Frenois *et al.*, 2004). *In vitro* experiments demonstrated synergy of benzylacetone and ETH on *M. smegmatis* growth (Fraaije *et al.*, 2004). Whereas benzylacetone itself did not display antimycobacterial activity, its addition to ETH used at subinhibitory concentrations (5 µg ml-1) produced significant inhibition of mycobacterial growth (Frenois *et al.*, 2004).

As an intracellular pathogen, *M. tuberculosis* resides within phagosomal compartments of host macrophages (Nguyen & Pieters, 2005). Therefore, EthR inhibitors not only have to specifically target the repressor but must be able to reach the macrophages' cytosol (Weber *et al.*, 2008). To screen for drug-like ETH potentiators, an EthR-based reporter system was first developed by the Fussenegger group (Weber *et al.*, 2008). This elegant mammalian-based system allows for assessment of not only specificity and bioavailability of tested molecules, but also their cytotoxicity to the host cell. A library of hydrophilic esters, the primary products of EthA-catalyzed Baeyer-Villiger oxidation of ETH, was synthesized and tested for their ability to release EthR from its O_{ethR} operator within a mammalian cell, using the therein described reporter system. A licensed food additive, 2-phenylethyl-butyrate, was found to effectively regulate EthR activity as well as to increase *M. tuberculosis* susceptibility to ETH (Weber *et al.*, 2008). *In vitro* analysis of *ethA* transcripts by quantitative real time PCR verified that 2-phenylethyl-butyrate dissociates EthR from the *ethA* promoter in a dose-dependent manner. To assess bioavailability, the reporter system was transfected into human embryonic kidney (HEK) cells that were subsequently implanted into mice. In this animal model, orally administered 2-phenylethyl-butyrate effectively reached the target cells to activate the reporter gene. Most importantly, 2-phenylethyl-butyrate displayed synergistic effects with ETH on the growth inhibitory activity against pathogenic mycobacteria (Weber *et al.*, 2008).

From previous analyses of ligand-binding EthR crystal structures (Dover *et al.*, 2004, Frenois *et al.*, 2006, Frenois *et al.*, 2004), the hydrophobic interactions and hydrogen-bonding properties of the amphiphilic binding cavity was utilized to design a pharmacophore model as a means of isolating moderately lipophilic compounds that could potentially interfere with the repressor function of EthR (Willand *et al.*, 2009). The novel pharmacophore model was designed as a low-molecular weight structure consisting of two hydrophobic ends connected by a 4-6 Å linker. This would, in turn, allow for hydrogen bonding interactions with the tunnel's uncharged polar surface formed by Asparagine 179 and Asparagine 176 side-chains. From a library of drug-like compounds, 131 compounds fitting the pharmacophore model were selected and analyzed for properties relevant for drug development such as molecular weight, rotatable bonds, polar surface area, hydrogen bond donors and acceptors, etc. (Willand *et al.*, 2009). Surface plasmon resonance and co-crystallization assays emphasized several compounds with the ability to inhibit EthR-DNA interaction. Using this approach, BDM14500, a lead compound comprised of a 1,2,4-oxadiazole linker, was identified to inhibit EthR-DNA interaction by more than 50%. More importantly, inhibition activity of ETH on *M. tuberculosis* growth is significantly boosted by BDM14500 (Willand *et al.*, 2009). The primary data obtained from studies of BDM14500 allowed further development of improved EthR ligands. Two thiophen-2-yl-1,2,4-oxadiazole analogs of BDM14500, BDM31343 and BDM31381, were synthesized and subjected to surface plasmon resonance, co-crystallization, and ETH potentiation assays (Flipo *et al.*, 2011, Willand *et al.*, 2009). Kinetic analysis showed that BDM31343 and BDM31381 inhibit the interaction of EthR and O_{ethR} with IC_{50} values in the nanomolar to micromolar range, indicating their potentially high efficacy. Indeed, in *M. bovis* BCG culture, BDM31381 treatment results in a 35-fold increase in the level of *ethA* mRNA. It is suggested that the efficacy of BDM31381 resides in its ability to form an energetically favorable orientation by generating a new hydrogen bond between the carbonyl of the ligand and the carboxamide of the Asparagine 179 side chain. In fact, MIC assays later confirmed that BDM31343 and BDM31381 are both more effective potentiators of ETH activity (Flipo *et al.*, 2011, Willand *et al.*, 2009). The addition of BDM31343 or BDM31381 (25 µM) respectively allows a 10 (0.1 vs 1 µg ml^{-1}) or 20 (0.025 vs 0.5 µg ml^{-1}) fold reduction in ETH concentration yet retains identical *M. tuberculosis* growth inhibition activity. In other words, BDM31343 and BDM31381 are able to potentiate ETH antimycobacterial activity by factors of 10 and 20, respectively (Willand *et al.*, 2009). *In vivo*, mice infected with *M. tuberculosis* were treated for 3 weeks with ETH alone or in conjunction with BDM31343 or BDM31381. Following treatment, the mycobacterial load in mouse lungs was quantified. Whereas the BDM31381/ETH combination had only a minor effect on bacterial load compared to control mice treated with ETH alone, the combination of BDM31343 with ETH resulted in a significant decrease of *M. tuberculosis* load with three times more efficiency than with ETH treatment alone. TB treatment with reduced ETH dosages by combining it with BDM31343 may thus allow for efficient elimination of the bacillus without severe side effects (Willand *et al.*, 2009).

3.3 Summary and future perspectives

Through the implementation of strategies including X-ray crystallography, pharmacophore modeling (Willand *et al.*, 2009), and synthetic mammalian gene circuits (Weber *et al.*, 2008), effective potentiators of ETH have been identified. While further *in vitro* and *in vivo* analyses of these compounds will need to be performed, it is expected that such potential molecules will boost activity and allow ETH to be reconsidered as a first-line anti-TB antibiotic (Weber *et al.*, 2008, Willand *et al.*, 2009). In addition, because ETH and INH inhibit the same target, InhA (Banerjee *et al.*, 1994), ETH potentiation might create an exponential boost for the anti-TB activity of INH and hence their combination. As the attrition rate of the developmental process is enormous (Bolten & DeGregorio, 2002), much work remains to be done in preclinical and clinical development and product approval stages in order to bring this concept to the clinics. Regardless of this risky process, the results obtained from these studies have showcased the potential of this approach in improving the efficacy of existing TB-drugs, thus extending their lifespan in TB treatment. Similar studies with other TB-drugs need to be encouraged, which will not only help to better understand their mechnisms of action and resistance, but also reveal further targets for the drug potentiation approach.

4. Antifolates

Folate is a generic name referring to a large group of chemically similar B vitamins that are essential for the existence of cells in all kingdoms of life. Whereas the synthetic form, widely used as a nutritional supplement, is called folic acid or vitamin B9 (pteroylmonoglutamic acid, PteGlu), most naturally occurring folate forms are derived from the reduced molecule tetrahydrofolate (H₄PteGlu, Figure 4). All of these compounds are comprised of three molecular components: a two-ring pteridine nucleus, a para-aminobenzoic acid (pABA) group, and one or more glutamate residues attached via amide linkages. These molecules vary by the C1 groups attached to the N-5 or/and N-10 positions of H₄PteGlu (Figure 4B).

Folates are important metabolites indispensable for the development and propagation of all organisms. $H_4PteGlu$ derivatives are required in reactions that involve the transfer of one-carbon units (C_1 reactions, Figure 4A). These reactions are essential for the biosynthesis of purines, thymidine, glycine, panthotenate, methionine, and formyl-methionyl-tRNA, the initiator of protein synthesis in bacteria (Blakley, 1969, Green et al., 1996, Selhub, 2002). Because these molecules are required for the synthesis of the building blocks of macromolecules such as nucleic acids and proteins, folate deficiency hinders cell division and consequently results in cell death. In addition, lack of folate derivatives also leads to defects in the recycling of homocysteine (Hcy, Figure 4) and S-adenosine methionine (SAM), which result in elevated homocysteine concentration (homocysteinemia) and reduced cellular methylation activities, respectively. Folates are particularly important during periods of rapid cell division and growth (Blakley, 1969, Green et al., 1996).

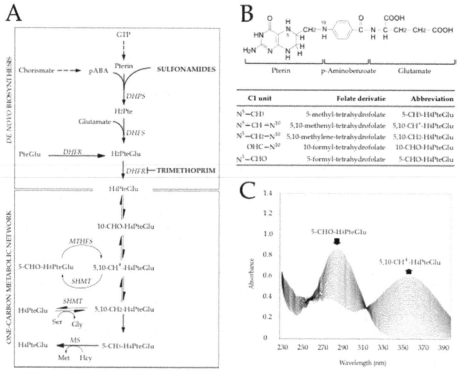

Fig. 4. Folate metabolism and antagonism in bacteria. (A) Simplified interconversions of folate derivatives in de novo folate synthesis and one-carbon metabolic network. DHFS, dihydrofolate synthase; Gly, glycine; Met, methionine; MS, methionine synthase; Pte, pteroate; Ser, serine. (B) Chemical structure of monoglutamylated tetrahydrofolate and its derivatives carrying C1 groups at various levels of oxidation attached to N-5 or/and N-10. Redrawn from (Waller et al., 2010). (C) Scanning spectrophotometric analysis of MTHFS reaction, which converts 5-CHO-H4PteGlu (Abs, 285nm) to 5,10-CH+-H4PteGlu (Abs, 360 nm), catalyzed by the M. tuberculosis MTHFS homolog, Rv0992c, a novel determinant of antifolate resistance.

Folate metabolism is generally divided into two stages: biosynthesis (upstream) and utilization (downstream) (Figure 4A). The upstream *de novo* folate biosynthesis involves: (i) pterin branch synthesizing the pteridine group from guanosine triphosphate (GTP), (ii) synthesis of pABA from chorismate, (iii) condensation of pteridine and pABA to form dihydropteroate (H_2Pte) and (iv) glutamylation which adds one or more glutamate groups to form dihydrofolate (H_2PteGlu) that is reduced to form H_4PteGlu. The downstream folate utilization is usually called one-carbon metabolism in which different active forms of H_4PteGlu participate in distinct reactions donating or accepting one-carbon units for the formation of purines, thymidine, glycine, panthotenate, methionine, and formyl-methionyl tRNA (Figure 4).

Because of the vital role of folates in multiple metabolic processes of the cell, folate antagonism has been used successfully in chemotherapeutic treatments of multiple diseases including cancers, malaria, psoriasis, rheumatoid arthritis, graft-versus-host disease, and bacterial infections (Bertino, 1971, Gorlick *et al.*, 1996, Vinetz, 2010). Folate antagonists (antifolates or *antifols*) have been used extensively for the treatment of infectious diseases from the late 1930s till 1960s, but their use has declined because of the emergence of resistant strains, their cytotoxicity, and most importantly the introduction of more effective drugs (Bertino, 1971, Libecco & Powell, 2004). Nevertheless, combination therapies using trimethoprim and sulfonamides to create synergistic effects are still used effectively today to treat some infectious diseases such as urinary tract infection, *Pneumocystis jiroveci* pneumonia, shigellosis, and for prophylaxis against recurrent and drug-resistant infections (Grim *et al.*, 2005, Libecco & Powell, 2004, Proctor, 2008). The absence of enzymes required for a complete *de novo* folate biosynthesis in humans and other mammals makes this pathway an attractive and potential target for the development of novel antimicrobial agents (Bermingham & Derrick, 2002). Whereas proteins participating in folate metabolism are well known, most current folate antagonists are thought to act on either the biosynthesis or the reduction of folate (Bermingham & Derrick, 2002, Gangjee *et al.*, 2007, 2008). Whereas trimethoprim and folate analogs such as methotrexate inhibit the reduction step through inhibition of dihydrofolate reductases (DHFR), sulfonamides and sulfone drugs are pABA analogs that outcompete pABA in the condensation with the pteridin group, catalyzed by dihydropteroate synthase (DHPS) (Bermingham & Derrick, 2002, Gangjee *et al.*, 2007, 2008).

4.1 Folate antagonism in chemotherapies of mycobacterial infections and antifolate resistance

The essentiality of folate-mediated one-carbon metabolism in fundamental metabolic and cellular processes has been recognized since the 1940s. Almost immediately after folates had been identified as essential metabolic cofactors, antifolate drugs that interfere with the folate pathway were developed and found to be effective antimicrobial and antineoplastic agents. As seen with other antibiotics, acquired resistance to antifolates in pathogenic bacteria also occurred rapidly following their introduction. These resistant forms are typically caused by mutations that alter either expression levels or protein structures of the targeted enzymes (Bertino, 1971, Libecco & Powell, 2004). DHFR can acquire resistance through point mutations of active-site residues, thus altering its affinity for trimethoprim (Adrian & Klugman, 1997, Volpato & Pelletier, 2009). While clinical resistant strains frequently show a diversity of mutations, residues that are most important for trimethoprim affinity are highly conserved among the isolates (Adrian & Klugman, 1997). For example, a point mutation in the DHFR gene that changes a conserved Isoleucine residue (Isoleucine 94 in *M. tuberculosis*

DHFR) to Leucine, confers 50-fold higher trimethoprim resistance in *Streptococcus pneumoniae* (Adrian & Klugman, 1997). This mutation is commonly found in DHFR from mammalian, parasitic and bacterial resistant isolates (Volpato & Pelletier, 2009). For sulfonamide and sulfone drugs, single point mutations at the Serine 53 or Proline 55 residues within DHPS are found in resistant isolates of *M. leprae* (Baca *et al.*, 2000, Kai *et al.*, 1999). The two affected residues are located in the drug binding region of *M. tuberculosis* DHPS and are highly conserved throughout bacteria and protozoa (Baca *et al.*, 2000). Combined mutations in DHFR and DHPS encoding genes have been known to confer resistance to all available antifolates (Bermingham & Derrick, 2002, Gangjee *et al.*, 2007, 2008). It is important to note that most current knowledge of trimethoprim and sulfonamide resistance comes from studies of bacteria distantly related to *M. tuberculosis*, and very limited information on mechanisms involved in antifolate resistance is available for mycobacterial species. With the increasing use of antifolates (Date *et al.*, 2010), a better understanding of antifolate resistance mechanisms in *M. tuberculosis* is urgently needed (Koser *et al.*, 2010).

Although much remains unknown about resistance mechanisms, antifolate drugs have been used to treat mycobacterial infections. For example, PAS (p-aminosalicilic acid) is currently used as a second-line drug for TB (Rengarajan *et al.*, 2004); the sulfone drug Dapsone has been used in monodrug regimens to treat leprosy for many decades (Doull, 1963). Interestingly, a recent study suggested that the frontline TB-drug INH may also target folate metabolism through the inhibitory action of its adducts on DHFR (Argyrou *et al.*, 2006). In addition, recent *in vitro* studies and a case report proposed that antifolate combinations such as those of co-trimoxazole (trimethoprim plus sulfamethoxazole) might be effective against TB, thus renewing much interest in the exploitation of antifolates to treat MDR and XDR-TB (Forgacs *et al.*, 2009, Ong *et al.*, 2010, Young, 2009). *M. tuberculosis* clinical strains isolated from TB patients were shown to be widely susceptible to clinically achievable concentrations of co-trimoxazole (Forgacs *et al.*, 2009), or sulfamethoxazole alone (Ong *et al.*, 2010). Importantly, the World Health Organization has recently called for widespread use of co-trimoxazole in the prophylactic treatment of HIV-AIDS patients to prevent opportunistic infections (Date *et al.*, 2010). While this practice shows promise, it is likely to expose infectious agents, including *M. tuberculosis*, to antifolates more frequently, which could lead to selection of resistant strains, thus shortening the lifespan of this powerful family of drugs (Vinetz, 2010). As in the case of β–lactams, strategies for potentiation of antifolates should be readily available to counterattack upcoming resistant strains, thereby extending their utility for TB treatment.

4.2 Potentiation of antifolates in mycobacteria

A method for boosting antifolate efficacy by utilizing combinations of drugs that target individual steps in folate biosynthesis is already in place. Trimethoprim is commonly coadministered with sulfonamides, for example sulfamethoxazole in the co-trimoxazole combination, to achieve synergy (Libecco & Powell, 2004) (Figure 4). However, in many cases including that of *M. tuberculosis*, the synergistic effect of trimethoprim on sulfonamides remains questioned and inconclusive (Forgacs *et al.*, 2009, Ong *et al.*, 2010, Suling *et al.*, 1998). In addition, bacterial strains resistant to both trimethoprim and sulfonamides have readily been isolated (Bermingham & Derrick, 2002, Gangjee *et al.*, 2007, 2008). Therefore, novel potentiation approaches targeting resistance mechanisms might be more effective in both potentiating available antifolates and preventing the emergence of resistant strains.

A recent study aimed at targeting intrinsic antifolate resistance in mycobacteria might reveal valuable targets for such resistance-targeted potentiation approaches (Ogwang *et al.*, 2011). To identify novel antifolate resistance determinants, a genetic screen was first employed using a saturated transposon-insertion library of *M. smegmatis*. These mutants are systematically tested for increased antifolate susceptibility, followed by chemical complementation using folate derivatives of both the *de novo* synthesis and the one-carbon interconversion network. This chemogenomic profiling approach allows for identification of novel determinants previously unknown to function in mycobacterial intrinsic antifolate resistance (Ogwang *et al.*, 2011). Using this non-bias screen, the genome-wide collection of antifolate resistance determinants in mycobacteria (mycobacterial antifolate resistome) was found to be composed of fifty resistance determinants (unpublished data).

A novel determinant identified from this screen was further characterized in a recent report (Ogwang *et al.*, 2011). The *M. smegmatis* mutant presented in this report exhibits hypersusceptibility to several combinations of trimethoprim/sulfonamides tested (Ogwang *et al.*, 2011). For example, its MIC to trimethoprim/sulfachloropyridazine is 64 fold lower than that of the parental *M. smegmatis* strain. The transposon insertion was mapped to a gene encoding a hypothetical protein with low homologies to 5,10-methenyl-tetrahydrofolate synthases (MTHFS, also called 5-formyl-tetrahydrofolate cyclo-ligase, EC.6.3.3.2) from other organisms, including the prototype MTHFS first described in humans (Ogwang *et al.*, 2011). Cross-species *in trans* expression of the human MTHFS was shown to restore antifolate resistance to the *M. smegmatis* mutant. A series of genetic knockout and complementation studies indicated that the disrupted gene encodes a MTHFS activity required for mycobacterial intrinsic antifolate resistance (Ogwang *et al.*, 2011). Absence of MTHFS enzymatic activity results in the inability to metabolize folinic acid (5-formyl-tetrahydrofolate, 5-CHO-H_4PteGlu) along with the reduced metabolism of 5-methyl-tetrahydrofolate (5-CH_3-H_4PteGlu), two major folate derivatives in the cell (Ogwang *et al.*, 2011). 5-CHO-H_4PteGlu is formed by the hydrolysis of 5,10-CH^+-H_4PteGlu catalyzed by serine hydroxymethyltransferase (SHMT, Figure 4A) (Holmes & Appling, 2002, Stover & Schirch, 1990), whereas MTHFS is the only enzyme known to recycle 5-CHO-H_4PteGlu back to 5,10-CH^+-H_4PteGlu in an irreversible, ATP-dependent reaction (Figure 4C). As a consequence of MTHMS absence in mycobacterial cells, polyglutamylated forms of 5-CHO-H_4PteGlu are elevated up to 80 fold, whereas the corresponding polyglutamylated forms of 5-CH_3-H_4PteGlu are reduced (Ogwang *et al.*, 2011). Interestingly, 5-CHO-H_4PteGlu is the only H_4PteGlu derivative whose biological function remains largely unknown (Stover & Schirch, 1993). Although it is well known chemically and widely used as a medical agent, 5-CHO-H_4PteGlu does not appear to function as a cofactor in any of the one-carbon metabolic reactions thus far known (Stover & Schirch, 1993). Because 5-CHO-H_4PteGlu is known as the most stable form of reduced folate species in nature, and its presence is increased in plant seeds and fungal spores, it was suggested that it might function as a folate storage form required for these dormant states of life (Kruschwitz *et al.*, 1994, Shin *et al.*, 1975, Stover & Schirch, 1993). In mammals and yeasts, 5-CHO-H_4PteGlu comprises 3-10% of total folate, whereas its presence may account for up to 50% of total folate in plant mitochondria during photorespiration when the glycine to serine flux is accelerated (Goyer *et al.*, 2005, Roje *et al.*, 2002). *In vitro*, 5-CHO-H_4PteGlu is also a potential inhibitor of SHMT and other enzymes of the one-carbon metabolism, thus it may potentially serve to regulate these metabolic reactions (Roje *et al.*, 2002, Stover & Schirch, 1991). Deletion of MTHFS in *Arabidopsis* leads to a 2-8-fold increased accumulation of total 5-CHO-H$_4$PteGlu, 46-fold accumulation of glycine, reduced growth and delayed flowering (Goyer *et al.*, 2005). In human cells, overexpression of MTHFS lowers folate levels and increases folate turnover, suggesting that MTHFS may also function as a folate-degrading enzyme (Anguera *et al.*, 2003).

The role of MTHFS in intrinsic antifolate resistance was found not only in mycobacteria but also in *E. coli*, a Gram-negative bacterium (Nichols *et al.*, 2011, Ogwang *et al.*, 2011), suggesting that this determinant functions ubiquitously among bacteria. Indeed, further work confirmed that *rv0992c*, the gene that encodes the MTHFS homolog in *M. tuberculosis*, is also required for antifolate resistance via its MTHFS enzymatic activity (Figure 4C). Pharmaceutical inactivation of MTHFS activity is therefore expected to sensitize *M. tuberculosis* to classical antifolates, including those current TB-drugs that happen to target folate pathways (PAS, INH, etc.). This intervention may also allow for reduction of effective therapeutic doses, thereby minimizing the cytotoxicity of classical antifolates which has been an issue for their widespread use in the clinics. Work is underway to identify specific inhibitors of *M. tuberculosis* MTHFS by rational design and high throughput screening, as well as to characterize their antifolate potentiation activity against *M. tuberculosis*.

4.3 Future perspectives

Fundamental studies of molecular mechanisms conferring both acquired and intrinsic antifolate resistance in *M. tuberculosis* and related mycobacteria should be further conducted. Knowledge obtained from these studies will be essential for strategic implementations of antifolate use for TB, and will reveal valid targets for the resistance-targeted potentiation of classical antifolates.

A potential problem for the development of MTHFS inhibitors might be their nonspecific inhibition towards human MTHFS. However, the low homologies of MTHFS proteins indicate the possibility to identify species-specific inhibitors. Trimethoprim, which specifically inhibits bacterial DHFR but not the human counterpart, represents an encouraging example for such possibilities. Interestingly, a recent work showed that *ygfA*, the gene that encodes the MTHFS homolog in *E. coli*, is required for the formation of drug persisters during antibiotic treatments (Hansen *et al.*, 2008). Although it remains to be characterized if the function of *ygfA* in antibiotic persister formation is related to its MTHFS activity, a similar role for *M. tuberculosis* *rv0992c* during TB latent infection is under investigation.

Although *in vitro* studies and a case report suggested that co-trimoxazole could be used for TB treatment (Forgacs *et al.*, 2009, Ong *et al.*, 2010, Young, 2009), more comprehensive well-designed trials with TB patients should be done to evaluate the efficacy of this antifolate combination. These trials should also address if these drugs may help to shorten the current TB regimens. In addition, new combinations using co-trimoxazole and PAS and/or INH should be tested against *M. tuberculosis* both *in vitro* and in patients.

5. Conclusions and future prospects

The primary goal of this chapter is to assess an emerging approach in TB drug development that uses knowledge of resistance mechanisms to sensitize *M. tuberculosis* to available, approved antibiotics (Figure 1) (Wright, 2000, Wright & Sutherland, 2007). Specific inhibitors that suppress resistance mechanisms would boost the efficacy of current anti-TB drugs, or potentiate the antimycobacterial activity of currently non-TB antibiotics, thus making use of drugs that are already available but have never been used for TB treatment before. Proofs of concept have been made in recent years to demonstrate the feasibility of this approach in potentiating the antimycobacterial activity of important antibiotics such as β–lactams, ethionamide, and antifolates. It is anticipated that this trend will become increasingly important in the future of drug development, not only for TB but any disease treated by chemotherapies. As the rate of drug resistance expansion appears far beyond that of the current drug developmental process, it is logical that such sustainable approaches should be promoted to improve the utility and protection of those effective agents.

Besides targeting antibiotic resistance mechanisms, currently approved drugs should be tested systematically against *M. tuberculosis*, especially drug resistant strains. Recent work showed that many antibiotics that had been thought to be inactive against TB might be effective as chemotherapeutic agents for the disease (Forgacs *et al.*, 2009, Hugonnet *et al.*, 2009, Ong *et al.*, 2010). In addition, drug-drug interactions among current combinatorial regimens for TB need to be further investigated. Most of the antibiotic combinations developed thus far are mainly aimed at minimizing the development of resistance, but disregard possible synergistic or antagonistic effects. Future drug combinations that minimize antagonistic effects but maximize synergy among the drugs used may not only reduce harmful clinical doses but also shorten treatment schedules, which would help to prevent the evolution and spread of antibiotic resistance.

6. Acknowledgments

We thank Hoa Nguyen for providing the data of *M. tuberculosis* MTHFS activity, Michael R. Jacobs, Sebastian Kurz, and Kien Nguyen for critical reading and comments on the manuscript. Work in the laboratory of L.N. is supported by the U.S. National Institutes of Health (Grant No. R01AI087903), the Case Western Reserve University School of Medicine, the Case/UHC Center For AIDS Research (AI36219), and the STERIS Corporation Award for Infectious Diseases Research.

7. References

Adrian, P. V. & Klugman, K. P., (1997) Mutations in the dihydrofolate reductase gene of trimethoprim-resistant isolates of *Streptococcus pneumoniae*. *Antimicrob Agents Chemother* 41: 2406-2413.

Anguera, M. C., Suh, J. R., Ghandour, H., Nasrallah, I. M., Selhub, J. & Stover, P. J., (2003) Methenyltetrahydrofolate synthetase regulates folate turnover and accumulation. *J Biol Chem* 278: 29856-29862.

Argyrou, A., Vetting, M. W., Aladegbami, B. & Blanchard, J. S., (2006) *Mycobacterium tuberculosis* dihydrofolate reductase is a target for isoniazid. *Nat Struct Mol Biol* 13: 408-413.

Baca, A. M., Sirawaraporn, R., Turley, S., Sirawaraporn, W. & Hol, W. G., (2000) Crystal structure of *Mycobacterium tuberculosis* 7,8-dihydropteroate synthase in complex with pterin monophosphate: new insight into the enzymatic mechanism and sulfa-drug action. *J Mol Biol* 302: 1193-1212.

Banerjee, A., Dubnau, E., Quemard, A., Balasubramanian, V., Um, K. S., Wilson, T., et al., (1994) inhA, a gene encoding a target for isoniazid and ethionamide in Mycobacterium tuberculosis. Science 263: 227-230.

Baulard, A. R., Betts, J. C., Engohang-Ndong, J., Quan, S., McAdam, R. A., Brennan, P. J., et al., (2000) Activation of the pro-drug ethionamide is regulated in mycobacteria. J Biol Chem 275: 28326-28331.

Bermingham, A. & Derrick, J. P., (2002) The folic acid biosynthesis pathway in bacteria: evaluation of potential for antibacterial drug discovery. Bioessays 24: 637-648.

Bertino, J. R., (1971) Folate antagonists as chemotherapeutic agents. In: Annals of the New York Academy of Sciences. New York: New York Academy of Sciences, pp. 519.

Beveridge, T. J., (1999) Structures of gram-negative cell walls and their derived membrane vesicles. J Bacteriol 181: 4725-4733.

Blakley, R. L., (1969) The biochemistry of folic acid and related pteridines, p. 569. North-Holland Publishing Co., Amsterdam, London.

Bolten, B. M. & DeGregorio, T., (2002) From the analyst's couch. Trends in development cycles. Nat Rev Drug Discov 1: 335-336.

Brennan, P. J. & Nikaido, H., (1995) The envelope of mycobacteria. Annu Rev Biochem 64: 29-63.

Brossier, F., Veziris, N., Truffot-Pernot, C., Jarlier, V. & Sougakoff, W., (2011) Molecular investigation of resistance to the antituberculous drug ethionamide in multidrug-resistant clinical isolates of Mycobacterium tuberculosis. Antimicrob Agents Chemother 55: 355-360.

Burns, M., (1999) Management of narrow therapeutic index drugs. J Thromb Thrombolysis 7: 137-143.

Chambers, H. F., Kocagoz, T., Sipit, T., Turner, J. & Hopewell, P. C., (1998) Activity of amoxicillin/clavulanate in patients with tuberculosis. Clin Infect Dis 26: 874-877.

Chambers, H. F., Moreau, D., Yajko, D., Miick, C., Wagner, C., Hackbarth, C., et al., (1995) Can penicillins and other beta-lactam antibiotics be used to treat tuberculosis? Antimicrob Agents Chemother 39: 2620-2624.

Chambers, H. F., Turner, J., Schecter, G. F., Kawamura, M. & Hopewell, P. C., (2005) Imipenem for treatment of tuberculosis in mice and humans. Antimicrob Agents Chemother 49: 2816-2821.

Date, A. A., Vitoria, M., Granich, R., Banda, M., Fox, M. Y. & Gilks, C., (2010) Implementation of co-trimoxazole prophylaxis and isoniazid preventive therapy for people living with HIV. Bull World Health Organ 88: 253-259.

Dauby, N., Muylle, I., Mouchet, F., Sergysels, R. & Payen, M. C., (2011) Meropenem/Clavulanate and Linezolid Treatment for Extensively Drug-Resistant Tuberculosis. Pediatr Infect Dis J. [puplished online ahead of print]

DeBarber, A. E., Mdluli, K., Bosman, M., Bekker, L. G. & Barry, C. E., 3rd, (2000) Ethionamide activation and sensitivity in multidrug-resistant Mycobacterium tuberculosis. Proc Natl Acad Sci U S A 97: 9677-9682.

Doull, J. A., (1963) Sulfone Therapy of Leprosy. Background, Early History and Present Status. Int J Lepr 31: 143-160.

Dover, L. G., Corsino, P. E., Daniels, I. R., Cocklin, S. L., Tatituri, V., Besra, G. S. & Futterer, K., (2004) Crystal structure of the TetR/CamR family repressor Mycobacterium tuberculosis EthR implicated in ethionamide resistance. J Mol Biol 340: 1095-1105.

Drawz, S. M. & Bonomo, R. A., (2010) Three decades of beta-lactamase inhibitors. *Clin Microbiol Rev* 23: 160-201.

Drug Information Online, (2011) Antibiotic Combo Fights Resistant TB. In: Drugs.com, Date of access: 28.02.2011, Available from: http://www.drugs.com/news/antibiotic-combo-fights-resistant-tb-16398.html

Dye, C., (2000) Tuberculosis 2000-2010: control, but not elimination. *Int J Tuberc Lung Dis* 4: S146-152.

Engohang-Ndong, J., Baillat, D., Aumercier, M., Bellefontaine, F., Besra, G. S., Locht, C. & Baulard, A. R., (2004) EthR, a repressor of the TetR/CamR family implicated in ethionamide resistance in mycobacteria, octamerizes cooperatively on its operator. *Mol Microbiol* 51: 175-188.

Flipo, M., Desroses, M., Lecat-Guillet, N., Dirie, B., Carette, X., Leroux, F., *et al.*, (2011) Ethionamide Boosters: Synthesis, Biological Activity, and Structure-Activity Relationships of a Series of 1,2,4-Oxadiazole EthR Inhibitors. *J Med Chem* 54: 2994-3010.

Flores, A. R., Parsons, L. M. & Pavelka, M. S., Jr., (2005) Genetic analysis of the beta-lactamases of *Mycobacterium tuberculosis* and *Mycobacterium smegmatis* and susceptibility to beta-lactam antibiotics. *Microbiology* 151: 521-532.

Forgacs, P., Wengenack, N. L., Hall, L., Zimmerman, S. K., Silverman, M. L. & Roberts, G. D., (2009) Tuberculosis and trimethoprim-sulfamethoxazole. *Antimicrob Agents Chemother* 53: 4789-4793.

Fraaije, M. W., Kamerbeek, N. M., Heidekamp, A. J., Fortin, R. & Janssen, D. B., (2004) The prodrug activator EtaA from *Mycobacterium tuberculosis* is a Baeyer-Villiger monooxygenase. *J Biol Chem* 279: 3354-3360.

Frenois, F., Baulard, A. R. & Villeret, V., (2006) Insights into mechanisms of induction and ligands recognition in the transcriptional repressor EthR from *Mycobacterium tuberculosis. Tuberculosis (Edinb)* 86: 110-114.

Frenois, F., Engohang-Ndong, J., Locht, C., Baulard, A. R. & Villeret, V., (2004) Structure of EthR in a ligand bound conformation reveals therapeutic perspectives against tuberculosis. *Mol Cell* 16: 301-307.

Gandhi, N. R., Moll, A., Sturm, A. W., Pawinski, R., Govender, T., Lalloo, U., *et al.*, (2006) Extensively drug-resistant tuberculosis as a cause of death in patients co-infected with tuberculosis and HIV in a rural area of South Africa. *Lancet* 368: 1575-1580.

Gangjee, A., Jain, H. D. & Kurup, S., (2007) Recent advances in classical and non-classical antifolates as antitumor and antiopportunistic infection agents: part I. *Anticancer Agents Med Chem* 7: 524-542.

Gangjee, A., Jain, H. D. & Kurup, S., (2008) Recent advances in classical and non-classical antifolates as antitumor and antiopportunistic infection agents: Part II. *Anticancer Agents Med Chem* 8: 205-231.

Gorlick, R., Goker, E., Trippett, T., Waltham, M., Banerjee, D. & Bertino, J. R., (1996) Intrinsic and acquired resistance to methotrexate in acute leukemia. *N Engl J Med* 335: 1041-1048.

Goyer, A., Collakova, E., Diaz de la Garza, R., Quinlivan, E. P., Williamson, J., Gregory, J. F., 3rd, *et al.*, (2005) 5-Formyltetrahydrofolate is an inhibitory but well tolerated metabolite in *Arabidopsis* leaves. *J Biol Chem* 280: 26137-26142.

Green, J., Nichols, B. & Matthews, R., (1996) Folate biosynthesis, reduction, and polyglutamylation. In: *Escherichia coli* and *Salmonella typhimurium* - Cellular and Molecular Biology. F. Neidhardt, R. Curtiss III, J. Ingraham, E. Lin, J. K. Low, B. Magasanik, W. Reznikoff, M. Riley, M. Schaechter & H. Umbarger (eds). Washington, DC: ASM Press, pp. 665-673.

Grim, S. A., Rapp, R. P., Martin, C. A. & Evans, M. E., (2005) Trimethoprim-sulfamethoxazole as a viable treatment option for infections caused by methicillin-resistant *Staphylococcus aureus*. *Pharmacotherapy* 25: 253-264.

Hansen, S., Lewis, K. & Vulic, M., (2008) Role of global regulators and nucleotide metabolism in antibiotic tolerance in *Escherichia coli*. *Antimicrob Agents Chemother* 52: 2718-2726.

Holmes, W. B. & Appling, D. R., (2002) Cloning and characterization of methenyltetrahydrofolate synthetase from *Saccharomyces cerevisiae*. *J Biol Chem* 277: 20205-20213.

Hugonnet, J. E. & Blanchard, J. S., (2007) Irreversible inhibition of the *Mycobacterium tuberculosis* beta-lactamase by clavulanate. *Biochemistry* 46: 11998-12004.

Hugonnet, J. E., Tremblay, L. W., Boshoff, H. I., Barry, C. E., 3rd & Blanchard, J. S., (2009) Meropenem-clavulanate is effective against extensively drug-resistant *Mycobacterium tuberculosis*. *Science* 323: 1215-1218.

Jarlier, V., Gutmann, L. & Nikaido, H., (1991) Interplay of cell wall barrier and beta-lactamase activity determines high resistance to beta-lactam antibiotics in *Mycobacterium chelonae*. *Antimicrob Agents Chemother* 35: 1937-1939.

Jarlier, V. & Nikaido, H., (1990) Permeability barrier to hydrophilic solutes in *Mycobacterium chelonei*. *J Bacteriol* 172: 1418-1423.

Jassal, M. & Bishai, W. R., (2009) Extensively drug-resistant tuberculosis. *Lancet Infect Dis* 9: 19-30.

Kai, M., Matsuoka, M., Nakata, N., Maeda, S., Gidoh, M., Maeda, Y., et al., (1999) Diaminodiphenylsulfone resistance of *Mycobacterium leprae* due to mutations in the dihydropteroate synthase gene. *FEMS Microbiol Lett* 177: 231-235.

Kasik, J. E., (1979) Mycobacterial Beta-Lactamases. In: Beta-Lactamases. J. M. T. Hamilton-Miller & J. T. Smith (eds). 0123215501, London: Academic Press, pp. 500.

Kasik, J. E. & Peacham, L., (1968) Properties of beta-lactamases produced by three species of mycobacteria. *Biochem J* 107: 675-682.

Koch, A. L., (2003) Bacterial wall as target for attack: past, present, and future research. *Clin Microbiol Rev* 16: 673-687.

Koser, C. U., Summers, D. K. & Archer, J. A., (2010) Role of the dihydrofolate reductase DfrA (Rv2763c) in trimethoprim-sulfamethoxazole (co-trimoxazole) resistance in *Mycobacterium tuberculosis*. *Antimicrob Agents Chemother* 54: 4951-4952; author reply 4952.

Kruschwitz, H. L., McDonald, D., Cossins, E. A. & Schirch, V., (1994) 5-Formyltetrahydropteroylpolyglutamates are the major folate derivatives in *Neurospora crassa* conidiospores. *J Biol Chem* 269: 28757-28763.

Lee, W., McDonough, M. A., Kotra, L., Li, Z. H., Silvaggi, N. R., Takeda, Y., et al., (2001) A 1.2-A snapshot of the final step of bacterial cell wall biosynthesis. *Proc Natl Acad Sci U S A* 98: 1427-1431.

Libecco, J. A. & Powell, K. R., (2004) Trimethoprim/sulfamethoxazole: clinical update. *Pediatr Rev* 25: 375-380.

Liu, J., Rosenberg, E. Y. & Nikaido, H., (1995) Fluidity of the lipid domain of cell wall from *Mycobacterium chelonae*. *Proc Natl Acad Sci U S A* 92: 11254-11258.

LoBue, P., (2009) Extensively drug-resistant tuberculosis. *Curr Opin Infect Dis* 22: 167-173.

McDonough, J. A., Hacker, K. E., Flores, A. R., Pavelka, M. S., Jr. & Braunstein, M., (2005) The twin-arginine translocation pathway of *Mycobacterium smegmatis* is functional and required for the export of mycobacterial beta-lactamases. *J Bacteriol* 187: 7667-7679.

Morlock, G. P., Metchock, B., Sikes, D., Crawford, J. T. & Cooksey, R. C., (2003) *ethA*, *inhA*, and *katG* loci of ethionamide-resistant clinical *Mycobacterium tuberculosis* isolates. *Antimicrob Agents Chemother* 47: 3799-3805.

Mukherjee, T., Basu, D., Mahapatra, S., Goffin, C., van Beeumen, J. & Basu, J., (1996) Biochemical characterization of the 49 kDa penicillin-binding protein of *Mycobacterium smegmatis*. *Biochem J* 320 (Pt 1): 197-200.

Nampoothiri, K. M., Rubex, R., Patel, A. K., Narayanan, S. S., Krishna, S., Das, S. M. & Pandey, A., (2008) Molecular cloning, overexpression and biochemical characterization of hypothetical beta-lactamases of *Mycobacterium tuberculosis* H37Rv. *J Appl Microbiol* 105: 59-67.

Nguyen, L. & Pieters, J., (2005) The Trojan horse: survival tactics of pathogenic mycobacteria in macrophages. *Trends Cell Biol* 15: 269-276.

Nguyen, L. & Pieters, J., (2009) Mycobacterial subversion of chemotherapeutic reagents and host defense tactics: challenges in tuberculosis drug development. *Annu Rev Pharmacol Toxicol* 49: 427-453.

Nguyen, L. & Thompson, C. J., (2006) Foundations of antibiotic resistance in bacterial physiology: the mycobacterial paradigm. *Trends Microbiol* 14: 304-312.

Nichols, R. J., Sen, S., Choo, Y. J., Beltrao, P., Zietek, M., Chaba, R., et al., (2011) Phenotypic landscape of a bacterial cell. *Cell* 144: 143-156.

Ogwang, S., Nguyen, H. T., Sherman, M., Bajaksouzian, S., Jacobs, M. R., Boom, W. H., et al., (2011) Bacterial conversion of folinic acid is required for antifolate resistance. *J Biol Chem* 286: 15377-15390.

Ong, W., Sievers, A. & Leslie, D. E., (2010) *Mycobacterium tuberculosis* and sulfamethoxazole susceptibility. *Antimicrob Agents Chemother* 54: 2748; author reply 2748-2749.

Prabhakaran, K., Harris, E. B. & Randhawa, B., (1999) Bactericidal action of ampicillin/sulbactam against intracellular mycobacteria. *Int J Antimicrob Agents* 13: 133-135.

Proctor, R. A., (2008) Role of folate antagonists in the treatment of methicillin-resistant *Staphylococcus aureus* infection. *Clin Infect Dis* 46: 584-593.

Quinting, B., Reyrat, J. M., Monnaie, D., Amicosante, G., Pelicic, V., Gicquel, B., et al., (1997) Contribution of beta-lactamase production to the resistance of mycobacteria to beta-lactam antibiotics. *FEBS Lett* 406: 275-278.

Rengarajan, J., Sassetti, C. M., Naroditskaya, V., Sloutsky, A., Bloom, B. R. & Rubin, E. J., (2004) The folate pathway is a target for resistance to the drug para-aminosalicylic acid (PAS) in mycobacteria. *Mol Microbiol* 53: 275-282.

Roje, S., Janave, M. T., Ziemak, M. J. & Hanson, A. D., (2002) Cloning and characterization of mitochondrial 5-formyltetrahydrofolate cycloligase from higher plants. *J Biol Chem* 277: 42748-42754.

Sala, C., Haouz, A., Saul, F. A., Miras, I., Rosenkrands, I., Alzari, P. M. & Cole, S. T., (2009) Genome-wide regulon and crystal structure of BlaI (Rv1846c) from *Mycobacterium tuberculosis*. *Mol Microbiol* 71: 1102-1116.

Science Centric, (2009) Antibiotic combination defeats extensively drug-resistant TB. In: ScienceCentric.com, Date of access: 28.02.2011, Available from: http://www.sciencecentric.com/news/09022702-antibiotic-combination-defeats-extensively-drug-resistant-tb.html

Selhub, J., (2002) Folate, vitamin B12 and vitamin B6 and one carbon metabolism. *J Nutr Health Aging* 6: 39-42.

Severin, A., Severina, E. & Tomasz, A., (1997) Abnormal physiological properties and altered cell wall composition in *Streptococcus pneumoniae* grown in the presence of clavulanic acid. *Antimicrob Agents Chemother* 41: 504-510.

Shin, Y. S., Kim, E. S., Watson, J. E. & Stokstad, E. L., (1975) Studies of folic acid compounds in nature. IV. Folic acid compounds in soybeans and cow milk. *Can J Biochem* 53: 338-343.

Sood, A. & Panchagnula, R., (2003) Design of controlled release delivery systems using a modified pharmacokinetic approach: a case study for drugs having a short elimination half-life and a narrow therapeutic index. *Int J Pharm* 261: 27-41.

Stover, P. & Schirch, V., (1990) Serine hydroxymethyltransferase catalyzes the hydrolysis of 5,10-methenyltetrahydrofolate to 5-formyltetrahydrofolate. *J Biol Chem* 265: 14227-14233.

Stover, P. & Schirch, V., (1991) 5-Formyltetrahydrofolate polyglutamates are slow tight binding inhibitors of serine hydroxymethyltransferase. *J Biol Chem* 266: 1543-1550.

Stover, P. & Schirch, V., (1993) The metabolic role of leucovorin. *Trends Biochem Sci* 18: 102-106.

Suling, W. J., Reynolds, R. C., Barrow, E. W., Wilson, L. N., Piper, J. R. & Barrow, W. W., (1998) Susceptibilities of *Mycobacterium tuberculosis* and *Mycobacterium avium* complex to lipophilic deazapteridine derivatives, inhibitors of dihydrofolate reductase. *J Antimicrob Chemother* 42: 811-815.

Tremblay, L. W., Fan, F. & Blanchard, J. S., (2010) Biochemical and structural characterization of *Mycobacterium tuberculosis* beta-lactamase with the carbapenems ertapenem and doripenem. *Biochemistry* 49: 3766-3773.

Tremblay, L. W., Hugonnet, J. E. & Blanchard, J. S., (2008) Structure of the covalent adduct formed between *Mycobacterium tuberculosis* beta-lactamase and clavulanate. *Biochemistry* 47: 5312-5316.

Vannelli, T. A., Dykman, A. & Ortiz de Montellano, P. R., (2002) The antituberculosis drug ethionamide is activated by a flavoprotein monooxygenase. *J Biol Chem* 277: 12824-12829.

Vilcheze, C., Av-Gay, Y., Attarian, R., Liu, Z., Hazbon, M. H., Colangeli, R., *et al.*, (2008) Mycothiol biosynthesis is essential for ethionamide susceptibility in *Mycobacterium tuberculosis*. *Mol Microbiol* 69: 1316-1329.

Vilcheze, C., Weisbrod, T. R., Chen, B., Kremer, L., Hazbon, M. H., Wang, F., et al., (2005) Altered NADH/NAD+ ratio mediates coresistance to isoniazid and ethionamide in mycobacteria. *Antimicrob Agents Chemother* 49: 708-720.

Vinetz, J. M., (2010) Intermittent preventive treatment for malaria in sub-saharan African: a halfway technology or a critical intervention? *Am J Trop Med Hyg* 82: 755-756.

Voladri, R. K., Lakey, D. L., Hennigan, S. H., Menzies, B. E., Edwards, K. M. & Kernodle, D. S., (1998) Recombinant expression and characterization of the major beta-lactamase of *Mycobacterium tuberculosis*. *Antimicrob Agents Chemother* 42: 1375-1381.

Volpato, J. P. & Pelletier, J. N., (2009) Mutational 'hot-spots' in mammalian, bacterial and protozoal dihydrofolate reductases associated with antifolate resistance: sequence and structural comparison. *Drug Resist Updat* 12: 28-41.

Waller, J. C., Alvarez, S., Naponelli, V., Lara-Nunez, A., Blaby, I. K., Da Silva, V., et al., (2010) A role for tetrahydrofolates in the metabolism of iron-sulfur clusters in all domains of life. *Proc Natl Acad Sci U S A* 107: 10412-10417.

Wang, F., Cassidy, C. & Sacchettini, J. C., (2006) Crystal structure and activity studies of the *Mycobacterium tuberculosis* beta-lactamase reveal its critical role in resistance to beta-lactam antibiotics. *Antimicrob Agents Chemother* 50: 2762-2771.

Wang, F., Langley, R., Gulten, G., Dover, L. G., Besra, G. S., Jacobs, W. R., Jr. & Sacchettini, J. C., (2007) Mechanism of thioamide drug action against tuberculosis and leprosy. *J Exp Med* 204: 73-78.

Watt, B., Edwards, J. R., Rayner, A., Grindey, A. J. & Harris, G., (1992) *In vitro* activity of meropenem and imipenem against mycobacteria: development of a daily antibiotic dosing schedule. *Tuber Lung Dis* 73: 134-136.

Waxman, D. J., Yocum, R. R. & Strominger, J. L., (1980) Penicillins and cephalosporins are active site-directed acylating agents: evidence in support of the substrate analogue hypothesis. *Philos Trans R Soc Lond B Biol Sci* 289: 257-271.

Weber, W., Schoenmakers, R., Keller, B., Gitzinger, M., Grau, T., Daoud-El Baba, M., et al., (2008) A synthetic mammalian gene circuit reveals antituberculosis compounds. *Proc Natl Acad Sci U S A* 105: 9994-9998.

Willand, N., Dirie, B., Carette, X., Bifani, P., Singhal, A., Desroses, M., et al., (2009) Synthetic EthR inhibitors boost antituberculous activity of ethionamide. *Nat Med* 15: 537-544.

World Health Organization, (2006) Questions : XDR-TB. In: www.who.int, Date of access: 26.02.2011, Available from:
http://www.who.int/tb/challenges/xdr/faqs/en/index.html

World Health Organization, (2010) Tuberculosis Fact Sheet. In: www.who.int Date of access: 26.02.2011, Available from:
http://www.who.int/mediacentre/factsheets/fs104/en/index.html

Wright, G. D., (2000) Resisting resistance: new chemical strategies for battling superbugs. *Chem Biol* 7: R127-132.

Wright, G. D. & Sutherland, A. D., (2007) New strategies for combating multidrug-resistant bacteria. *Trends Mol Med* 13: 260-267.

Xu, X., Vilcheze, C., Av-Gay, Y., Gomez-Velasco, A. & Jacobs, W. R., Jr., (2011) Precise null deletion mutations of the mycothiol synthetic genes reveal their role in isoniazid and ethionamide resistance in *Mycobacterium smegmatis*. *Antimicrob Agents Chemother* 55: 3133-3139.

Young, L. S., (2009) Reconsidering some approved antimicrobial agents for tuberculosis. *Antimicrob Agents Chemother* 53: 4577-4579.

Zhang, Y., (2005) The magic bullets and tuberculosis drug targets. *Annu Rev Pharmacol Toxicol* 45: 529-564.

Zimmerman, T. J., Kooner, K. S., Kandarakis, A. S. & Ziegler, L. P., (1984) Improving the therapeutic index of topically applied ocular drugs. *Arch Ophthalmol* 102: 551-553.

10

Insight into the Key Structural Features of Potent Enoyl Acyl Carrier Protein Reductase Inhibitors Based on Computer Aided Molecular Design

Auradee Punkvang[1], Pharit Kamsri[1], Kodchakon Kun-asa[1],
Patchreenart Saparpakorn[2], Supa Hannongbua[2],
Peter Wolschann[3] and Pornpan Pungpo[1]
[1]*Ubon Ratchathani University*
[2]*Kasetsart University*
[3]*University of Vienna*
[1,2]*Thailand*
[3]*Austria*

1. Introduction

Tuberculosis (TB) caused by *Mycobacterium tuberculosis* (*M. tuberculosis*) is one of the leading reason of mortality and is still spread worldwide, indicated by more than 9 million incident cases of TB in 2009 (World Health Organization, 2010). Current standard treatment regimens of TB are severely hampered by multidrug resistant tuberculosis (MDR-TB), extensively drug-resistant tuberculosis (XDR-TB) and HIV co-infection with TB (WHO, 2010). This fact prompts the research to develop novel and more potent drug candidates to treat *M. tuberculosis* strains resistant to existing drugs. The enoyl acyl carrier protein reductase (InhA) of *M. tuberculosis* catalyzing the NADH-specific reduction of 2-trans-enoyl-ACP (Quemard et al., 1995) is an attractive target for designing novel antibacterial agents (Campbell et al., 2001; Heath et al., 2004; White et al., 2005; Zhang et al., 2004; Wen et al., 2009; Wright et al., 2007). InhA has been identified as the primary target of isoniazid (INH), one of the most effective first-line anti-TB drugs (Rozwarski et al., 1998; Vilcheze et al., 2006; Dessen et al., 1995; Lei et al., 2000; Johnsson et al., 1995; Quemard et al., 1996). InhA is inhibited by the active adduct of INH (INH-NAD) (Timmins et al., 2006; Johnsson et al., 1997) which is covalently formed between NAD+ and the reactive acyl radical of INH generated by the activation of catalase-peroxidase (KatG) (Saint-Joanis et al., 1999; Zhao et al., 2006; Metcalfe et al., 2008; Sinha et al., 1983; Nguyen et al., 2001; Heym et al., 1993; Johnsson et al., 1994). The mutations in KatG have been linked to the major mechanism of INH resistance (de la Iglesia et al., 2006; Banerjee et al., 1994). To overcome the INH resistance associated with mutations in KatG, compounds that directly inhibit the InhA enzyme without requiring activation of KatG have been developed as new promising agents against tuberculosis (Freundlich et al., 2009; am Ende et al., 2008; Boyne et al., 2007; Sullivan et al., 2006; He et al., 2006; He et al., 2007; Kuo et al., 2003). Triclosan, 5-chloro-2-(2,4-

dichlorophenoxy)phenol as shown in Fig.1, has been shown to inhibit InhA without the requirement for KatG-mediated activation (Parikh et al., 2000; Kuo et al., 2003). Because of the remarkable properties of triclosan, a series of triclosan derivatives with modifications at the 5-chloro of triclosan, 5-substituted triclosan derivatives shown in Fig.1, was synthesized in order to optimize the potency of triclosan against InhA (Freundlich et al., 2009). Furthermore, using structure-based drug design, three lipophilic chlorine atoms of triclosan were removed, and one chlorine atom of ring A was replaced by an alkyl chain of varying length resulting in the alkyl diphenyl ethers shown in Fig. 1 (Sullivan et al., 2006). The most efficacious triclosan derivatives in the two classes of 5-substituted triclosan and alkyl diphenyl ether derivatives are more potent than the parent compound triclosan. Importantly, a subset of these triclosan analogues displays high efficacy against both INH-sensitive and INH-resistant strains of *M. tuberculosis* more than those of isoniazid. Because of the remarkable property of 5-substituted triclosan derivatives and alkyl diphenyl ethers, their structural requirements for a better therapeutic activity against tuberculosis in both cases of drug-sensitive and drug-resistant strains of *M. tuberculosis* are fascinating and need to be thoroughly examined. Therefore, in the present study, a structure based drug design using molecular docking calculations was applied to investigate the important drug-enzyme interactions of 5-substituted triclosan derivatives and the related alkyl diphenyl ethers in the InhA binding pocket. Moreover, approaches based on 2D and 3D QSAR methods, HQSAR (Hologram QSAR), CoMFA (Comparative Molecular Field Analysis) and CoMSIA (Comparative Molecular Similarity Indices Analysis) (Cramer et al., 1998; Klebe et al., 1994; Tong et al., 1998) have been used to elucidate the relationship between the structures and the activities of these compounds. A powerful guideline for designing novel and highly effective antitubercular agents is the consequence of these investigations.

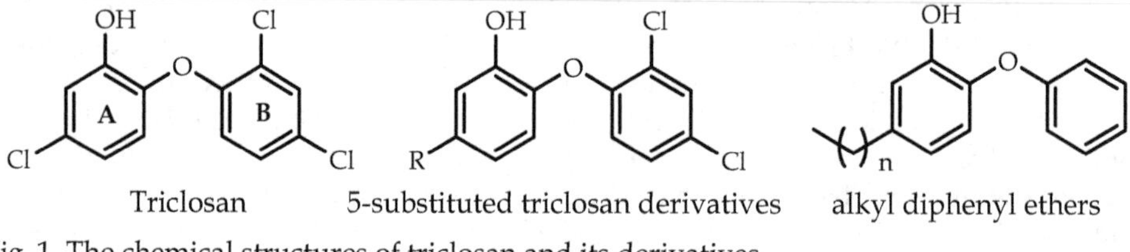

Triclosan   5-substituted triclosan derivatives   alkyl diphenyl ethers

Fig. 1. The chemical structures of triclosan and its derivatives

2. Materials and methods of calculations

2.1 Data sets and InhA inhibitory activity

Chemical structures and experimental biological activities expressed as IC_{50} (the half maximal inhibitory concentration) of 17 compounds of 5-substituted triclosan derivatives (Freundlich et al., 2009) and 12 alkyl diphenyl ether derivatives (am Ende et al., 2008; Sullivan et al., 2006) were selected for the present study. All chemical structures of these compounds were constructed using standard tools available in GaussView 3.07 program (Gaussian, Inc., 2006) and were then fully optimized using an *ab initio* quantum chemical method (HF/3-21G) implemented in the Gaussian 03 program (Gaussian, Inc., 2004). The compounds were divided into a training set of 25 compounds and a test set of 4 compounds for the model development and model validation, respectively. The representatives of the test set were manually selected and are covering the utmost range of activity and structural diversity of direct InhA inhibitors in the data set.

Cpd.	R_1	R_2	R_3	R_4	IC_{50} [nM]	$Log(1/IC_{50})$
1	Cl	Cl	H	Cl	1100	2.96
2*	CH_3	Cl	H	Cl	800	3.10
3	$CH_2(C_6H_{11})$	Cl	H	Cl	110	3.96
4	CH_2CH_3	Cl	H	Cl	120	3.92
5	$(CH_2)_2CH_3$	Cl	H	Cl	91	4.04
6*	$(CH_2)_3CH_3$	Cl	H	Cl	55	4.26
7	$CH_2CH(CH_3)_2$	Cl	H	Cl	96	4.02
8	$(CH_2)_2CH(CH_3)_2$	Cl	H	Cl	63	4.20
9	$CH_2CH(CH_3)CH_2CH_3$	Cl	H	Cl	130	3.89
10	CH_2(2-pyridyl)	Cl	H	Cl	29	4.54
11	CH_2(3-pyridyl)	Cl	H	Cl	42	4.38
12	CH_2(4-pyridyl)	Cl	H	CN	75	4.12
13	o-CH_3-C_6H_5	Cl	H	Cl	1300	2.89
14	m-CH_3-C_6H_5	Cl	H	Cl	870	3.06
15	$CH_2C_6H_5$	Cl	H	Cl	51	4.29
16	$(CH_2)_2C_6H_5$	Cl	H	Cl	21	4.68
17	$(CH_2)_3C_6H_5$	Cl	H	Cl	50	4.30
18	$(CH_2)_5CH_3$	H	H	H	11	4.96
19	CH_2CH_3	H	H	H	2000	2.70
20*	$(CH_2)_3CH_3$	H	H	H	80	4.10
21	$(CH_2)_4CH_3$	H	H	H	17	4.77
22	$(CH_2)_7CH_3$	H	H	H	5	5.30
23	$(CH_2)_{13}CH_3$	H	H	H	150	3.82
24*	$(CH_2)_5CH_3$	NO_2	H	H	180	3.74
25	$(CH_2)_5CH_3$	H	NO_2	H	48	4.32
26	$(CH_2)_5CH_3$	H	H	NO_2	90	4.05
27	$(CH_2)_5CH_3$	NH_2	H	H	62	4.21
28	$(CH_2)_5CH_3$	H	NH_2	H	1090	2.96
29	$(CH_2)_5CH_3$	H	H	NH_2	55	4.26

*The test set compounds

Table 1. The chemical structures and IC_{50} values of 5-substituted triclosan and alkyl
diphenyl ether derivatives against InhA

2.2 Molecular docking calculations

The X-ray crystal structures of InhA complexed with 2-(2,4-dichlorophenoxy)-5-(2-phenylethyl)phenol (5-substituted triclosan derivative) and 5-octyl-2-phenoxyphenol (alkyl diphenyl ether derivative) with pdb codes of 3FNH and 2B37, respectively, were employed for molecular docking calculations of compounds 1-17 and compounds 18-29, respectively. Docking calculations of the data set were carried out by the Autodock 3.05 program using Lamarckian Genetic Algorithm (LGA) (Morris et al., 1998). Docking parameters were used as default values, except for the number of docking runs which was set to 50. The docking calculation was validated by reproducing the X-ray conformation of the ligand as well as the orientation in its pocket. The root mean-square deviation (RMSD) value between the original and docked coordinates lower than 1Å is acceptable. The ligand pose with the lowest final docked energy was selected as the best binding mode of 5-substituted triclosan and alkyl diphenyl ether derivatives. Then, the conformations of all compounds were used according to this binding mode for CoMFA and CoMSIA setups.

2.3 CoMFA and CoMSIA techniques

CoMFA and CoMSIA, 3D-QSAR methods, are successfully used to derive a correlation between the biological activities of a set of compounds with a special alignment and their three-dimensional descriptors. In both CoMFA and CoMSIA, a set of compounds is aligned and the structurally aligned molecules are represented in terms of fields around the molecule (three-dimensional descriptors). CoMFA and CoMSIA are based on the assumption that changes in biological activities of compounds are related to changes in molecular properties represented by fields around the molecule. Therefore, the structural alignment of compounds is an important prerequisite for the setup of appropriate CoMFA and CoMSIA models. In the present study, the reasonable binding modes of the compounds in the data set obtained from the validated docking calculations were employed for the molecular alignment. SYBYL 8.0 molecular modeling software (Tripos, Inc, 2007) was used to construct CoMFA and CoMSIA models. CoMFA descriptors, steric and electrostatic fields, were calculated using a sp^3 carbon probe atom with a formal charge of +1 which was placed at the intersections in a grid with the spacing of 2Å. The maximum steric and electrostatic energies were truncated at 30 kcal/mol. Five CoMSIA descriptors, steric, electrostatic, hydrophobic, hydrogen bond donor and hydrogen bond acceptor fields, were derived with the same grid as used for the CoMFA field calculation. There are no energy cutoffs necessary for CoMSIA calculations because a distance-dependent Gaussian type potential was used in contrary to the procedure of CoMFA calculations. CoMFA and CoMSIA descriptors were set as independent variables and log $(1/IC_{50})$ values were used as dependent variables in the partial least square (PLS) analysis to derive a linear relationship between molecular descriptors and activities. The cross-validation was performed using the leave-one-out method with a 2.0 kcal/mol column filter to minimize the influence of noisy columns. A final non cross-validated analysis with the optimal number of components was sequentially performed and was then employed to analyze the results. The non-cross-validated correlation coefficient (r^2) and the leave-one-out (LOO) cross-validated correlation coefficient (q^2) were used to evaluate the predictive ability of the CoMFA and CoMSIA models. Contour maps were created to visualize the molecular areas responsible for the biological effects.

2.4 HQSAR

Hologram QSAR (HQSAR) does not require information about the three-dimensional geometry of the inhibitors. Hence, in contrary to CoMFA and CoMSIA methods, HQSAR needs no molecular alignment. Each compound of the data set was converted into all possible molecular fragments including linear, branched, cyclic, and overlapping fragments in the size of 4-7 atoms. Molecular fragment generation utilizes the fragment distinction parameters including atoms (A), bonds (B), connections (C), hydrogen atoms (H), chirality (Ch) as well as hydrogen donor and acceptor properties (DA). The generated molecular fragments are counted in bins of a fixed length array to produce a molecular hologram. PLS statistical method was employed to establish a correlation of the molecular hologram descriptors with the biological data. The HQSAR module of SYBYL 8.0 was employed for the HQSAR study. The same training and test sets as for CoMFA and CoMSIA studies were used. The most convenient model was selected based on the best cross-validated r^2 to determine these structural subunits which are important for the biological activities.

3. Result and discussion

3.1 The X-ray crystal structures of 5-substituted triclosan and alkyl diphenyl ether derivatives

To probe the interaction of 5-substituted triclosan and alkyl diphenyl ether derivatives with InhA, the X-ray crystal structures of these compounds complexed with InhA have been solved (Freundlich et al., 2009; Sullivan et al., 2006). To compare the conformational change of InhA complexed with the different ligands, the ligand-unbound InhA (pdb code 1ENY) and InhA bound with 2-(2,4-dichlorophenoxy)-5-(2-phenylethyl)phenol (pdb code 3FNH) and 5-octyl-2-phenoxyphenol (pdb code 2B37), compounds 16 and 22, respectively, are superimposed as shown in Fig. 2.

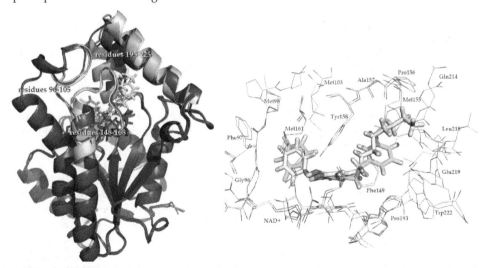

Fig. 2. Superimposition of ligand unbound InhA, InhA bound with compound 16 (cyan) and compound 22 (yellow) with pdb codes of 1ENY, 3FNH and 2B37, respectively. InhAs are colored by purple, whereas residues 96-105, 148-168 and 195-225 complexed with compounds 16 and 22 are colored by cyan and yellow, respectively.

The binding residues within 6Å apart from compounds 16 and 22 consist of residues 96-105, 148-168 and 195-225. As compared with the ligand-unbound InhA, only positions of residues 195-225 including two α-helixes and one loop of the InhA bound with compounds 16 and 22 have been changed to accommodate the binding of two different ligands. On the other hand, the binding residues 96-105 and 148-168 of the InhA bound with these compounds are located in the same position compared to those of the ligand-unbound InhA as shown in Fig. 2. These results imply that residues 195-225 could be sufficiently flexible for the binding of different ligands, whereas residues 96-105 and 148-168 are more rigid, which are consistent with the mobility of these residues investigated by means of molecular dynamics simulations performed in one of our previous investigations (Punkvang et al., 2010). With regard to the binding modes of compounds 16 and 22 in InhA binding site, the B rings of these compounds are bound in a similar orientation and buried with the rigid residues 96-105, 148-168 and the pyrophosphate group of NAD+. The aromatic B ring of compound 22 interacts with the methyl side chain of Met161 to form the methyl-π interaction, whereas that of compound 16 loses this interaction. The hydroxyl group at the A ring of compounds 16 and 22 form two hydrogen bonds with Tyr158 as well as the 2´-hydroxyl group of NAD+. The substituents at the A rings of compounds 16 and 22, the ethyl phenyl and the octyl chain, respectively, are occupied with the flexible residues 195-225. The first four carbons of the octyl chain of compound 22 superimpose well with the ethyl phenyl of compound 16 and interact with the flexible residues of Phe149, Tyr158, Pro193, Met199, Ile215, Leu218, Glu219 and Trp222, respectively. The last four carbons of the octyl chain of compound 22 interact with Met155, Pro156, Ala157, Gln214, whereas these interactions are lost for binding of compound 16. The presence of the methyl-π interaction and more interactions with the flexible residues 195-225 of the substituents at the A rings of compound 22 may be accounted for higher activity of compound 22 as compared with that of compound 16.

3.2 Docking calculations of 5-substituted triclosan and alkyl diphenyl ether derivatives

Molecular docking calculations using the Autodock 3.05 program have been successfully applied to investigate the binding modes of all 5-substituted triclosan and alkyl diphenyl ether derivatives in the InhA binding pocket. The RMSD between the docked and crystallographic conformations is lower than 1Å, indicating that molecular docking calculations are rendering high reliability for reproducing the binding mode of all 5-substituted triclosan and alkyl diphenyl ether derivatives. All predicted binding modes of these inhibitors that are similar to the binding modes as those of the above X-ray crystal structures are shown in Fig. 3.

The B rings are surrounded by the more rigid residues 96-105 and 148-168, whereas the A rings and their substituents are surrounded by the flexible residues 195-225. The hydroxyl groups at the A ring of all 5-substituted triclosan and alkyl diphenyl ether derivatives could create the same hydrogen bonding pattern with NAD+ and Tyr158. The major modification of 5-substituted triclosan and alkyl diphenyl ether derivatives is the variation of substituent R_1 at the A ring. The increasing length of an alkyl chain at the substituent R_1 results in the decreasing IC_{50} values for InhA inhibition of both 5-substituted triclosan and alkyl diphenyl ether derivatives, compounds 2, 4-6, 19-22. Compound 22 bearing the octyl chain at the A ring is the most active compound in the data set. To compare the binding modes of compounds containing alkyl chains of different lengths at the position R_1, the predicted

binding modes of compounds 18-20 containing C6, C2 and C4 alkyl chains, respectively, are
superimposed on the X-ray binding mode of compound 22 as shown in Fig. 4.

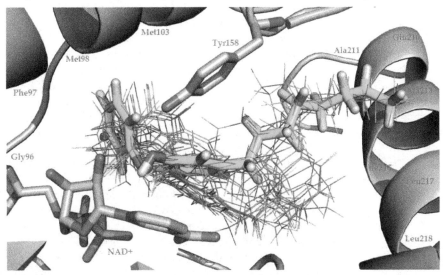

Fig. 3. Superposition of all predicted binding modes of 5-substituted triclosan and alkyl
diphenyl ether derivatives (green line) in InhA (pink) derived from molecular docking
calculations and the X-ray structure of compound 22 (green stick)

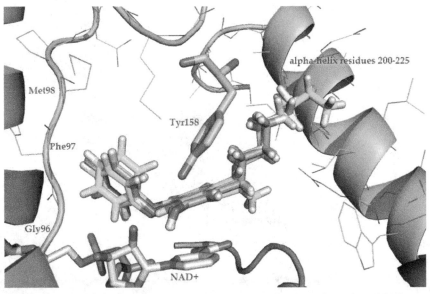

Fig. 4. The predicted binding modes of compounds 18 (yellow), 19 (green) and 20 (orange)
containing C6, C2 and C4 chains at the substituent R_1, respectively, and the X-ray binding
mode of compound 22 (cyan) in the InhA binding pocket (cyan)

The longer octyl chain of compound 22 could more closely interact with α-helix residues 200-225, whereas C6, C2 and C4 alkyl chains of compounds 18-20 are far from these residues, particularly the C2 alkyl chain of compound 19. This result may explain the higher activity of compound 22 bearing the longer alkyl chain at the position R_1 as compared with those of compounds 18-20. However, when the octyl chain of compound 22 was enlarged to a C14 chain resulting in compound 23, there is a corresponding increase in IC_{50} value for InhA inhibition from 5 nM to 150 nM. In contrast to the C8 chain of compound 22 which lies in a linear conformation in InhA binding pocket, the C14 chain of compound 23 forms a U-like shape within InhA binding pocket and slightly interacts with α-helix residues 200-225 as shown in Fig. 5. Moreover, the B ring of this compound loses the methyl-π interaction with Met161. These results may be accounted for the lower potency of compound 23. In the case of compounds 13 and 14, where phenyl rings are directly attached to the A ring at position R_1, the activity against InhA of these compounds are lower than those of compounds 15-17 which have a linker between the A ring and the phenyl ring at substituent R_1. Based on molecular docking calculations, the phenyl substituents of compounds 13 and 14 overlap with an ethyl linker of compound 16 and are surrounded by the rigid residues 148-168. To avoid the steric clash with these residues, a change of the binding conformation of compounds 13 and 14 has occurred, leading to a loss of the π-π stacking of the A ring with nicotinamide ring of NAD+ as compared with that of compound 16. Moreover, a linker phenyl substituent of compound 16 could create more hydrophobic interactions with the hydrophobic residues in the flexible residues 195-225. These results may explain why compounds 13 and 14 are of lower potency compared to compounds 15-17.

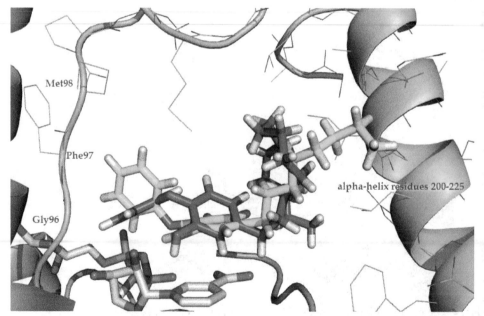

Fig. 5. The predicted binding modes of compound 23 (pink) and the X-ray binding mode of compound 22 (cyan) in InhA binding pocket (cyan)

The presence of NO_2 and NH_2 groups at the B ring of the alkyl diphenyl ether derivatives giving compounds 24-29 results in lower activities (increasing of IC_{50} values) for InhA inhibition of these compounds as compared with that of compound 18. Based on molecular docking calculations, the A rings and hexyl substituents of compounds 24-29 overlap well with that of compound 18 as shown in Fig. 6. However, the NO_2 and NH_2 substituents at the B ring of compounds 24-29 induce the position change of B rings of these compounds to avoid the steric conflict with the rigid residues Gly96, Phe97, Met98, Met161 and the pyrophosphate group of NAD+. Because of this reorientation, the B rings of compounds 24-29 lose the methyl-π interaction with Met161 as compared with compound 27. Therefore, the lower activities against InhA of alkyl diphenyl ether derivatives which contain the NO_2 and NH_2 groups at the B ring may be a consequence of the loss of the methyl-π interaction of the B rings of these compounds.

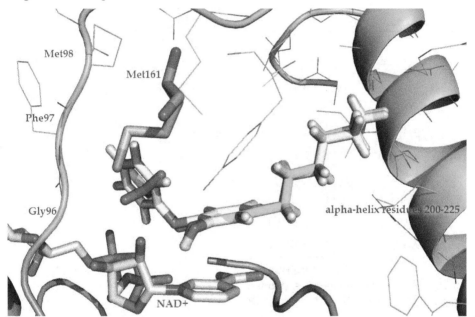

Fig. 6. Superposition of the predicted binding modes of compounds 18 (yellow) and 24 (green)

3.3 CoMFA, CoMSIA and HQSAR models

The results of the PLS analyses of CoMFA, CoMSIA and HQSAR models are summarized in Table 2. QSAR models 1, 3 and 5 derived from the PLS analyses of all compounds in the training set show a poor q^2. To improve the quality of these QSAR models, compound 19 was considered as an outlier resulting in better q^2 values of models 2, 4 and 6. However, HQSAR model 6 still shows a poor q^2 of 0.27. To modify this model, compounds 23 and 28 were omitted from the training set which yields the satisfying HQSAR, model 7. Based on a good q^2, models 2, 4 and 7 were selected as the final CoMFA, CoMSIA and HQSAR models, respectively. The final CoMFA model composing the steric and electrostatic fields gives q^2 of 0.66 and r^2 of 0.99. In the case of the final CoMSIA model including the steric, electrostatic and hydrophobic fields, a higher q^2 value of 0.73 as compared with that of the final CoMFA model was obtained. This result indicates that the final CoMSIA model performs better in the prediction than the final CoMFA model, which is an indication for the fact that beyond steric and electrostatic effects, hydrogen bonding may be an additional contribution. Among the considered descriptors of the final CoMSIA and CoMFA models, the electrostatic fields of both models are the most important parameter influencing the IC_{50} values of the 5-substituted triclosan and alkyl diphenyl ether derivatives in the training set. With regard to the best HQSAR model generated based on the combination of the different fragment types, atom (A), bond (B) and connection (C), this model shows q^2 value of 0.74 with r^2 value of 0.97 which are in the same level with those of the final CoMSIA model.

Models		Statistical parameters						Fraction
		q^2	r^2	N	s	SEE	F	
	CoMFA							
1	S/E	0.38	0.91	3	0.56	0.21	73.19	48/52
2	S/E	0.66	0.99	6		0.05	698.63	39/61
	CoMSIA							
3	S/E/H	0.45	0.89	4	0.54	0.24	39.27	24/46/30
4	S/E/H	0.73	0.99	6		0.07	277.19	19/57/24
	HQSAR							
5	A/B/C	0.14	0.32	1	0.63	0.56	-	-
6	A/B/C	0.27	0.43	1	0.54	0.47	-	-
7	A/B/C	0.74	0.97	6		0.12	-	-

Table 2. Summary of statistical results of CoMFA, CoMSIA and HQSAR models, N, optimum number of components; s, standard error of prediction, SEE, standard error of estimate; F, F-test value; S, steric field; E, electrostatic field; H, hydrophobic field; A, atom; B, bond; C, connection

3.4 Validation of the QSAR models

Satisfyingly good correlations between actual and predicted activities of the training set based on the final CoMFA, CoMSIA and HQSAR models are depicted in Fig. 7. The predicted activities of the training set derived from the final QSAR models are close to the experimental activities indicating the high degree of correlation between the actual and predicted activities. In order to assess the external predictive ability of selected QSAR models, InhA inhibition activities of the test set were predicted. The IC_{50} values of test set compounds predicted by the final CoMFA, CoMSIA and HQSAR models are within one logarithmic unit difference from the experimental values except those of compound 2 as presented in Fig. 7. This result reveals that all selected QSAR models are reliable to predict the activity of external data set. Therefore, the final CoMFA, CoMSIA, and HQSAR models can be utilized for designing new direct InhA inhibitors with improved activity.

Insight into the Key Structural Features of Potent Enoyl Acyl Carrier Protein Reductase Inhibitors Based on
Computer Aided Molecular Design

253

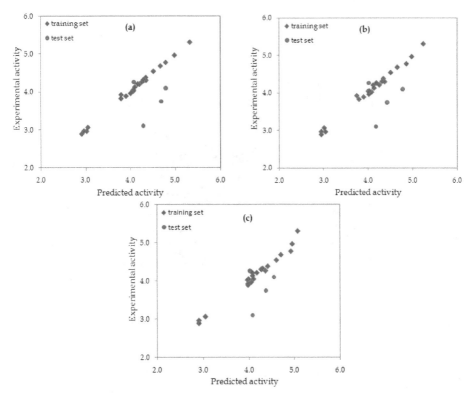

Fig. 7. Plots between the actual and predicted activities of the training and test sets derived
from the final CoMFA (a), CoMSIA (b) and HQSAR (c) models, respectively

3.5 CoMFA and CoMSIA contour maps

To reveal the importance of molecular descriptor fields, steric, electrostatic and hydrophobic
fields, on the InhA inhibition activities of 5-substituted triclosan and alkyl diphenyl ether
derivatives, CoMFA and CoMSIA contour maps were established and depicted in Fig. 8 and
9, respectively. CoMFA and CoMSIA contour maps are merged with the InhA pocket
complexed with compounds 16 and 22 in order to link the structural requirement for better
activity of 5-substituted triclosan and alkyl diphenyl ether derivatives visualized by CoMFA,
CoMSIA contour maps toward the interaction of these compounds in InhA binding pocket.
Green and yellow contours indicate areas where favorable and unfavorable steric bulks are
predicted to enhance the antitubercular activities of the direct InhA inhibitors. Blue and red
contours indicate regions where electropositive and electronegative groups lead to
increasing antitubercular activity, respectively. Purple and white contours represent areas
where the hydrophobic group and the hydrophilic group, are predicted to favour the
biological activities. Compounds 16 and 22 were selected as the template for graphic
interpretation of CoMFA and CoMSIA models. CoMFA model shows three yellow contours
surrounding the B rings of compounds 16 and 22 buried in the pocket consisting of the rigid
residues Gly96, Phe97, Met98, Met161 and NAD+ as shown in Fig. 8(a). These contours
indicate that the substituent of the B ring should be small in order to increase the enzyme

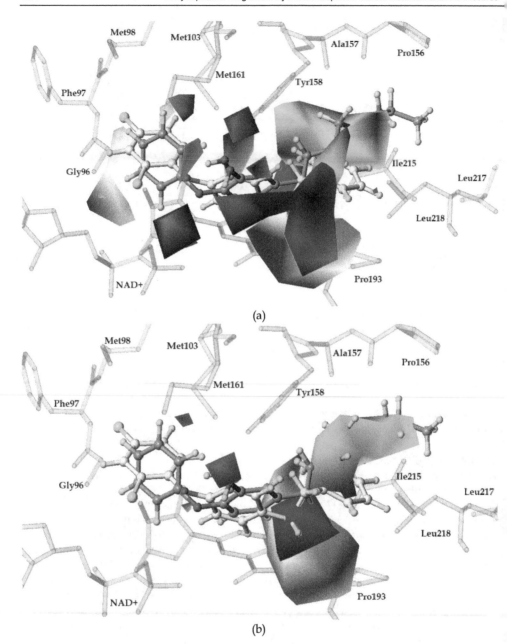

(a)

(b)

Fig. 8. Steric and electrostatic contours of CoMFA (a) and CoMSIA (b) models in combination with compounds 16 (yellow) and 22 (orange) in InhA binding pocket (cyan). Green and yellow contours represent favourable and unfavourable steric regions, respectively. Blue and red contours are favoured for electropositive and electronegative groups, respectively.

inhibitory activity of 5-substituted triclosan and alkyl diphenyl ether derivatives. Moreover, this structural requirement is preferable for the interaction of the B ring with the rigid moiety consisting of residues Gly96, Phe97, Met98, Met161 and NAD+. In addition, the B rings of compounds 16 and 22 are covered by a large purple contour and immediately flanked by two white contours as shown in Fig. 9. A large purple region conforms to the aromatic B rings of 5-substituted triclosan and alkyl diphenyl ether derivatives which are crucial for the forming of the methyl-π interaction with the methyl side chain of Met161. Furthermore, the presence of hydrophilic substituent with a small size at both sides of the B ring should enhance the activity against InhA of 5-substituted triclosan and alkyl diphenyl ether derivatives.

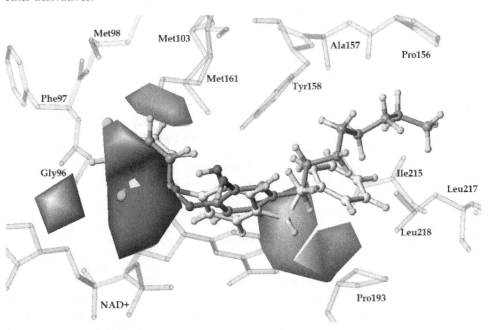

Fig. 9. CoMSIA hydrophobic contours in combination with compounds 16 (yellow) and 22 (orange) in InhA binding pocket (cyan). Purple and white contours show favourable and unfavourable hydrophobic regions, respectively.

With regard to the substituent R_1 of the A ring, CoMFA and CoMSIA models in Fig. 8 and 9 present the large blue, white and yellow contours near the ethyl linker of compound 16 and the first two carbons of the octyl side chain of compound 22 which are surrounded by the rigid residues 148-168. These contours suggest that the blue, white and yellow regions near those of compounds 16 and 22 favor the small moiety with the electropositive and hydrophilic properties. It is important to note that this favored small moiety could be helpful not only for the activities against InhA of 5-substituted triclosan and alkyl diphenyl ether derivatives but also for the binding of these compounds at a position where rigid residues 148-168 are presented. This finding agrees well with the experimental data that compounds with no linker and the methyl linker between the A ring and the analogues of phenyl and pyridyl at substituent R_1, compounds 10-15, show IC_{50} values higher than that of compound 16 containing the ethyl linker. Based on the obtained molecular docking results, the analogues of bulky phenyl and pyridyl at substituent R_1 of compounds 10-15 overlap with the ethyl linker of compound 16 located near the blue, white and yellow regions. Another interesting contour of CoMFA and CoMSIA models is the large green contour at the phenyl substituent of compound 16 and the last six carbons of the octyl chain of compound 22. The green contour indicates that the presence of the bulky substituent at this region should increase the InhA inhibitory activities of 5-substituted triclosan and alkyl diphenyl ether derivatives. This result is in line with the experimental results that compounds 1-2, 4-9, 19-21 presenting the shorter chain of substituent R_1 display lower activities as compared with that of compound 22 bearing the longer octyl chain. Remarkably, based on the large green area, the combination between substituents R_1 of 5-substituted triclosan derivatives and alkyl diphenyl ether derivatives, the phenyl substituent of compound 16 and the last six carbons of the octyl chain of compound 22, may generate the optimal substituent R_1 such as the phenyl incorporated with alkyl chain. Therefore, the designed compounds should display the better profile against InhA.

3.6 HQSAR contribution maps
HQSAR contribution maps are helpful to visualize the contributions of molecular fragments to the activities against InhA of 5-substituted triclosan and alkyl diphenyl ether derivatives in the present data. The color codes indicate the different contributions of all atoms in each compound to the biological activity. An atom with negative contributions is represented at the red end of the spectrum, whereas an atom with positive contributions is represented at the green end of the spectrum. The white colored atoms stand for intermediate contributions. Fig. 10 depicts the individual atomic contributions to the activity against InhA of compounds 13, 16 and 22. There are green and yellow atoms at the A ring of compounds 16 and 22 indicating the positive contributions of the A ring to the activity against InhA of these compounds. Moreover, the positive contributing fragments are presented at the ethyl linker of compound 16 and the first carbon of the octyl chain of compound 22 emphasizing the importance of these fragments. As previously shown by CoMFA and CoMSIA contours, these positively contributing moieties of compounds 16 and 22 are surrounded by yellow, blue and white contours implying that these fragments are optimal for steric, electrostatic and hydrophobic requirements. Obviously supporting this finding, the omission of the ethyl linker resulting in compound 13 induces the appearance of the negative contributing fragments at the A ring and the phenyl substituent leading to the lower activity of this compound as compared with that of compound 16. Considering the phenyl substituent of compound 16 and the last six carbons of the octyl chain of compound 22 buried in green CoMFA and CoMSIA contours as shown in Fig. 8, these fragments are colored by white indicating that these atoms have no contributions to the activity. Therefore, the modification of these white parts following the CoMFA and CoMSIA suggestions may improve the activity against InhA of 5-substituted triclosan and alkyl diphenyl ether derivatives. In case of the B rings of compounds 16 and 22, most atoms in the B ring and Cl substituents of compound 16 are colored by red and orange, suggesting the negative contributions of these fragments, whereas those of compound 22 are colored by white indicating no contribution of these fragments. This result may be accounted for the higher activity of compound 22 as compared with that of compound 16. Based on the obtained CoMFA and CoMSIA models, the B ring of compounds 16 and 22 are covered by a large purple contour and immediately flanked by two white contours. Therefore, the adjustment of the substituent at the B ring

based on the structural requirement suggested by CoMFA and CoMSIA models may induce the occurrence of the positive contribution on the B ring and its substituents resulting in the better activity against InhA. Noticeably, about the chlorine substituents at the B ring of 5-substituted triclosan derivatives, the precence of a positively contributing fragment at the substituent R_1 of the A ring induces the negative contribution on the chlorine substituents as shown by HQSAR contribution maps of compounds 13 and 16 in Fig. 10. This result implies that more interactions of substituent R_1 of the A ring reduce the role of the B ring chlorines on the activities. Consistent with this finding, alkyl diphenyl ether derivatives without the B ring chlorines, compounds 18, 21 and 22, display activities against InhA higher than those of triclosan and its derivatives bearing the B ring chlorines, compounds 1-17. On the other hand, the B ring chlorines can be more preferable for the activities in case of compounds with less interactions of substituent R_1 to InhA. As exemplified by compounds with shorter lenght of the alkyl chain (C2 and C4 chains at the substituent R_1), compounds 19 and 20 possess lower activites than those of compounds 4 and 6 containing the B ring chlorines. It is important to note that the influence of B ring chlorines on inhibitory activity of triclosan derivatives which is argued in Freundlich's work (Freundlich et al. 2009) and Sullivan's work (Sullivan et al., 2006) could be evaluated by our HQSAR model.

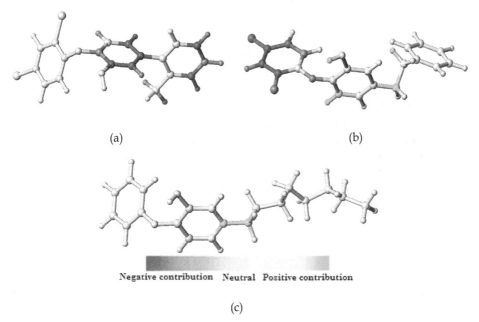

(a)   (b)

Negative contribution   Neutral   Positive contribution

(c)

Fig. 10. The final HQSAR contribution maps of compounds 13 (a), 16 (b) and 22 (c)

4. Conclusion

Molecular docking calculations were successfully applied to determine the potential binding modes of 5-substituted triclosan and alkyl diphenyl ether derivatives in the InhA binding pocket. The B rings of these compounds are occupied in the rigid pocket consisting of residues 96-105 and 148-168, whereas the A rings and their substituents are buried in the flexible residues 195-225. The B ring substituents that could perturb the methyl-π interaction of the B ring with Met161 produce the poor activities of alkyl diphenyl ether derivatives. On the other hand, the substituent R_1 at the A ring that could interact more with the flexible residues 195-225 and avoid the steric conflict with the rigid residues 148-168 might result in the better activities of 5-substituted triclosan and alkyl diphenyl ether derivatives against InhA. Besides, the key structural elements for a good activity against InhA of these compounds based on CoMFA, CoMSIA and HQSAR were clearly elucidated in the present study. Based on CoMFA and CoMSIA guidelines, compounds with the combination of substituents R_1 of 5-substituted triclosan derivatives and alkyl diphenyl ether derivatives should display the better profile against InhA. In agreement with CoMFA and CoMSIA results, the HQSAR contribution maps show the individual contribution of the atoms to IC_{50} values of 5-substituted triclosan and alkyl diphenyl ether derivatives. Moreover, HQSAR contribution maps could reveal the contribution of two chlorine atoms on the B ring of 5-substituted triclosan derivatives to their IC_{50} values. Consequently, the integrated results from the structure-based design using molecular docking calculations and the ligand-based design using various QSAR approaches provide insights into key structural features that can be utilized for designing novel and more active InhA inhibitors in the series of 5-substituted triclosan and alkyl diphenyl ether derivatives. Particularly, the modified compound suggested in the present study might be a member of a next drug generation of InhA inhibitor. These results demonstrate that computer aided molecular design approaches are fruitful for rational design and for possible syntheses of novel and more active InhA inhibitors that might be next generation of antitubercular agents.

5. Acknowledgment

This research was supported by the Thailand Research Fund (DBG5380006, DBG5380042, RTA53800010). A. Punkvang is grateful to the grant from under the program Strategic Scholarships for Frontier Research Network for the Ph.D. K. Kun-asa is grateful to Science Achievement Scholarship of Thailand (SAST). Faculty of Science, Ubon Ratchathani University, University of Vienna and ASEA-Uninet are gratefully acknowledged for supporting this research.

6. References

am Ende, C.W.; Knudson, S.E.; Liu, N.; Childs, J.; Sullivan, T.J.; Boyne, M.; Xu, H.; Gegina, Y.; Knudson, D.L.; Johnson, F.; Peloquin, C.A.; Slayden, R.A. & Tonge, P.J. (2008). Synthesis and in vitro antimycobacterial activity of B-ring modified diaryl ether InhA inhibitors. *Bioorganic & Medicinal Chemistry Letters*, Vol.18, No.10, (May 2008), pp. 3029-3033

Banerjee, A.; Dubnau, E.; Quemard, A.; Balasubramanian, V.; Um, K.S.; Wilson, T.; Collins, D.; de Lisle, G. & Jacobs, W.R., Jr. (1994). inhA, a gene encoding a target for isoniazid and ethionamide in Mycobacterium tuberculosis. *Science*, Vol.263, No.5144, (January 1994), pp. 227-230

Boyne, M.E.; Sullivan, T.J.; am Ende, C.W.; Lu, H.; Gruppo, V.; Heaslip, D.; Amin, A.G.; Chatterjee, D.; Lenaerts, A.; Tonge, P.J. & Slayden, R.A. (2007). Targeting fatty acid biosynthesis for the development of novel chemotherapeutics against Mycobacterium tuberculosis: evaluation of A-ring-modified diphenyl ethers as high-affinity InhA inhibitors. *Antimicrobial Agents and Chemotherapy*, Vol.51, No.10, (October 2007), pp. 3562-3567

Campbell, J.W. & Cronan, J.E., Jr. (2001). Bacterial fatty acid biosynthesis: Targets for antibacterial drug discovery. *Annual Review of Microbiology*, Vol.55, pp. 305-332

Cramer, R.D. III; Patterson, D.E. & Bunce, J.D. Comparative molecular field analysis (CoMFA). 1. Effect of shape on binding of steroids to carrier proteins. *Journal of the American Chemical Society*, Vol.110, No.18, (August 1998), pp. 5959-5967

De La Iglesia, A.I. & Morbidoni, H.R. (2006). Mechanisms of action of and resistance to rifampicin and isoniazid in Mycobacterium tuberculosis: new information on old friends. *Revista Argentina de microbiología*, Vol.38, No.2, (April-June 2006), pp. 97-109

Dessen, A.; Quemard, A.; Blanchard, J.S.; Jacobs, W.R., Jr. & Sacchettini, J.C. (1995). Crystal structure and function of the isoniazid target of Mycobacterium tuberculosis. *Science*, Vol.267, No.5204, (March 1995), pp. 1638-1641

Freundlich, J.S.; Wang, F.; Vilcheze, C.; Gulten, G.; Langley, R.; Schiehser, G.A.; Jacobus, D.P.; Jacobs, W.R., Jr. & Sacchettini, J.C. (2009). Triclosan derivatives: Towards potent inhibitors of drug-sensitive and drug-resistant Mycobacterium tuberculosis. *ChemMedChem*, Vol.4, No.2, (February 2009), pp. 241-248

GaussView 03, Revision 3.07 (2006) Gaussian, Inc., Wallingford CT

Gaussian 03 (2004) Gaussian, Inc., Wallingford CT

Heath, R.J. & Rock, C.O. (2004). Fatty acid biosynthesis as a target for novel antibacterials. *Current Opinion in Investigational Drugs*, Vol.5, No.2, (February 2004), pp.146-153

He, X.; Alian, A.; Stroud, R. & Ortiz de Montellano, P.R. (2006). Pyrrolidine carboxamides as a novel class of inhibitors of enoyl acyl carrier protein reductase from Mycobacterium tuberculosis. *Journal of Medicinal Chemistry*, Vol.49, No.21, (October 2006), pp. 6308-6323

He, X.; Alian, A. & Ortiz de Montellano, P.R. (2007). Inhibition of the Mycobacterium tuberculosis enoyl acyl carrier protein reductase InhA by arylamides. *Bioorganic & Medicinal Chemistry*, Vol.15, No.21, (2007), pp. 6649-6658

Heym, B.; Zhang, Y.; Poulet, S.; Young, D. & Cole, S.T. (1993). Characterization of the katG gene encoding a catalase-peroxidase required for the isoniazid susceptibility of Mycobacterium tuberculosis. *Journal of Bacteriology*, Vol.175, No.13, (July 1993), pp. 4255-4259

Johnsson, K.; King, D.S. & Schultz, P.G. (1995). Studies on the mechanism of action of isoniazid and ethionamide in the chemotherapy of tuberculosis. *Journal of the American Chemical Society*, Vol.117, No.17, (May 1995), pp. 5009-5010

Johnsson, K. & Schultz, P.G. (1994). Mechanistic studies of the oxidation of isoniazid by the catalase peroxidase from Mycobacterium tuberculosis. *Journal of the American Chemical Society*, Vol.116, No.16, (August 1994), pp. 7425-7426

Johnsson, K.; Froland, W.A. & Schultz, P.G. (1997). Overexpression, purification, and characterization of the catalase-peroxidase KatG from Mycobacterium tuberculosis. *Journal of Biological Chemistry*, Vol.272, No.5, (January 1997), pp. 2834-2840

Klebe, G.; Abraham, U. & Mietzner, T. Molecular similarity indices in a comparative analysis (CoMSIA) of drug molecules to correlate and predict their biological activity. *Journal of Medicinal Chemistry*, Vol.37, No.24, (November 1994), pp. 4130-4146

Kuo, M.R.; Morbidoni, H.R.; Alland, D.; Sneddon, S.F.; Gourlie, B.B.; Staveski, M.M.; Leonard, M.; Gregory, J.S.; Janjigian, A.D.; Yee, C.; Musser, J.M.; Kreiswirth, B.; Iwamoto, H.; Perozzo, R.; Jacobs, W.R., Jr.; Sacchettini, J.C. & Fidock, D.A. (2003). Targeting tuberculosis and malaria through inhibition of Enoyl reductase: compound activity and structural data. *Journal of Biological Chemistry*, Vol.278, No.23, (June 2003), pp. 20851-20859

Lei, B.; Wei, C.J. & Tu, S.C. (2000). Action mechanism of antitubercular isoniazid. Activation by Mycobacterium tuberculosis KatG, isolation, and characterization of inha inhibitor. *Journal of Biological Chemistry*, Vol.275, No.4, (January 2000), pp. 2520-2526

Metcalfe, C.; Macdonald, I.K.; Murphy, E.J.; Brown, K.A.; Raven, E.L. & Moody, P.C. (2008). The tuberculosis prodrug isoniazid bound to activating peroxidises. *Journal of Biological Chemistry*, Vol.283, No.10, (March 2008), pp. 6193-6200

Morris, G.M.; Goodshell, D.S.; Halliday, R.S.; Huey, R.; Hart, W.E.; Belew, R.K. & Olson, A.J. (1998). Automated docking using a lamarckian genetic algorithm and empirical binding free energy function. *Journal of Computational Chemistry*, Vol.19, No.14, (November 1998), pp.1639-1662

Nguyen, M.; Claparols, C.; Bernadou, J. & Meunier, B. A fast and efficient metal-mediated oxidation of isoniazid and identification of isoniazid-NAD(H) adducts. *ChembioChem*, Vol.2, No.12, (December 2001), pp. 877-883

Punkvang, A.; Saparpakorn, P.; Hannongbua, S.; Wolschann, P.; Beyer, A. & Pungpo, P. (2010). Investigating the structural basis of arylamides to improve potency against M. tuberculosis strain through molecular dynamics simulations. *European Journal of Medicinal Chemistry*, Vol.45, No.12, (December 2010), pp.5585-5593

Quemard, A.; Sacchettini, J.C.; Dessen, A.; Vilcheze, C.; Bittman, R.; Jacobs, W.R., Jr & Blanchard, J.S. (1995). Enzymatic characterization of the target for isoniazid in Mycobacterium tuberculosis. *Biochemistry*, Vol.34, No.26, (July 1995), pp. 8235-8241

Quemard, A.; Dessen, A.; Sugantino, M.; Jacobs, W.R., Jr. & Sacchetini, J.C. (1996). Blanchard JS. Binding of catalase-peroxidase-activated isoniazid to wild-type and mutant Mycobacterium tuberculosis enoyl-ACP reductases. *Journal of the American Chemical Society*, Vol.118, No.6, (February 1996), pp. 1561-1562

Rozwarski, D.A.; Grant, G.A.; Barton, D.H.; Jacobs, W.R., Jr & Sacchettini, J.C. (1998). Modification of the NADH of the isoniazid target (InhA) from Mycobacterium tuberculosis. *Science*, Vol.279, No.5347, (January 1998), pp. 98-102

Sullivan, T.J.; Truglio, J.J.; Boyne, M.E.; Novichenok, P.; Zhang, X.; Stratton, C.F.; Li, H.J.; Kaur, T.; Amin, A.; Johnson, F.; Slayden, R.A.; Kisker, C. & Tonge, P.J. (2006). High affinity InhA inhibitors with activity against drug-resistant strains of Mycobacterium tuberculosis. *ACS Chemical Biology*, Vol.1, No.1, (February 2006), pp.43-53

SYBYL 8.0 (2007) Tripos, Inc.

Saint-Joanis, B.; Souchon, H.; Wilming, M.; Johnsson, K.; Alzari, P.M. & Cole, S.T. (1999). Use of site-directed mutagenesis to probe the structure, function and isoniazid activation of the catalase/peroxidase, KatG, from Mycobacterium tuberculosis. *Biochemical Journal*, Vol.338, No.Pt.3, (March 1999), pp. 753-760

Sinha, B.K. (2001). (1983). Enzymatic activation of hydrazine derivatives. *Journal of Biological Chemistry*, Vol.258, No.2, (January 1983), pp. 796-801

Sullivan, T.J.; Truglio, J.J.; Boyne, M.E.; Novichenok, P.; Zhang, X.; Stratton, C.F.; Li, H.J.; Kaur, T.; Amin, A.; Johnson, F.; Slayden, R.A.; Kisker, C. & Tonge, P.J. (2006). High affinity InhA inhibitors with activity against drug-resistant strains of Mycobacterium tuberculosis. *ACS Chemical Biology*, Vol.17, No.1, (February 2006), pp. 43-53

Timmins, G.S. & Deretic, V. (2006). Mechanisms of action of isoniazid. *Molecular Microbiology*, Vol.62, No., (December 2006), pp. 1220-1227

Tong, W.; Lowis, D.R.; Perkins, R.; Chen ,Y.; Welsh, W.J.; Goddette, D.W.; Heritage, T.W. & Sheehan, D.M. (1998). Evaluation of quantitative structure–activity relationship methods for large-scale prediction of chemicals binding to the estrogen receptor. *Journal of Chemical Information and Modeling*, Vol.38, No.4, (July-August 1998), pp. 669-677

Vilcheze, C.; Wang, F.; Arai, M.; Hazbon, M.H.; Colangeli, R.; Kremer, L.; Weisbrod, T.R.; Alland, D.; Sacchettini, J.C. & Jacobs, W.R., Jr. (2006). Transfer of a point mutation in Mycobacterium tuberculosis inhA resolves the target of isoniazid. *Nature Medicine*, Vol.12, No.9, (September 2006), pp. 1027-1029

World Health Organization (WHO). (2010). Global tuberculosis control 2010, WHO report 2010, pp. 5, ISBN 9789241564069, Geneva, Switzerland

WHO. (2010). Multidrug and extensively drug-resistant TB (M/XDR-TB), 2010 Global report on surveillance and response, ISBN 9789241599191, Geneva, Switzerland

Wen, L.; Chmielowski, J.N.; Bohn, K.C.; Huang, J.K.; Timsina, Y.N.; Kodali, P. & Pathak, A.K. (2009). Functional expression of Francisella tularensis FabH and FabI, potential antibacterial targets. *Protein Expression and Purification*, Vol.65, No.1, (May 2009), pp.83-91

White, S.W.; Zheng, J.; Zhang, Y.M. & Rock, C.O. (2005). The structural biology of type II fatty acid biosynthesis. *Annual Review of Biochemistry*, Vol.74, (2005), pp.791-831

Wright, H.T. & Reynolds, K.A. (2007). Antibacterial targets in fatty acid biosynthesis. *Current Opinion in Microbiology*, Vol.10, No.5, (October 2007), pp.447-453

Zhang, Y.M.; Lu, Y.J. & Rock, C.O. (2004). The reductase steps of the type II fatty acid synthase as antimicrobial targets. *Lipids*, Vol.39, No.11, (November 2004), pp.1055-1060

Zhao, X.; Yu, H.; Yu, S.; Wang, F.; Sacchettini, J.C. & Magliozzo, R.S. (2006). Hydrogen peroxide-mediated isoniazid activation catalyzed by Mycobacterium tuberculosis catalase-peroxidase (KatG) and its S315T mutant. *Biochemistry*, Vol.45, No.13, (April 2006), pp. 4131-4140

Permissions

The contributors of this book come from diverse backgrounds, making this book a truly international effort. This book will bring forth new frontiers with its revolutionizing research information and detailed analysis of the nascent developments around the world.

We would like to thank Chris Rundfeldt, Ph.D., DVM, for lending his expertise to make the book truly unique. He has played a crucial role in the development of this book. Without his invaluable contribution this book wouldn't have been possible. He has made vital efforts to compile up to date information on the varied aspects of this subject to make this book a valuable addition to the collection of many professionals and students.

This book was conceptualized with the vision of imparting up-to-date information and advanced data in this field. To ensure the same, a matchless editorial board was set up. Every individual on the board went through rigorous rounds of assessment to prove their worth. After which they invested a large part of their time researching and compiling the most relevant data for our readers. Conferences and sessions were held from time to time between the editorial board and the contributing authors to present the data in the most comprehensible form. The editorial team has worked tirelessly to provide valuable and valid information to help people across the globe.

Every chapter published in this book has been scrutinized by our experts. Their significance has been extensively debated. The topics covered herein carry significant findings which will fuel the growth of the discipline. They may even be implemented as practical applications or may be referred to as a beginning point for another development. Chapters in this book were first published by InTech; hereby published with permission under the Creative Commons Attribution License or equivalent.

The editorial board has been involved in producing this book since its inception. They have spent rigorous hours researching and exploring the diverse topics which have resulted in the successful publishing of this book. They have passed on their knowledge of decades through this book. To expedite this challenging task, the publisher supported the team at every step. A small team of assistant editors was also appointed to further simplify the editing procedure and attain best results for the readers.

Our editorial team has been hand-picked from every corner of the world. Their multi-ethnicity adds dynamic inputs to the discussions which result in innovative outcomes. These outcomes are then further discussed with the researchers and contributors who give their valuable feedback and opinion regarding the same. The feedback is then collaborated with the researches and they are edited in a comprehensive manner to aid the understanding of the subject.

Apart from the editorial board, the designing team has also invested a significant amount of their time in understanding the subject and creating the most relevant covers. They scrutinized every image to scout for the most suitable representation of the subject and create an appropriate cover for the book.

The publishing team has been involved in this book since its early stages. They were actively engaged in every process, be it collecting the data, connecting with the contributors or procuring relevant information. The team has been an ardent support to the editorial, designing and production team. Their endless efforts to recruit the best for this project, has resulted in the accomplishment of this book. They are a veteran in the field of academics and their pool of knowledge is as vast as their experience in printing. Their expertise and guidance has proved useful at every step. Their uncompromising quality standards have made this book an exceptional effort. Their encouragement from time to time has been an inspiration for everyone.

The publisher and the editorial board hope that this book will prove to be a valuable piece of knowledge for researchers, students, practitioners and scholars across the globe.

List of Contributors

Jakyung Yoo and José L. Medina-Franco
Torrey Pines Institute for Molecular Studies, USA

Rahul Aggarwal and Charles J. Ryan
University of California San Francisco, United States of America

Vanina A. Medina, Diego J. Martinel Lamas, Pablo G. Brenzoni, Noelia Massari, Eliana Carabajal and Elena S. Rivera
Laboratory of Radioisotopes, School of Pharmacy and Biochemistry, University of Buenos Aires, Argentina

Vanina A. Medina
National Scientific and Technical Research Council (CONICET), Argentina

Karolina Gluza and Paweł Kafarski
Department of Bioorganic Chemistry, Faculty of Chemistry, Wrocław University of Technology, Wrocław
Poland

Ethirajulu Kantharaj and Ramesh Jayaraman
S*BIO Pte Ltd, Singapore

Elizabeth Hong-Geller and Nan Li
Bioscience Division, Los Alamos National Laboratory, Los Alamos, NM, USA

Isidro Palos
Universidad Autónoma de Tamaulipas, Reynosa, México

Abraham García
Facultad de Ciencias Químicas, Universidad Autónoma de Nuevo León, Monterrey, México

Jose Prisco Palma-Nicolás
Instituto de Fisiología Celular, Universidad Nacional Autónoma de México DF, México

Virgilio Bocanegra-García and Gildardo Rivera
Centro de Biotecnología Genomica, Instituto Politécnico Nacional, Reynosa, México

Mario Zucca, Sara Scutera and Dianella Savoia
University of Torino, Italy

Kerstin A. Wolff, Marissa Sherman and Liem Nguyen
Case Western Reserve University School of Medicine, Cleveland, Ohio, United States of America

Auradee Punkvang, Pharit Kamsri, Kodchakon Kun-asa and Pornpan Pungpo
Ubon Ratchathani University, Thailand

Patchreenart Saparpakorn and Supa Hannongbua
Kasetsart University, Thailand

Peter Wolschann
University of Vienna, Austria

Printed in the USA
CPSIA information can be obtained
at www.ICGtesting.com
JSHW011447221024
72173JS00004B/975